HEALTH HAZARDS OF THE HUMAN ENVIRONMENT

Mary L Sevesney

HEALTH HAZARDS

OF

THE HUMAN ENVIRONMENT

Prepared by 100 specialists
in 15 countries

WORLD HEALTH ORGANIZATION

GENEVA

1972

Reprinted, 1973
(Chapter 14 revised)

PRINTED IN BELGIUM

CONTENTS

PREFACE

In July 1972 the United Nations Conference on the Human Environment held in Stockholm focused worldwide attention on the environmental hazards that threaten human health. These hazards have been of constant concern to the World Health Organization throughout the twenty-five years of its existence. In 1971 the Twenty-fourth World Health Assembly carried out an extensive review of the problems involved and indicated several areas where action is particularly needed: [1]

➤ *Basic environmental health and sanitation must be improved in all countries, and especially in the developing countries; special emphasis should be placed on the provision of adequate quantities of potable water and on the sanitary disposal of wastes.*

➤ *International agreement should be reached on criteria, guides, and codes of practice concerning known environmental influences on health.*

➤ *The development and coordination of epidemiological health surveillance should be stimulated in order to provide basic information on adverse effects on human health attributable to the environment; one method of achieving this is through environmental monitoring systems.*

➤ *Knowledge of the effects of environmental factors on human health should be extended by collecting and disseminating information, by stimulating, supporting, and coordinating research, and by assisting in the training of personnel.*

To facilitate work in these areas, WHO has compiled this wide-ranging survey of environmental hazards to human health for the benefit of health authorities and others concerned with environmental problems. The vast field covered by the subject, coupled with the purposely condensed treatment of the technical components, precludes anything but a synoptic review of the highlights, and the reader is referred to other sources for details and specialized treatment of individual topics. Most of the material was prepared by the technical staff of WHO, but a number of experts outside the Organization were also invited to submit contributions. Each chapter was submitted to several reviewers, selected for their special competence in the subject matter. This procedure was considered to be more appropriate than asking experts to review the book as a whole, since it covers such a wide range of disciplines. The names of the contributors and reviewers are listed on pages 371-374; their invaluable advice and assistance are gratefully acknowledged.

---

[1] Resolution WHA24.47 (*Off. Rec. Wld Hlth Org.*, 1971, No. 193).

Some of the subjects discussed in this book are still of a controversial nature and the views expressed are not necessarily shared by all the contributors and reviewers. It is also emphasized that these views should not be construed as representing decisions or the policy of the World Health Organization.

INTRODUCTION

General Considerations

This publication is addressed primarily to health authorities called upon to deal with environmental problems, although it is hoped that much of it will be of interest to others concerned with deterioration of the environment. The human environment is considered here as comprising those external physical, chemical, biological, and social influences that have a significant and detectable effect on the health and well-being of the individual or of communities of people.

The World Health Organization, since its inception in 1947, has been actively concerned with environmental factors and their effects on human health. This concern is largely based on the simple fact that poor sanitary conditions and the accompanying communicable diseases are the greatest causes of morbidity and mortality in the developing countries, where the majority of the world's people live. Such conditions are characterized by water supplies that are inadequate in both quality and quantity, poor or non-existent waste disposal systems, abundant insect and animal reservoirs and vectors of disease agents, and insufficient health education, to which is often added the resistance-sapping factor of malnutrition.

These conditions have been largely eliminated in the economically advanced and industrialized countries, but other environmental hazards to human health often exert their effects more subtly than do communicable diseases, and take their toll in both industrialized and developing countries. They include physical and chemical factors and psychosocial influences, and together with microbiological agents they make up that part of the ecosystem most directly affecting man's health. WHO's concern with the environment thus extends far beyond sanitation, in the traditional sense of this term.

It has become increasingly clear in recent years that environmental degradation, if allowed to proceed unchecked, could result in serious and sometimes irreversible damage to life on this planet. It is of crucial importance to define as clearly as possible, and then to control, adverse effects of the environment on human health. Frequently, however, the precise definition of such effects is not yet possible, mainly because of our lack of knowledge of many of the components involved.

This ignorance on our part, allied to the highly complex inter-relationships between environmental factors and health, results in appreciable uncertainty on many issues on which judgements and decisions are required daily. The situation is all the more confused because such judgements and decisions are influenced not only by the availability of scientific knowledge but also by economic, political, cultural, and other considerations. Thus, any general prescriptions for action to protect human health and well-being will have to be adapted to the conditions existing in different countries.

Under these circumstances, the course adopted in preparing this publication has been to document as clearly as possible what is and what is not known about environmental hazards to human health, thus revealing important areas where further research is required. The information presented should assist health officials in making decisions appropriate to their particular circumstances. It should also contribute to the development of a rational and integrated approach, both short-term and long-term, to environmental health problems in many countries and at the international level.

Much is known, and much remains to be learned, about environmental hazards to human health. These hazards cover so vast a range that they can be dealt with here only in a highly synoptic form. It is hoped that this publication, despite its inevitable limitations, may serve as a concise reference work for health officials and other interested authorities. More detailed information on particular topics can be obtained by consulting the references listed at the end of each chapter and in the recently published bibliography of selected publications of the UN system 1946–1971. [1]

Arrangement of the Publication

Part I

In Part I, environmental hazards are considered from the standpoint of the media, e.g., air, water, food, and insect and rodent vectors, and other community influences, e.g., home, workplace, and culture, that are involved in the exposure of man to actual and potential hazards. Obviously, such hazards are the concern and responsibility of many sections of society and government, but the focus on health components characterizes the approach adopted by WHO in order to assist health authorities.

Part II

To deal with health problems from the standpoint of the environment, it is sometimes necessary to fix arbitrary and possibly artificial boundaries

---

[1] Winton, H.N.M., ed., (1972) *Man and the environment—a bibliography of selected publications of the UN system 1946-1971*, New York and London, R.R.Bowker.

between the components of what is really an inseparable whole. The triad of host, environment, and parasite, for example, are linked inseparably in any consideration of infectious diseases. The same is true of the inter-relationships between host and environment from the point of view of the effects on health of physical, chemical, and social factors.

In general, each specific environmental contaminant and hazard is considered separately in Part II. Because of the special problems they pose, however, the various agents that act as mutagens, carcinogens, and teratogens are dealt with as groups.

The general discussion of toxicological problems and the interpretation of the results of laboratory tests on specific substances are intended to under-line certain serious difficulties. As already pointed out, judgements and decisions by health and other government authorities are seldom based strictly on the available scientific evidence concerning the possible health hazard associated with a specific chemical or other agent. Political, cultural, and economic considerations cause local, regional, and national authorities to come to quite different policy conclusions when faced with the same scientific evidence (or lack of evidence) concerning a particular hazard. Some governments, for example, may adopt the attitude that it would take too long to accumulate sufficient knowledge as to the precise toxicity for man of substance "X"; they therefore restrict industrial or other uses of this substance solely on the basis of any carcinogenicity observed in laboratory animals, regardless of the dosage or routes of administration and the consequent limitations of many of the procedures used (see Chapter 12). Other governments may find such decisions inappropriate because of the resulting interference with economic development, and because they have assessed the risk involved as relatively low. Knowledge of the risk of harmful effects is inadequate for nearly all potentially toxic substances; the technical principles of certain laboratory procedures and the judgements based on them are therefore dealt with at some length in Chapter 11.

Part III

In view of the rapid development and increasing influence of science and technology, it is especially urgent to define and to integrate from an operational viewpoint the wide range of components involved in environ-mental health hazards. A prime need is the development of a system of integrated surveillance and monitoring of man's health and well-being in relation to environmental factors, so that steps may be taken to avoid major dangers that would otherwise take him by surprise. A fundamental require-ment of any such system is built-in flexibility, so that both orderly change and unexpected developments can be readily and profitably accommodated without compromising the entire structure.

For some years WHO has been engaged in surveillance and monitoring activities (see Chapters 21 and 25 on communicable diseases and adverse drug reactions respectively), and is gradually developing, within the limits of its financial resources, additional operations along the lines described in Part III. Surveillance and monitoring is a relatively new field, and great methodological and operational problems have yet to be solved. The success of WHO's work in this area depends, of course, on the efforts of national and local agencies, and on collaboration between these agencies, WHO, and other international organizations concerned with environmental problems. WHO's immediate practical aim is to develop an early warning system for the adverse effects of the environment on human health, the ultimate goal being a comprehensive health information network linking all countries of the world.

Although surveillance and monitoring activities are already in progress in several health and environmental fields, they are still fragmentary. Future needs can be met only by a much more systematic and integrated effort that will take advantage of the remarkable achievements in communications theory and practice, notably with regard to the accumulation, organization, and handling of data, in turn served by systems theory, automated instrumentation, and electronic computers.

Part IV

Part IV approaches environmental health hazards from the standpoint of public health operations and the principles and practice of intervention and control procedures. Political, economic, and cultural differences make it difficult to formulate criteria and standards that could be generally applied to problems such as air and water pollution and food contamination.

Nevertheless, experience has shown this to be possible and useful in certain instances. Consideration is given to particular problems and segments of the community environment, such as basic sanitation, where methods for the control of communicable disease are readily available. The application of advanced technology for the control of environmental pollutants and nuisances is discussed. Part IV also outlines the experience gained by some authorities in dealing with certain pressing problems despite lack of knowledge of the mechanism, nature and extent of the effects of some environmental influences on the health of man.

PART I

THE COMMUNITY ENVIRONMENT

CHAPTER 1

AIR

Three dramatic episodes in this century, in the Meuse Valley (1930), Donora, Pennsylvania (1948), and London (1952), have demonstrated that, in extreme cases, community air pollution can result in considerable loss of life and serious illness (see pp. 24-25). However, the exact nature and extent of the associations between air pollution and community health have not been fully established. Current knowledge of the health effects of air pollution will be reviewed in this chapter, and the difficulty of reaching definitive conclusions and making generalizations that may be useful and warranted will be emphasized.

General Considerations

Introduction

The average adult male exchanges about 15 kg of air a day (Goldsmith, 1968b), compared to less than 1.5 kg of food or about 2.5 kg of water. Air itself is a mixture of gases consisting of roughly 78 % nitrogen, 21 % oxygen, and a little less than 1 % argon. Together with 0.03 % carbon dioxide, these elements make up 99.99 % of dry air; a number of minor gaseous elements (neon, helium, methane, krypton, and some others) complete the total. In the usual range of absolute humidities, water vapour adds another 1–3 % by volume.

Ambient air is more than a mixture of these gases. When sampled close to ground level, it contains other gases, vapours and particulate matter derived either from natural sources, such as volcanoes, or from man's activities. Some components, such as spores, seeds, and pollen grains, for example, are not pollutants; they are natural constituents frequently found in the atmosphere. Plant pollen may cause ill health in some people (hay fever and asthma); although it is a natural and essential constituent of air, it is not one to which all individuals are equally sensitive. Air pollution is the result of the discharge into the atmosphere of foreign gases, vapours, droplets and particles, or of excessive amounts of normal constituents, such as the carbon dioxide and suspended particulate matter produced by the burning of fossil fuels. Fears have been expressed that the resulting increased levels of carbon dioxide, through their effect on the radiation of heat on a global scale, may lead to calamitous climatic changes, but comprehensive discussions of these problems (Study of Critical Environmental Problems, 1970; Study of Man's Impact on Climate, 1971) now suggest that such fears are premature.

In a discussion of the possible direct health hazards from community air pollution, it should be remembered that a complex relationship exists between biological phenomena and the content of the earth's atmosphere. Thus while airborne pollen causes allergic reactions in some individuals, it is essential for plant fertilization.   Another example is the effect of night air on certain pathogenic bacteria and viruses; downwind of urban areas in the United Kingdom, this air is rapidly lethal to these infective agents whereas upwind of such areas they can survive for long periods or indefinitely (Druett & May, 1968; May et al., 1969).

Sources and types of pollutant

The general concept of pollution as a consequence of human activity suggests a classification based on the type of activity resulting in pollution. Atmospheric pollutants will be considered in this chapter in relation to their production by combustion sources, specific industrial activities, certain community activities, and personal habits, such as smoking.   Combustion sources include: (i) power plants and domestic heating equipment, whether coal- or oil-fired; these produce sulfur oxides, nitrogen oxides, and particulates, which may differ from place to place with respect to physical composition and chemical characteristics; and (ii) motor vehicles, which produce both the photochemical oxidant type of pollution, first noted and most severe in Los Angeles, and pollution by carbon monoxide and lead, as found in many cities.   In addition to common pollutants, such as sulfur dioxide and particulate matter, specific industrial activities produce pollutants related to the processes and products of the industry concerned.

Historical conditions have affected the degree of importance accorded to the pollution problem and the kinds of air pollution data available. In western society, man-made contamination of community air had its origins in the 14th century with the change-over from wood to coal as a source of energy.   Until well into this century " air pollution" was synonymous for most people with smoke and sulfur dioxide (Halliday, 1961; Chambers, 1962).   This form of air pollution from household heating probably represents the earliest recognizable form of such pollution, although its effects on indoor air have often been underestimated. [1]

---

[1] In developing countries with populations not familiar with urban conditions, it may be a most serious problem, as pointed out by Sofoluwe (1969) in studies of infant bronchitis in Lagos, Nigeria, and by Cleary & Blackburn (1968), who measured air pollution levels in native huts in New Guinea.

The substitution of petroleum products for coal in many regions reduced some of the concern caused by the visible nuisance of coal smoke. The tremendous increase in the use of petroleum products, particularly in petrol-powered motor vehicles, produced a new type of pollution. The internal combustion engine discharges carbon monoxide, lead, nitrogen oxides, and assorted hydrocarbons into the community air only a few feet from the breathing zone of the population. The local concentrations of these substances reach appreciable levels, which are greatest in urban centres where traffic density is greatest. Under conditions of poor natural ventilation and strong sunlight, a complex series of reactions takes place between the nitrogen oxides and hydrocarbons leading to the formation of ozone, peroxyacyl nitrates (PAN), and several other substances (usually grouped together as "photochemical oxidants"). This more extensive type of motor vehicle pollution affects the entire air environment of a community (Los Angeles "smog").

Air pollution from motor vehicles in developing countries does not yet present a problem of the magnitude reached in highly industrialized countries. However, as urbanization and industrialization develop in these countries, the contribution to air pollution from motor vehicle emissions could increase very rapidly, the more so since the vehicles in service will be on the average older and less well maintained, and have a high weight-to-horsepower ratio; the resulting pollution will be out of proportion to the number of vehicles. Diesel engines, an attractive alternative to petrol-powered motor vehicles in some developing countries, have the advantage that they produce virtually no hydrocarbons that can take part in photochemical reactions and no carbon monoxide. Unless correctly maintained, however, they can produce smoke, odour, and noise (WHO Expert Committee on Urban Air Pollution, 1969).

The combustion of fuel for heating and energy production represents the commonest and most widespread source of atmospheric pollution. In contrast, the emissions of specific pollutants by industry are much more restricted both in area and numbers of sources. However, industrial activities are a major source of pollutants in many places. The effects of point sources of pollutants, such as industrial plants, depend on many local factors, among which are topography, weather conditions, stack height, location, control equipment, raw materials used and type of process. In addition to sulfur dioxide, suspended particulate matter, and oxides of nitrogen, industrial air pollutants include lead, cadmium, mercury, beryllium, the mercaptans and hydrogen sulfide, fluorides, chlorine, asbestos, and many other wastes and by-products of technological processes.

Airborne biological agents such as pollens and micro-organisms, while not pollutants as defined here, are environmental factors that may have important health effects and will therefore be briefly discussed.

Effect of meteorological and topographical conditions

Not only the nature and source of the pollutants themselves, but also meteorological and topographical conditions are essential in determining the potential for the build-up of dangerous concentrations.

Turbulence in the atmosphere is a principal mechanism by which undesirable levels of contaminants are prevented from building up. For a given wind pattern, turbulence will be greater over steep hills or tall buildings than over a flat plain. The meteorological condition of temperature inversion, in which relatively warmer air overlies cold air, results in minimal turbulence and marked atmospheric stability. Inversions can affect the movement of air over a fairly wide region, and when they persist for a number of hours, or even days, pollutant concentrations tend to build up because of the absence of turbulence. For a fuller treatment, the reader is referred to one of the many excellent works on these subjects (Stern, 1968; Berljand, 1968; World Meteorological Organization, 1970).

Air Pollution and Health

General considerations

Interpretation of health reactions to pollution depend on evidence obtained from studies of two types: epidemiological studies and toxicological studies. Epidemiological studies are concerned with the effects occurring in human populations exposed under natural conditions. Experimental studies on man or animals, in which the level, duration and conditions of exposure are under the control of the investigator, are included in the term "toxicological".

Epidemiological evidence can quantify responses and provide the necessary link connecting air pollution and the health of the population. Toxicological evidence is complementary, in the sense that it can be gathered under well-controlled and defined conditions that permit conclusions as to causation, but its relevance to the natural setting is often in doubt. In addition, toxicological information permits better design of epidemiological studies. Both types of evidence are needed to form a reasonable judgement about the health effects of air pollution. When they lead to divergent conclusions, it seems more prudent to rely somewhat more on the epidemiological data. In discussing either type of evidence, the usual precautions concerning interpretation apply (Paul, 1966; Loomis, 1968).

In addition to general environmental exposure, specific exposure results from tobacco smoke, the air of work-places, and household heating and cooking fumes. This applies particularly to smoke, sulfur oxides, carbon monoxide, and nitrogen oxides, but the duration and levels of exposure differ, as do the associated pollutants and the relationships between exposure and effects. These additional sources should be carefully considered before any conclusions are drawn about the relationship between air pollution and health.

Cigarette smoking is an especially troublesome complication in the epidemiological analysis of community air pollution. It is a personal pollution of the inhaled air, which then contains a high concentration of carbon monoxide and polycyclic aromatic compounds, such as benzo[a]-pyrene. In view of the major causal role of cigarette smoking in chronic respiratory disease and possibly in cardiovascular disease, it is always necessary to adjust for the effects of smoking before the effects of community air pollution on health can be evaluated. However, studies of smoking and health can themselves point to reactions that are important to study in relation to community air pollution. Apart from the inhalation of tobacco smoke by smokers themselves, non-smokers may be exposed to significant air pollution from tobacco smoke in smoke-filled rooms. As recently pointed out, carbon monoxide concentrations in rooms filled with tobacco smoke may attain or even exceed both the permissible limit for the general population and that for occupational exposure; depending on the length of exposure, such concentrations may be harmful to health, particularly in the case of persons already suffering from chronic broncho-pulmonary and coronary heart disease (US Public Health Service, 1972).

Similarly, experience with pollutants under occupational conditions constitutes a limited source of information for assessing the harmfulness of various forms of community air pollution. Occupational exposures are limited to a certain number of hours per day or week, whereas community exposures fluctuate but may be continuous. Occupational exposure can be directly altered or controlled if damage to health appears to be occurring, whereas control of community exposures is a much more complex and difficult matter. Finally, whereas community exposures affect the entire population, occupational exposure affects a sector of the population that is of limited age range, predominantly male, relatively free from unhealthy and susceptible individuals, and possibly under surveillance through industrial health programmes.

Epidemiological evidence

A number of factors affect the sensitivity of the population. These include age, sex, general state of health and nutrition, concurrent exposures, pre-existing disease, and temperature and humidity at the time of exposure. In general, older persons, the very young, those in poor health, cigarette smokers, the occupationally exposed, and those with pre-existing chronic bronchitis, coronary heart disease and asthma are more vulnerable to pollutant exposures.

The multifactorial nature of certain diseases frequently used as indices in epidemiological studies, e.g., chronic bronchitis, asthma, emphysema, and lung cancer, combined with differences in methods of measurement, definitions of disease, and socio-economic factors, make the interpretation of differences between areas or countries difficult.   Nevertheless, a growing body of evidence seems to show a consistent association between air pollution and health impairment of varying degrees.   Such associations are found between: (1) acute pollution exposure and morbidity and mortality; (2) chronic lower-level exposure and morbidity and mortality; (3) exposure and impairment of function and performance; (4) exposure and symptoms of sensory irritation; and (5) exposure and other effects on well-being.

Acute air pollution episodes

(1) *Mortality*

One of the worst air pollution disasters occurred in December 1952 in London.   A dense cold fog settled on the city for four days, resulting in a sudden increase in the death rate above the expected value.   The excess amounted to an estimated 3500–4000 deaths in Greater London (population 8.3 million), either during the fog or shortly afterwards.   Figures recorded in the smaller area of the County of London are shown in Table 1. The increase in deaths from bronchitis was the largest single contributor to the rise in death rate.   Deaths from other diseases involving impairment of respiratory function were also increased.   There was a rise in the number of deaths from heart disease, which could be due to the additional strain placed on the heart by impairment of respiratory function or to a direct effect.   There was also a substantial increase in deaths from all other causes.   This residual excess mortality constituted a statistically significant increase, and it is unlikely that it was secondary, to any large extent, to impairment of respiratory function.   It may thus have been due to other potentially lethal effects of air pollution.   A close correlation was found, however, between excess mortality and atmospheric concentrations of smoke and sulfur dioxide.

Two other acute air pollution episodes occurred prior to the London fog of 1952 and directed attention to the fact that outbreaks of sickness and death were sometimes associated with dirty air.   The first occurred in the Meuse Valley in Belgium in the first week of December 1930, when a heavy fog associated with a very stable air mass trapped emissions from neighbouring industrial plants.   Within three days many residents complained of respiratory symptoms; over 60 died, 10 times the figure expected for that period.   No measurements of pollution were made either during or prior to the episode, and the inference that the cause of the increased mortality was a higher than normal concentration of air pollutants created by the weather abnormality was made retrospectively by the exclusion of other possibilities (Heimann, 1961).

TABLE 1

INCREASE IN MORTALITY IN THE LONDON FOG OF DECEMBER 1952[1]

Cause of death	Seasonal norm (deaths per week)	Deaths in week after fog	Excess deaths	Percentage of total excess deaths
Bronchitis	75	704	629	39
Other lung diseases	98	366	268	17
Coronary artery disease, myocardial degeneration	206	525	319	20
Other diseases	508	889	381	24
Total	887	2484	1597	100

Data from: Royal College of Physicians of London (1970).

[1] Statistics for the County of London (population 3.3 million).

Donora, Pennsylvania, located in another highly industrialized area, suffered a similar weather anomaly (unusually still and stable air) in October 1948. Again there was a striking increase in respiratory tract complaints with almost half of the town's 12 000 inhabitants noting some symptoms. Measurements of pollution were made after the event and epidemiological data were gathered some months later by questioning a household sample. Scrutiny of Donora's mortality statistics revealed that a similar large increase had taken place in 1945, but the possibility that environmental factors might be involved was not recognized at that time (Heimann, 1961).

These three examples show the variation in the quality and kinds of information available concerning acute episodes. Good data on pollutants and on morbidity and mortality are both lacking for the Meuse valley disaster. Mortality data were available for Donora, and morbidity was estimated from a sample survey carried out later; however, the nature of the pollutants present in the air during the emergency could only be inferred. London in 1952, in contrast, had a well-developed vital statistics system and a network of smoke and sulfur dioxide monitoring stations. The monitoring of smoke and sulfur dioxide has been carried out in the United Kingdom since 1912, but the choice of these substances for surveillance reflects the view, alluded to earlier, that these are the only important pollutants (Halliday, 1961). As a result, it is still not clear today what were, in fact, the toxic constituents of the London fog of 1952.

Subsequent studies in Europe, the United States, and Japan have confirmed that an abrupt rise in the concentrations of smoke *and* sulfur dioxide in the ambient air is positively associated with excess mortality, the magnitude of which is related to the level and duration of the rise in concentration of these pollutants. The individuals most severely affected are the aged, and patients with chronic obstructive pulmonary disease and/or heart disease (US National Air Pollution Control Administration, 1969a). [1] Smoke and sulfur dioxide are still the main pollutants measured in many epidemiological studies on the assumption that the variations in the concentrations of these substances set the pattern for other important pollutants. This assumption is of doubtful validity.

It was pointed out, in a review of published studies by the US National Air Pollution Control Administration (1969a,b), that abrupt increases to levels of over 175 μg/m³ (0.25 parts per million, ppm) of sulfur dioxide [2] and 750 μg/m³ of smoke [3] were associated in the United Kingdom with a small increase in daily mortality detectable in large populations. The rise in mortality was more pronounced when sulfur dioxide concentrations exceeded 1000 μg/m³ (0.35 ppm) *and* at the same time smoke reached 1200 μg/m³. By the time sulfur dioxide exceeded 1500 μg/m³ (0.5 ppm) with smoke greater than 2000 μg/m³, the increase in mortality over the base-line was 20 % or more (US National Air Pollution Control Administration, 1969a).

Attempts have been made, in a few studies, to link increased mortality with high photochemical oxidant concentrations in the Los Angeles area, but to date the evidence produced has not been convincing. A primary difficulty involves disentangling the effect of high temperatures on mortality. It is doubtful whether high oxidant levels help to step up the increase in mortality seen during "heat waves" (US National Air Pollution Control Administration, 1970).

A possible association between average carbon monoxide levels and variation in daily mortality from cardiovascular conditions in Los Angeles was recently suggested (Hexter & Goldsmith, 1971).

(2) Morbidity

Symptoms of patients with bronchitis in London were investigated by means of diaries in which each patient kept a daily record of changes in

---

[1] The US National Air Pollution Control Administration is now incorporated in the Environmental Protection Agency.

[2] Concentrations of sulfur dioxide can be expressed as parts by volume per million parts of air by volume, abbreviated to parts per million or ppm, or as micrograms/m³. The first has the advantage of being independent of atmospheric temperature and pressure, whereas the second has the advantage of being comparable to the smoke concentration units (see below). However, it has the disadvantage that the conversion factor is somewhat dependent on atmospheric temperature and pressure. The change in this factor is less than 10 % in the 0–25°C range at normal atmospheric pressure, so that the conversion factor for standard temperature and pressure (0°C and 760 mm Hg) would be adequate for most purposes. Under these conditions, the factor is 2857 μg/m³ = 1 ppm.

[3] Measured volumes of air are sucked through special filter papers or other trapping devices and the weight of particles is determined. Such measurements are expressed in micrograms/m³. Other methods involve determining the reflectance of stained filter paper or the light scattering effect of particles trapped on a white paper tape. This latter method gives "smoke shade" units (given as coh units, i.e., "coefficient of haze"). One coh unit is the quantity of light-scattering solids producing an optical density of 0.01 when measured by light transmission (Jacobs, 1962). For cities in the USA, where coh units are frequently used, the sulfur dioxide and smoke shade levels resulting in a small excess in mortality in large populations are, respectively, 1700 μg/m³ and 6 coh units. Conversion from "smoke shade" to absolute concentrations for purposes of comparison is thought to be unreliable, "smoke shade" being a relative rather than absolute measure (US National Air Pollution Control Administration, 1969a, b).

his condition, expressed in standard terms (Lawther, 1958). Levels of smoke greater than 300 µg/m³ *and* levels of sulfur dioxide greater than 600 µg/m³ (0.21 ppm) were associated with acute worsening of symptoms. An increase in morbidity, mainly of the respiratory type, was also an important feature of the Meuse Valley, Donora, and London disasters. Other analyses of increases in the frequency of clinic and emergency room visits during or shortly after acute pollution episodes in New York City, London, Rotterdam, Yokkaichi (Japan) and elsewhere have tended to show rises at or shortly after the commencement of such episodes (US National Air Pollution Control Administration, 1969a,b).

Although acute episodes of pollution involving loss of life and serious injury have fortunately been few, they have focused world opinion on the health effects of high concentrations of pollutants (and also on the potential hazard if acute episodes occur). The measurable health effects of long-term exposure to lower concentrations of pollutants are much less clear-cut.

Effects of chronic exposures on mortality and morbidity

Acute air pollution episodes represent abrupt and unusual exposures to high concentrations of air pollutants, and produce the most obvious health effects. It is still uncertain whether prolonged exposure to lower levels is also deleterious to the health of the community. A good deal of attention has been directed to this question (Royal College of Physicians of London, 1970; US National Air Pollution Control Administration, 1969a,b), but the difficulty of matching populations for important variables, such as smoking habits, age, sex, socio-economic status, occupation, pre-existing disease, and ethnic background, makes it difficult to draw conclusions that are generally applicable. Nevertheless, the studies mentioned below strongly suggest that long-term exposure to air pollution of moderate intensity impairs health. The prevalence and severity of such impairment have yet to be determined precisely.

(1) *Respiratory mortality and morbidity*

Aggravation and/or causation of chronic bronchitis, asthma, and pulmonary emphysema have all been considered in association with community air pollution. Several recent studies have shown that both overall mortality and mortality from respiratory disease are higher in areas of high atmospheric pollution than in otherwise similar areas of low atmospheric pollution (Wicken & Buck, 1964; Winkelstein, 1967, 1968; Zeidberg et al., 1967a,b). After adjustment for density of population and size of community, an association between chronic respiratory disease mortality and sulfur oxide and particulate pollution, by county, has been demonstrated in the United Kingdom (Buck & Brown, 1964). When density of population and domestic overcrowding were taken into account, the rates for premature death or disablement and for absence from work due to bronchitis were highest among postmen working in the most polluted areas in the country (Reid & Fairbairn, 1958). Similar findings concerning disability were reported for bus crews in London (Cornwall & Raffle, 1961). A survey among general practitioners showed that, after age, sex, social class, and tobacco smoking had been taken into account, bronchitis was twice as frequent in large towns as in rural areas (College of General Practitioners, 1961). It should be noted that chronic bronchitis in both high and low polluted areas is highest among cigarette smokers. While there is strong suggestive evidence that air pollution is a causal factor in chronic bronchitis, it may be more important as an aggravating factor.

The difficulty of matching populations for important secondary variables has led to the carrying out of a number of epidemiological studies on schoolchildren, so as to minimize the importance of smoking, occupation and previous medical history. The results of such studies in the United Kingdom indicate an increase in respiratory illness in schoolchildren in areas of high pollution, as compared to areas of low pollution. The fear has been expressed that such increased rates of infection may cause higher rates of chronic pulmonary disease in this population in later life (Douglas & Waller, 1966; Lunn et al., 1967; Paccagnella et al., 1969; Colley, 1971). Social class and housing conditions have also been associated with respiratory diseases of children.

Smoke and sulfur oxides have been the most commonly used indices of pollution in the attempts that have been made to relate respiratory morbidity and mortality to levels of pollution. Epidemiological evidence that photochemical oxidant concentrations in air can be correlated with exacerbation of symptoms in patients with chronic respiratory disease has been found in some studies but not in others.

(2) Mortality from cancer

The possibility that air pollution is a causal factor in cancer of the lung has given rise to considerable concern. The evidence in favour of a causal relationship is briefly: (a) the excess occurrence of the disease in urban areas; (b) the presence in polluted air of substances such as benzo[a]pyrene, which under experimental conditions can cause cancer; and (c) the general rise in lung cancer, which appears to follow certain assumed trends in pollution.

Early studies in the United Kingdom indicated that variations in lung cancer mortality in urban areas were associated with variations in pollutant concentrations. The Royal College of Physicians of London (1970) has reviewed the issue, and concluded that the evidence against the importance of community air pollution as a causal factor in cancer of the lung is stronger than the evidence for it.   The urban/non-urban differential in lung cancer is greatest in countries with the lowest urban air pollution (Sweden, Norway and Denmark).   No consistent association has been shown between variations in the benzo[a]pyrene content of air and lung cancer rates, and the experimental production of lung cancer with this agent requires other agents, biological or physical.   The upward trend as well as other experimental and epidemiological evidence are best explained by the causal role of cigarette smoking in lung cancer.   Finally, epidemiological studies in the USA (Winkelstein, 1967) and UK (Buck & Brown, 1964), which did show associations between air pollution and chronic respiratory disease, failed to show an association with lung cancer (though one study did show an association with bladder cancer).

Nevertheless, in a comparable review by Cleary (1967), evidence is presented to show that, in the USA, South Africa, New Zealand and Australia, immigrants from the United Kingdom have a higher lung cancer death rate than those born in these countries; immigrants from Norway have a lower rate than native-born citizens of the USA; and the lung cancer mortality rates for all these migrants are intermediate between those of their countries of origin and destination, strongly suggesting an environmental factor in early life.   Other studies show that lung cancer rates among urban non-smokers are 14–163 % higher than in mixed or rural areas.   Similar urban-rural differences are found in many industrialized countries.

While the existence of an urban excess of lung cancer has been proved, it is uncertain that air pollution is the "urban factor" responsible.   In contrast, recent work incriminates cigarette smoking more strongly than ever; there is also a small contribution from occupational exposure.

The Royal College of Physicians also notes (citing Stocks, 1960) that deaths from cancer of the stomach and intestine are significantly related to levels of smoke pollution in 30 English county boroughs.   Another study of similar material (Gardner et al., 1969) showed that adjustment of death rates from these causes to allow for differences in social class reduced the correlation between air pollution and stomach cancer for men and abolished it for women.   However, Winkelstein (1969) and Zeidberg et al. (1967b) have demonstrated that the higher incidence of stomach cancer in areas of high pollution was maintained even when economic differences were taken into account.   In none of these studies, however, was any allowance made for possible differences in smoking habits, although these are known to affect death rates from stomach cancer.

Pollution exposure and impairment of function and performance

Impairment of lung function is often associated with the chronic respiratory conditions that air pollution aggravates.   One measure of function, the resistance to air flow into and out of the lung, gives some idea of the work required to breathe. Spicer (1967) and Spicer et al. (1962) studied chronic bronchitis patients in Baltimore, and found that changes in airway resistance occurred at the same time and were correlated with sulfur dioxide concentration peaks measured 38 hours earlier. In another study, male chronic bronchitis and emphysema patients were placed in a hospital environment for three weeks; airway resistance was measured at frequent intervals (Remmers & Balchum, 1965). During the first and third weeks the room air was unfiltered and was essentially the same as the community air. During the second week the air was specially filtered to remove as many irritants as possible. The investigators found that airway resistance was higher in the first and third weeks as compared to the second week. An effect was present even when smoking was adjusted for (Ury & Hexter, 1969). In contrast, workers in Los Angeles (Rokaw & Massey, 1962; Schoettlin, 1962) and Cincinnati (Carey et al., 1958) have not found convincing evidence that changes in respiratory function are associated with low levels of oxidants. The populations studied may have been so ill that disease-associated factors swamped environmental factors as sources of variability in pulmonary function.

Some pollutants produce demonstrable changes in airway resistance in human volunteers. The experimentally demonstrable effects of sulfur dioxide occur only at concentrations (2–5 ppm) higher than those likely to occur in community exposures, which are almost always considerably below 1 ppm. However, concentrations of ozone capable of increasing airway resistance in the laboratory (0.1–1 ppm) are not much higher than those reported in the Los Angeles area (up to 0.15 ppm).

A second type of functional impairment is due to the binding of haemoglobin by carbon monoxide. This interferes with the transfer of oxygen from the blood to crucial tissues, such as the heart muscle and brain. The effect on heart muscle has suggested that carbon monoxide exposures might be particularly harmful for persons with far-advanced coronary artery disease or recent myocardial infarction. Suggestive results have been reported in Los Angeles (Cohen et al., 1969), but it is premature to draw any conclusions at this time.

The most readily observable impact of such functional effects is probably on performance. Photochemical pollution was associated with impaired performance of student athletes (Wayne et al., 1967) and with increased likelihood of motor vehicle accidents in California (Ury, 1968). Work and school absenteeism has been related to pollutant exposures in several countries (Goldsmith, 1968b). However, a systematic effort to observe impairment in performance has not yet begun. Such studies should provide a sound basis for assessing the cost of air pollution in terms of well-being and productivity.

Air pollution exposure and symptoms of sensory irritation

Since eye and respiratory irritation, and objectionable odours, are readily and frequently observed by private citizens, they are likely to be major factors in political responsiveness to air pollution. In addition, such symptoms may be of importance as indicators of more serious health effects.

In general, community complaints are more likely to be made because of pollutants that are irritating, subject to wide fluctuations (e.g., discharges from point sources), or odoriferous.

Research on odour effects is carried out in relatively few countries, notable among which are Sweden (Cederlöf et al., 1964; Lindvall, 1970; Jonsson et al., 1970) and the USA (Stockman & Anderson, 1966; Kendall & Lindvall, 1971). Classification and identification of odours and monitoring for air pollution odours are hampered by the relative insensitivity of laboratory instruments as compared to the human nose.

Probably the most common sensory effect of air pollution is eye irritation from cinders, smoke, fly ash, and photochemical oxidants (Goldsmith, 1968b). Toxicological evidence based on exposures to irradiated automobile exhaust shows that irritation of the nose, throat and eyes can result from oxidant concentrations of 0.10–0.15 ppm, levels common in the Los Angeles area (US National Air Pollution Control Administration, 1970).

Other air pollution effects on well-being

Interference with visibility, obscuration of sunlight, persistence of fog, and damage to plants and materials are other pollutant effects that also affect human well-being (Stern, 1968). The effects of living in a murky neighbourhood are depressing and dehumanizing. Such oppressive effects are a major basis for objections to air pollution. It is reasonable to assume that mental well-being is adversely affected by such phenomena as impaired visibility, pollution-stained buildings and fabrics, and loss of sunlight.

Chemicals potentially hazardous as community air pollutants

The epidemiological evidence as to the effects of air pollution on man, as presented in the preceding pages, refers to the common urban air pollutants, such as sulfur dioxide and suspended particulate matter, and to some extent carbon monoxide and "oxidants". A large number of other pollutants are found in urban air, particularly in the vicinity of specific industries. At present, however, there is little or no epidemiological evidence as to the effects of such pollutants on human health; in addition, the information that is available relates solely to populations in the neighbourhood of pollution sources. The pollutants in question include a variety of chemical substances (toxic metals, other inorganic compounds and organic compounds) known to be harmful to health, on the basis either of occupational exposure studies or of animal experiments, usually conducted at much higher concentration levels than those found in community air. The discussion that follows is by no means exhaustive. Its purpose is to illustrate the variety of substances that may occur as air pollutants; for additional information on some of these pollutants, the reader is referred to Chapter 12.

Lead and other toxic metals

Airborne toxic metals are found mainly in suspended particulate matter. The data supplied by the US Department of Health, Education, and Welfare (1966) show that arithmetic mean and maximum concentrations of some metals found in biweekly samples of urban air in the USA in 1964-1965 usually did not exceed 0.1 $\mu g/m^3$ and 1.0 $\mu g/m^3$ respectively, except for lead, copper, iron, magnesium, titanium, vanadium and zinc. Similar results were obtained in Japan (Osaka Prefectural Government, 1970). Marked diurnal variations in concentrations were observed (Rahm et al., 1971), and the presence of certain metals may be related to characteristic community activities. For example, high average concentrations of vanadium or arsenic may be found in communities using a specific type of fuel; iron and manganese are present in high concentrations in the neighbourhood of ferromanganese plants, and lead concentrations vary with the intensity of vehicular traffic and the distance from the road concerned. In general, however, air does not seem to be an important source of intake of these substances.

Lead. Mining and industrial processes, such as lead smelting and the manufacture of lead storage batteries, in certain localities, may discharge lead into the air in addition to the airborne lead emitted by motor vehicles. Based on a typical concentration of airborne lead of 2–4 $\mu g/m^3$, the average inhaled intake is estimated at 20–30 μg per day. There seems to be no consensus of opinion as to the significance to human health of the levels of exposure now encountered in community air (Committee on Biologic Effects of Atmospheric Pollutants, 1971).

Because of difficulties in measurement, no systematic monitoring of *mercury* in air has so far been carried out. Mercury may appear in air as a vapour or as an aerosol or in both forms. Some early measurements in Germany (Stock & Cucuel, 1934) gave average values of 0.02 $\mu g/m^3$ of total mercury; similar measurements in the USA (Cholak, 1952; Williston, 1968) gave values for particulate mercury ranging from 0.03 to 0.21 $\mu g/m^3$ and for mercury vapour from 0.001 to 0.0050 $\mu g/m^3$, with marked seasonal variations. In large industrial cities, total concentrations of 1 $\mu g/m^3$ may be approached, on a 24-hour basis (US Environmental Protection Agency, 1971b). The sources of mercury in air are not well understood. Industrial emissions from alkali plants may be significant; it has also been suggested, however, that the bulk of atmospheric mercury is due to evaporation from soil and water, and that the atmosphere plays a major role in the global and regional transport of mercury (Study Group on Mercury Hazards, 1971). Another possible source of atmospheric mercury is the combustion of coal and petroleum products (Hammond, 1971). Although only few data are available at present, it does not seem likely that airborne mercury would be a significant source of intake for man (US Environmental Protection Agency, 1971b).

Yearly average values of *cadmium* in air are of the order of 0.002 $\mu g/m^3$ (US Department of Health, Education, and Welfare, 1966). Much higher values, up to weekly means of 0.3 $\mu g/m^3$, were recorded in Sweden near factories using copper cadmium alloys. Similar values were found in Japan in the neighbourhood of a zinc smelter (Friberg et al., 1971). No data are available at present as to the chemical state in which cadmium appears in air, but it is certainly associated with airborne particles that gradually settle and deposit on land or water surfaces. Measurements of cadmium deposition were made in the area surrounding certain factories, and it seems that this may be an important source of cadmium in soil and plants (Rühling, 1969; Rühling & Tyler, 1970; Olofsson, 1970; Yamagata & Shigematsu, 1970). In general, airborne cadmium is a minor source of intake for man.

The use of *beryllium* has increased markedly in the last 30 years; contamination of neighbourhood air is most likely from metallurgical plants, lamp manufacture, and from production for different uses in the nuclear power industry. Both acute and chronic forms of beryllium poisoning have been found in "neighbourhood cases", the chronic forms predominating (Stokinger, 1966; Hardy, 1965). Of the 60 people with non-occupational berylliosis on the file of the Beryllium Registry, 18 were exposed to beryllium contained in polluted air in the vicinity of beryllium plants (Hardy et al., 1967). Together with mercury and asbestos, beryllium is considered as a "hazardous air pollutant", for which national emission standards have been proposed in the USA (US Environmental Protection Agency, 1971a).

Available data on *manganese* concentrations in urban air show values up to 10 $\mu g/m^3$ with an average of the order of 0.1 $\mu g/m^3$ (Sullivan, 1969a). In addition to industrial sources (iron and steel, ferromanganese, dry cell batteries, the chemical industry), the burning of coal and residual fuel oil may contribute to airborne manganese. Fuel additives used as anti-knock compounds (e.g., methylcyclopentadienyl manganese tricarbonyl) and smoke inhibitors, constitute an additional source. In at least two instances, airborne manganese was considered to be associated with an increased incidence of pneumonia in populations living in industrial areas (Elstad, 1939; Pancheri, 1955). Surveys made in the USSR (Dokučaev & Skvorceva, 1962) indicated adverse effects of manganese air pollution on the health of children living in the vicinity of a manganese production plant.

Atmospheric emissions of *arsenic* [1] are associated with metal smelters refining arsenical ores and with the use of arsenic-containing pesticides; reports from Czechoslovakia and India indicate that coal burning is another possible source (Bencko, 1970; Dave, personal communication, 1972). Ambient air concentrations of arsenic are of the order of 0.02 $\mu g/m^3$; these values may be much higher in the vicinity of arsenic-emitting sources (Sullivan, 1969b). Rosenstein (1970) has recently made a toxicological evaluation of low concentrations of arsenic in air. Two air pollution episodes involving high concentrations of arsenic have been recorded in the USA. In one case, local irritation of skin and mucosa was observed in children in the neighbourhood of a gold mine and smelter (Birmingham et al., 1954, 1965). In the other case (Sullivan, 1969b), a large number of animals were killed by eating plants contaminated with arsenic trioxide, but no effects on human health were recorded. Another episode occurred in Chile (Oyanguren & Perez, 1966) in the vicinity of a copper mine; urine analysis showed a significant degree of absorption of arsenic in all individuals in the area. In Czechoslovakia, increased amounts of arsenic were found in the hair of children living near a power station (Bencko, 1970); this was accompanied by a decrease in haemoglobin and in the number of red cells.

Hydrogen sulfide and mercaptans

The mercaptans (general formula R-SH) and hydrogen sulfide are toxic and strongly odorous substances formed in a number of industrial processes, notably petroleum refining, manufacture of pulp and paper, tanning, and sulfur dye manufacture. Because of their disagreeable odour, both are detectable at concentrations far below those considered toxic. Some mercaptans have a noticeable odour at concentrations of 3×10^{-5} ppm, while the threshold limit value for occupational exposure to one of the most potent (perchloromethyl mercaptan) is 0.1 ppm. Hydrogen sulfide is detectable by odour at concentrations of 0.04–0.1 ppm, i.e., about one tenth of the concentration at which, for example, sulfur dioxide is perceived by smell. Disastrous exposure of a community in Poza Rica, Mexico, occurred in 1950 when the failure of a natural gas sulfur removal unit released hydrogen sulfide into the surrounding air for about 20 minutes during a temperature inversion. This incident caused the death of 22 persons, while 320 others were hospitalized; all those concerned lived near the

---

[1] Arsenic occupies a position intermediate between the metals and the non-metals; it is conveniently considered here with the metals.

stack of the sulfur removal unit (Heimann, 1961; McCabe & Clayton, 1952). Hydrogen sulfide released from industrial sources has been a frequent cause of public complaint.

Fluorides, chlorine, and hydrogen chloride

Fluorides are present in the air of both rural and urban communities; the sources may be natural, coal burning (e.g., Indian coal contains 10–20 g per ton (Dave, personal communication, 1972)), or industrial (aluminium plants, brick and pottery kilns, phosphate fertilizer production, and some metallurgical processes). Fluoride concentrations in urban air range from less than 0.05 $\mu g/m^3$ up to about 2 $\mu g/m^3$; outside urban areas, concentrations rarely exceed 0.1 $\mu g/m^3$ (Thompson et al., 1971). Airborne fluorides may have adverse effects on agriculture (Weinstein & McCune, 1971). There have been reports of mottling of teeth and reduced incidence of dental caries in the vicinity of aluminium plants and similar installations (Macúch et al., 1963) and of fluorosis in children as a result of exposure to airborne fluorides (Sadilova, 1957).

Communities have been exposed to *chlorine* gas through accidents connected mainly with the transportation of liquefied chlorine (Kowitz et al., 1967; Joyner & Durel, 1962; Chasis et al., 1947). Similarly, a number of episodes of plant damage as a result of the accidental release of chlorine in the environment have been reported (Stahl, 1969). Among the important sources of atmospheric emission of chlorine are chlorine and caustic soda production plants.

A potentially hazardous chlorine compound emitted by industrial sources is hydrogen chloride.

Asbestos

The use of *asbestos* for protection against fire, for insulation purposes, in brake and clutch linings, flooring and building materials, and in other applications has expanded rapidly during the last 20 years. The possible sources of airborne asbestos are numerous, therefore, ranging from natural processes of weathering, to asbestos mining and the processing and manufacturing of asbestos-containing products. Data on asbestos concentrations in the ambient air are very scarce. According to some recent measurements, concentrations in the urban air are of the order of 10–100 nanograms per cubic metre (ng/m³) [1] (Selikoff et al., 1971). The asbestos air pollution problem is difficult to define, both because of our ignorance of the actual levels and because of the uncertainty as to the relationship between exposure and the possible health effects (Langmuir et al., 1961; Royall, 1967; Martin, 1970).

---

[1] 1 nanogram = 1×10^{-9} g.

Organochlorine pesticides

Measurements of concentrations of airborne organochlorine pesticides in the ambient air have been made in areas both near to and remote from those where these products have been used in agriculture. These measurements have shown that the distribution of such concentrations depends heavily on meteorological conditions, on proximity to the site of application, and on the time that has elapsed since application. For example, values obtained by Tabor (1966) for DDT were mainly in the range 0.1–400 ng/m^3. The level found in London air was of the order of 10 ng/m^3 (Abbot et al., 1966). In agricultural areas, typical values are in the range 0.1–22 ng/m^3 (Galley, 1971). This shows that ambient air is certainly not an important source of exposure of the general population to such compounds as DDT. Nevertheless, air may be an important vehicle for the transport of DDT—on a global scale—from the continents to the oceans (IMCO/FAO/WMO/WHO/IAEA/UN Joint Group of Experts on the Scientific Aspects of Marine Pollution, 1971).

Biological air pollutants

Aeroallergens

A wide range of airborne materials are capable of eliciting a hypersensitive (allergic) response in susceptible individuals. Moulds, dusts, paints, vegetable fibres, and, most importantly, pollens of wind-pollinated plants, are some of the materials known to produce such reactions. They may occur naturally, be associated with a particular occupational activity, or both. Seasonal allergic syndromes provided, in fact, early and dramatic evidence that certain health effects may be related to specific air pollutants. Despite some recent advances in this field, the nature and method of transport of aeroallergens, as well as other determinants of clinical responses, remain obscure to a large extent (Solomon, 1970).

For many possible allergens in ambient air, even the preliminary surveys have yet to be carried out. Data are particularly scarce as to the prevalence of bacteria in free air or in association with agricultural and industrial operations. The information available concerning airborne actinomycetes is also inadequate (Lloyd, 1969). Some data are available on insect-derived material, necessarily limited to larger body fragments recognizable microscopically (Solomon, 1970).

Aeroallergen-induced rhinitis and asthma are most commonly seen in North America and Western Europe (Williams, 1959) but such manifestations also occur elsewhere (Solomon, 1969; Lawther, 1965). A group of allergic pneumotides are now recognized that differ in their manifestations from bronchial asthma as seen in atopic persons; hypersensitivity develops to components of various organic dusts sufficiently small to penetrate to the alveolar level (Pepys, 1969). Examples of such conditions are "farmer's lung", involving thermophilic actinomycetes present in the dust of mouldy hay (Gregory et al., 1963), and bagassosis, which is known to follow exposure to the dust of mouldy sugar cane (Sakula, 1967).

Airborne micro-organisms

The transmission of infections through the air is a controversial subject; much of the confusion is due to the lack of precise definitions of such terms as "airborne infections" and "droplet infections". Although droplets travel short distances in the air, they transmit infections only between persons in close proximity; engineering methods of air purification in enclosed spaces therefore have little influence on the incidence of such infections. The term "airborne infections" is thus appropriate only if it refers to the transmission of infectious diseases by droplet nuclei, i.e., particles small enough [1] to remain suspended in the air for a long period (Langmuir, 1965). Such airborne infections appear to occur in enclosed spaces, such as schools, hospitals and laboratories (Wells, 1955; Langmuir et al., 1961). A study was recently carried out in two types of dwelling in Upper Volta and Mali (Chipponi et al., 1970) to determine the relationship between bacterial air pollution and the spread of cerebrospinal meningitis. In homes and schools in Upper Volta, the total number of airborne bacteria, including those of oral origin, was found to be much higher during the dry season, when epidemics of cerebrospinal meningitis occur, than in the rainy periods. In Mali, two districts of the city of Bamako, differing in the incidence of this disease, were examined. The number of airborne bacteria in the high-incidence district was found to be ten times greater than in the low-incidence district. The measurements were carried out during an epidemic of cerebrospinal meningitis. Examples of airborne outbreaks of infectious diseases are few and not always well documented. The diseases include, for example, Q-fever (Wellock, 1960), histoplasmosis (Furcolow, 1961), anthrax (Brachmann et al., 1960), and coccidioidomycosis. The case of coccidioidomycosis is perhaps the most convincing. This condition is endemic in arid regions of the south-western USA, and cases have been reported in Europe, the Hawaian islands and Argentina (Smith & Conant, 1960). Man and animals are infected by contaminated dust in areas where *Coccidioides imitis* spores are present.

Viruses can remain infectious for long periods of time if airborne in closed spaces (Benbough, 1969, 1971). The open air appears to have a bactericidal as well as a viricidal activity, associated by some authors with the air pollution complex of oxidants and ozone (Druett & May, 1968).

---

[1] Of the order of 5 µm or less.

Recent measurements of the viricidal activity of the open air (Benbough & Hood, 1971) show that its sterilizing power increases with decreasing size of the particles containing viruses.

Air Quality Criteria, Guides, and Standards [1]

At present air quality standards differ considerably from country to country. These differences have to be interpreted in relation to the criteria on which they are based, the recommended methods of sampling and measurement, and the legal background for implementing these standards. They reflect not only what a community can or will afford to control air pollution, but also the different philosophies on which control programmes are based.

Criteria and guides

A WHO Expert Committee on Air Quality Criteria and Guides for Urban Air Pollutants (1972) reviewed the available information and developed criteria and guides on which to base air quality standards. The specific substances reviewed were sulfur oxides and particulates (taken together), carbon monoxide, photochemical oxidants, and nitrogen dioxide. The remainder of this chapter is based on the report of the Committee.

TABLE 2

EXPECTED ADVERSE EFFECTS OF SULFUR DIOXIDE AND
SMOKE ON SELECTED POPULATION GROUPS

Concentration [a] ($\mu g/m^3$)		Adverse effect
Sulfur dioxide	Smoke	
500 (daily average)	500 (daily average)	Excess mortality and hospital admissions
500-250 [b] (daily average)	250 (daily average)	Deterioration of patients with pulmonary disease
100 (annual arithmetic mean)	100 (annual arithmetic mean)	Respiratory symptoms
80 (annual geometric mean)	80 (annual geometric mean) [c]	Visibility and/or human annoyance effects

[a] Measured by the method recommended by the British Standards Institution (1963), whereby both pollutants are measured at the same time. These values may have to be adjusted when other procedures are used.

[b] The range reflects differences of opinion within the Committee.

[c] Based on high-volume samplers.

Sulfur oxides and suspended particulates

These substances may be indicators of effects on human health rather than the causal factors *per se*; in addition, it is difficult to relate the various

---

[1] See also Chapter 32.

studies with each other because of the different methods used to measure the levels of these compounds.   Nevertheless, there is a need to develop criteria and guides, and the Committee agreed that certain levels can be related to certain adverse effects (see Table 2).   It should be emphasized that these effects apply to the simultaneous occurrence of the two pollutants; the relative effect of varying the concentration of one or the other could not be assessed.

Carbon monoxide

Both the concentration and the duration of exposure are important. Equilibrium is not rapidly attained: it takes about 3 hours for the blood to reach 50 % saturation with carbon monoxide, assuming that the individual starts with low basal carboxyhaemoglobin (approximately 0.5 %) and engages in light activity.   If he is a cigarette smoker or if carbon monoxide from other sources helps to raise his blood COHb, he will reach equilibrium sooner; if his blood COHb level is higher than the equilibrium value he will excrete CO until he reaches that equilibrium value.   Individuals should be protected from levels of 4 % COHb or more, since there is good evidence that measurable effects occur at about this level and that there is an increased risk to persons who already have cardiovascular disease.   Table 3 shows, for selected levels of CO in the ambient air, the time it takes for the COHb level of an individual engaged in light activity to rise from a low or basal level to 4 % COHb.

TABLE 3
CO CONCENTRATIONS IN AMBIENT AIR AND TIME
REQUIRED TO REACH 4 % CARBOXYHAEMOGLOBIN IN MAN *

Ambient CO		Time (hours)
mg/m³	ppm	
29	25	24
35	30	8
117	100	1

* Starting from "basal" values,
and assuming light activity at sea level.

Photochemical pollution

This type of pollution tends to be regional and requires sunlight as the source of energy to allow the photochemical reactions to take place. The eye, nose, and throat irritation associated with this type of pollution is felt almost instantaneously, so it is necessary to set maximum permissible values for short periods.   The probable effects on health of photochemical oxidants and the levels of exposure at which they appear to occur are shown below:

Health effect	Level and duration of exposure
Increased mortality	Not reported to date
Increased asthmatic attacks	250 μg/m^3 for 1 hour [a]
Pulmonary dysfunction	200 μg/m^3 for 1 hour
Annoyance and eye irritation	200 μg/m^3 for 1 hour

[a] Oxidant as measured by the neutral buffered KI method and expressed as ozone.

Nitrogen dioxide

Despite its demonstrated biological activity in animals, it was not possible to develop any specific criteria or guides for this substance, because of the lack of relevant information.

Standards

When air quality criteria and guides, such as those outlined above, are used to evaluate risks and to set standards, the ideal would be to have a complete set of dose-response curves for the different air pollutants, for different effects, and for different types of population exposed. However, this information is not available for any single substance, and certainly not for the combinations of substances found in the ambient air. Owing to the uncertainty of the dose-response relationships, it is prudent to use a safety factor, even when standards are derived from air quality guides. The magnitude of such a safety factor is dependent upon many considerations. These considerations may be political, with the main emphasis on cost-benefit analysis; they may arise from the significance and reliability of the data, e.g., whether the experimental evidence was gathered from animals or human beings; or they may depend on the specific effect against which protection is sought—mortality or some lesser effect.

Such standards may vary from country to country and within a country in the course of time. The development of national air pollution standards should include both standards to be met in a few years and long-term goals. In some countries it may be necessary in the immediate future to base standards on tolerable levels, and to establish intermediate goals of preventing illness and death in susceptible sub-groups of the population. Certainly the long-term goal should be to protect against all effects of significance to human health, including somatic and genetic change. This means that the levels should be as low as possible and the number of persons exposed as small as possible. It should be pointed out, however, that the decision with regard to a standard to protect the population from significant harm must be based on statistical probability; as a result, it cannot be guaranteed that every individual will be protected from such harm.

Short-term goals

On the basis of present knowledge, the Committee could make only the general statement that severe effects should obviously be avoided. Standards may evolve differently in different countries, depending on exposure conditions as well as on the socio-economic situation and the importance of other health problems.

Long-term goals

A long-term goal should be to keep exposure to the air pollutants discussed here as low as possible; non-effect levels are not yet well-defined, and will probably not be defined with any great degree of certainty for a long time to come.

TABLE 4
RECOMMENDED LONG-TERM GOALS

Pollutant	Limit
Sulfur oxides [a]	Annual mean 60 μg/m^3 98 % of observations below 200 μg/m^3
Suspended particulates [a]	Annual mean 40 μg/m^3 98 % of observations below 120 μg/m^3
Carbon monoxide (non-dispersive infra-red)	8-hour average 10 mg/m^3 1-hour maximum 40 mg/m^3
Photochemical oxidants as measured by neutral buffered KI method and expressed as ozone	8-hour average 60 μg/m^3 1-hour maximum 120 μg/m^3

[a] Measured by the method recommended by the British Standards Institution (1963), whereby sulfur oxides and suspended particulates are measured in conjunction. Where other methods are used, an appropriate adjustment may be necessary.

Our knowledge of the health effects of the pollutants under discussion is markedly less at concentrations lower than those considered above. Any forecast of the possible effects of such concentrations must therefore be speculative. However, it is possible to set levels, intermediate between those concentrations and the natural background levels, as a goal to be aimed at, in the hope that, in the light of present knowledge, they will produce no ill effects at all. Taking into consideration all the available evidence, the Committee recommended the limits shown in Table 4 as long-term goals to prevent undesirable effects from air pollutants. It should be understood that these recommendations are tentative and subject to change as more data on dose-response relationships within different populations become available.

These guidelines should be considered as proposals for limiting values that will give a high probability of avoiding adverse effects on human health. The values may be reduced if requirements for animals, plants, or materials are more stringent. On the one hand, they should not be regarded as the lowest values allowable or the levels up to which pollution is necessarily allowed; on the other hand, they shôuld not be considered as levels above which an adverse effect will appear. The proposed values merely indicate a limit below which the risk can be considered negligible. Their purpose is to guide the responsible authorities in the establishment of long-term. goals.

REFERENCES

Abbot, D. C., Harrison, R. B., Tatton, J. O. G. & Thomson, J. (1966) *Nature*, **211**, 259-261

Benbough, J. E. (1969) *J. gen. Virol.*, **4**, 473-477

Benbough, J. E. (1971) *J. gen. Virol.*, **10**, 209-220

Benbough, J. E. & Hood, A. M. (1971) *J. Hyg. (Lond.)*, **69**, 619-626

Bencko, U. (1970) *Wiss. Z. Humboldt Univ. Berl.*, **19**, 499-500

Berljand, M. E., ed. (1968) [*Atmospheric diffusion and air pollution*], Leningrad, Gidrometeoizdat (*Glavnaja Geofizičeskaja Observatorija, Trudy*, vol. 234)

Birmingham, D. J., Key, M. M. & Holaday, D. A. (1954) *An outbreak of dermatitis in a mining community — report of environmental and medical surveys*, US Department of Health, Education, and Welfare (report TR-11)

Birmingham, D. J., Key, M. M., Holaday, D. A. & Perone, V. B. (1965) *Arch. Derm.*, **91**, 457-464

Brachman, P. S., Plotkin, S. A., Bumford, F. H. & Atchinson, M. M. (1960) *Amer. J. Hyg.*, **72**, 6-23

British Standards Institution (1963) *Standard No. B.S. 1747*, London, British Standards Institution, parts 2, 3, 4

Buck, S. F. & Brown, D. A. (1964) *Research Paper 7*, London, Tobacco Research Council

Carey, G. C. R., Phair, J. J., Shephard, R. J. & Thompson, M. L. (1958) *Amer. industr. Hyg. Ass. J.*, **19**, 363-377

Cederlöf, R., Friberg, L., Jonsson, E., Kaij, L. & Lindvall, T. (1964) *Nord. Hyg.*, **45**, 39-48

Chambers, L. A. (1962) In: Stern, A. C., ed., *Air pollution*, New York and London, Academic Press, vol. 1, pp. 3-22

Chasis, H., Zappi, J. A., Bannon, J. H., Whittenberger, J. L., Helm, J., Doherry, J. L. & MacLeod, C. M. (1947) *Occup. Med.*, **4**, 152-176

Chipponi, P., Darrigol, J., Skalova, R. & Cvjetanovic, B. (1970) *Study of bacterial air pollution in Sahelian region of Africa affected by cerebrospinal meningitis*, Geneva, WHO (unpublished document BD/CSM/70.10)

Cholak, J. (1952) *The nature of atmospheric pollution in a number of industrial communities. In: Proceedings of a National Air Pollution Symposium, Pasadena, Calif.*

Cleary, G. J. (1967) *Clean Air*, September, pp. 15-18

Cleary, G. J. & Blackburn, C. R. B. (1968) *Arch. environm. Hlth*, **17**, 785-794

Cohen, S. I., Deane, M. & Goldsmith, J. R. (1969) *Arch. environm. Hlth*, **19**, 510-517

College of General Practitioners (1961) *Brit. med. J.*, **2**, 973-978

Colley, J. R. T. (1971) *Brit. med. Bull.*, **27**, 1-13

Committee on Biologic Effects of Atmospheric Pollutants (1971) *Airborne lead in perspective*, National Research Council, National Academy of Sciences, Washington, D.C.

Cornwall, C. J. & Raffle, P. A. B. (1961) *Brit. J. industr. Med.*, **18**, 24-53

Dokučaev, V. F. & Skvorcova, N. N. (1962) *Atmospheric air pollution with manganese compounds and their effects on the organism.* In: *USSR literature on air pollution and related occupational diseases*, Washington, D.C., US Department of Commerce, vol. 9, p. 40

Douglas, J. W. B. & Waller, R. E. (1966) *Brit. J. prev. soc. Med.*, **20**, 1-8

Druett, H. A. & May, K. R. (1968) *Nature (Lond.)*, **220**, 395-396

Elstad, D. (1939) *Nord. Med.*, **3**, 2527-2533

Friberg, L., Piscator, M. & Nordberg, G. (1971) *Cadmium in the environment — a toxicological and epidemiological appraisal*, Stockholm, Karolinska Institute

Furculow, M. L. (1961) *Bact. Rev.*, **25**, 301-309

Galley, R. A. E. (1971) *The contribution of pesticides used in public health programmes to the pollution of the environment. I. General and DDT*, Geneva, World Health Organization (unpublished document WHO/VBC/21.32.6)

Gardner, M. J., Crawford, M. D. & Morris, J. N. (1969) *Brit. J. prev. Med.*, **23**, 133-140

Goldsmith, J. (1968a) *Science*, **162**, 1352-1359

Goldsmith, J., (1968b) In: Stern, A. C., ed., *Air pollution*, 2nd ed., New York and London, Academic Press, vol. 1

Gregory, P. H., Lacey, M. E., Fenstein, G. N. & Skinner, F. A. (1963) *J. gen. Microbiol.*, **33**, 147-174

Halliday, I. C. (1961) *A historical review of atmospheric pollution.* In: *Air pollution*, Geneva, World Health Organization (*Monograph Series*, No. 46), pp. 9-38

Hammond, A. L. (1971) *Science*, **171**, 788-789

Hardy, H. L., Rabe, E. W. & Lorch, S. (1967) *J. occup. Med.*, **9**, 271-276

Hardy, I. C. (1965) *New Engl. J. Med.*, **273**, 1188-1199

Heimann, H. (1961) *Effects of air pollution on human health.* In: *Air pollution*, Geneva, World Health Organization (*Monograph Series*, No. 46), pp. 159-220

Hexter, A. C. & Goldsmith, J. R. (1971) *Science*, **172**, 265-267

IMCO/FAO/WMO/WHO/IAEA/UN Joint Group of Experts on the Scientific Aspects of Marine Pollution (1971) *Report of the Third Session, Rome, 1971*, Geneva, World Health Organization (unpublished document WHO/W.POLL./71.8)

Jacobs, M. B. (1962) In: Stern, A. C., ed., *Air pollution*, New York and London, Academic Press, vol. 1, pp. 447-495

Jonsson, E., Deane, M. & Sanders, G. (1970) *Community reactors to odors from pulp mills: a pilot study in Eureka, California* (paper submitted for Conference on the Measurement and Evaluation of Odor Sources, Stockholm, Karolinska Institute)

Joyner, R. E. & Durel, E. G. (1962) *J. occup. Med.*, **4**, 152-157

Kendall, D. A. & Lindvall, T. (1971) *Evaluation of community odor exposure: a report of a symposium*, Cambridge, Mass., Little

Kowitz, T. A., Reba, R. C., Parker, T. R. & Spicer, S. W. (1967) *Arch. environm. Hlth*, **14**, 545-558

Langmuir, A. D. (1965) *Air-borne infection.* In: Rosenau, M. J., ed., *Preventive medicine and public health*, New York, Appleton-Century-Crofts

Langmuir, A. D. et al. (1961) *Bact. Rev.*, **25**, 173-377

Lawther, P. J. (1958) *Proc. roy. Soc. Med.*, **51**, 262-264

Lawther, P. J. (1965) *Assignment report: air pollution in Kuwait, 27 February-5 March 1965*, Geneva, World Health Organization (unpublished document EM/ES/71)

Lindvall, T. (1970) *Nord. Hyg.*, Suppl. No. 2, 1-181

Lloyd, A. B. (1969) *J. gen. Microbiol.*, 57, 35-40

Loomis, T. A. (1968) *Essentials of toxicology*, Philadelphia, Lea and Febiger

Lunn, J. E., Knowelden, J. & Handyside, A. J. (1967) *Brit. J. prev. soc. Med.*, 21, 7-16

Macúch, P., Balážová, G., Bartošová, L., Hluchán, E., Ambruš, J., Janovicová, J. & Kirilčuková, V. (1963) *J. Hyg. Epidem. (Praha)*, 7, 389-403

Martin, A. E. (1970) *Hlth Trends*, No. 1, 19-21

May, K. R., Druett, H. A. & Packman, L. P. (1969) *Nature (Lond.)*, 221, 1146-1147

McCabe, L. & Clayton, G. D. (1952) *A. M. A. Arch. industr. Hyg.*, 6, 199-213

Olofsson, A. (1970) [*Report on investigations of atmospheric emissions from Finspång plant*], Svenska Metallverken (unpublished report No. HL 757)

Osaka Prefectural Government (1970) *Environmental pollution control center*, Osaka

Oyanguren, H. & Pérez, E. (1966) *Arch. environm. Hlth*, 13, 185-189

Paccagnella, B., Pavanello, R. & Pesarin, F. (1969) *Arch. environm. Hlth*, 18, 495-502

Pancheri, G. (1955) *Industrial atmospheric pollution in Italy*. In: Mallette, F. S., ed., *Problems and control of air pollution*, New York, Reinhold

Paul, J. R. (1966) *Clinical epidemiology*, Revised ed., Chicago, University of Chicago Press

Pepys, J. (1969) *Hypersensitivity diseases of the lungs due to fungi and organic dusts*, Basle, Karger (*Monographs in Allergy*, Vol. 4)

Rahm, K., Wesolovski, J. J., John, W. & Ralston, H. R. (1971) *J. Air Pollut. Control Ass.*, 21, 406-409

Reid, D. D. & Fairbairn, A. S. (1958) *Lancet*, 1, 1147-1152

Remmers, J. E. & Balchum, O. J. (1965) *Effects of Los Angeles urban air pollution upon respiratory function of emphysematous patients*. In: *Proceedings of the 58th Meeting of the Air Pollution Control Association*, Toronto

Rokaw, S. N. & Maseey, F. (1962) *Amer. Rev. resp. Dis.*, 86, 703-704

Royal College of Physicians of London (1970) *Air pollution and health: a report for the Royal College of Physicians of London*, London, Pitman

Royall, H. J. (1968) *Roy. Inst. publ. Hlth Hyg. J.*, Nos. 4-6, 126-146

Rozenštejn, I.S. (1970) *Gig. i Sanit.*, No. 1, p. 15

Rühling, A. (1969) *Contamination by heavy metals in the Oskarsham Avla*, Lund, Lund University, Department of Ecological Botany

Rühling, A. & Tyler, G. (1970) *Regional differences in deposit of heavy metals in Scandinavia*, Lund, Lund University, Department of Ecological Botany (Report No. 10)

Sadilova, M.S. (1957) [*Fluorosis in children resulting from air pollution by fluorine*]. In: [*Maximum permissible concentrations of atmospheric pollutants*], vol. 3, pp. 108-116

Sakula, A. (1967) *Brit. med. J.*, 3, 708-710

Schoettlin, C. E. (1962) *Amer. Rev. resp. Dis.*, 86, 878-897

Selikoff, I. J., Hammond, E. C. & Heimann, H. (1971). In: Englung, H. M. & Beery, W. T., eds, *Proceedings of the Second International Clean Air Congress*, New York & London, Academic Press

Smith, D. T. & Conant, N. F. (1960) *Zinsser's microbiology*, 12th ed., New York, Appleton-Century-Crofts

Sofoluwe, G. O. (1969) *W. Afr. med. J.*, **18**, 35-42

Solomon, W. R. (1969) *Advanc. environm. Sci. Technol.*, **1**, 197-236

Solomon, W. R. (1970) *Allergenic substances in ambient air*, Geneva, World Health Organization (unpublished working paper)

Spicer, W. S. (1967) *Arch. environm. Hlth*, **14**, 185-188

Spicer, W. S., Storey, P. B., Morgan, W. K. C., Kerr, H. D. & Standiford, N. E. (1962) *Amer. Rev. resp. Dis.*, **86**, 705-712

Stahl, Q. R. (1969) *Peliminary air pollution survey of chlorine gas (a literature review)*, Raleigh, N. C., US Department of Health, Education, and Welfare

Stern, A. C., ed. (1968) *Air pollution*, 2nd ed., New York and London, Academic Press, vol. 1

Stock, A. & Cucuel, F. (1934) *Naturwissenschaften*, **22**, 390-393

Stockman, R. L. & Anderson, D. O. (1966) *Physiologic, economic and nuisance effects of emissions from sulfate pulping.* In: Hendrickson, E. R., ed., *Atmospheric emissions from sulfate pulping: Proceedings of an International Conference*, pp. 72-95

Stocks, P. (1960) *Brit. J. Cancer*, **14**, 397-418

Stokinger, H. E., ed. (1966) *Beryllium, its industrial hygiene aspects*, New York, Academic Press

Study Group on Mercury Hazards (1971) *Environm. Res.*, **4**, 1-69

Study of Critical Environmental Problems (1970) *Man's impact on the global environment*, Cambridge, Mass., MIT Press

Study of Man's Impact on Climate (1971) *Inadvertent climate modification*, Cambridge, Mass., MIT Press

Sullivan, R. J. (1969a) *Preliminary air pollution survey of manganese and its compounds (a literature survey)*, Raleigh, N. C., US Department of Health, Education, and Welfare

Sullivan, R. J. (1969b) *Preliminary air pollution survey of arsenic and its compounds (a literature review)*, Raleigh, N. C., US Department of Health, Education, and Welfare

Tabor, E. C. (1966) *Trans. N. Y. Acad. Sci. Ser. II*, **28**, 569-578

Thompson, R. J., McMullen, T. B. & Morgan, G. B. (1971) *J. Air Pollut. Control Ass.*, **21**, 484-487

Ury, H. K. (1968) *Arch. environm. Hlth*, **17**, 334-342

Ury, H. K. & Hexter, A. C. (1969) *Arch. environm. Hlth*, **18**, 473-480

US Department of Health, Education, and Welfare (1966) *Air quality data, 1964-1965*, Cincinnati, Ohio, Division of Air Pollution

US Environmental Protection Agency (1971a) *Federal Register*, **36**, 23239-23256

US Environmental Protection Agency (1971b) *Background information: proposed national emission standards for hazardous air pollutants: asbestos, beryllium, mercury*, Research Triangle Park, N. C.

US National Air Pollution Control Administration (1969a) *Air quality criteria for particulate matter*, Washington, D.C., US Public Health Service (Publication No. AP-49)

US National Air Pollution Control Administration (1969b) *Air quality criteria for sulfur oxides*, Washington, D.C., US Public Health Service (Publication No. AP-50)

US National Air Pollution Control Administration (1970) *Air quality criteria for photochemical oxidants*, Washington, D.C., US Public Health Service (Publication No. AP-63)

US Public Health Service (1972) *Health consequences of smoking: report to the Surgeon General*, Washington, D.C., US Department of Health, Education, and Welfare

Wayne, W. S., Wehrle, P. F. & Carroll, R. E. (1967) *J. Amer. med. Ass.*, **199**, 901-904

Weinstein, L. V. H. & McCune, D.C. (1971) *J. Air Pollut. Control Ass.*, **21**, 410-413

Wellock, C. E. (1960) *Calif. Hlth*, **18**, 73

Wells, W. F. (1955) *Airborne contagion and air hygiene: an ecological study of droplet infections*, Cambridge, Mass., Harvard University Press

WHO Expert Committee on Urban Air Pollution (1969) *Report*, Geneva (*Wld Hlth Org. techn. Rep. Ser.*, No. 410)

Wicken, A. M. & Buck, S. F. (1964) *Research Paper 8*, London, Tobacco Research Council

Williams, D. A. (1959)   In: Jamar, J. A., ed., *International text book of allergy*, Springfield, Ill., Thomas, Chapter 4

Williston, S. H. (1968) *J. geophys. Res.*, **73**, 7051-7055

Winkelstein, W. (1967) *Arch. environm. Hlth*, **14**, 162-169

Winkelstein, W. (1968) *Arch. environm. Hlth*, **16**, 401-405

Winkelstein, W. (1969) *Arch. environm. Hlth*, **18**, 544-547

World Meteorological Organization (1970) *Meteorological aspects of air pollution*, Geneva (*Technical Note* No. 106)

Yamagata, N. & Shigematsu, I. (1970) *Bull. Inst. publ. Hlth (Tokyo)*, **19**, 1-27

Zeidberg, L. D., Hagstrom, R. M., Sprague, H. A. & Landau, E. (1967a) *Arch. environm. Hlth*, **15**, 237-248

Zeidberg, L. D., Horton, R. J. M. & Landau, E. (1967b) *Arch. environm. Hlth*, **15**, 214-224

CHAPTER 2

WATER

In theory, man can exist on quantities of water as small as 5 litres or less per day; some nomadic peoples do, in fact, live for long periods on such quantities. However, 40 to 50 litres per day are required for personal and domestic hygiene, if he is to remain healthy, while still greater amounts are necessary in more sophisticated environments to enable him to engage in animal husbandry and rural industry; thus a villager will need 100 litres or more. In an industrialized country, or one in which irrigated agriculture is practised, it is not uncommon for 400 to 500 litres to be needed per head. Such needs are becoming increasingly difficult to meet, as pollution has reduced the quality of many water sources.

Water is considered polluted when it is altered in composition or condition so that it becomes less suitable for any or all of the functions and purposes for which it would be suitable in its natural state. This definition includes changes in the physical, chemical and biological properties of water, or such discharges of liquid, gaseous or solid substances into water as will or are likely to create nuisances or render such waters harmful to public health, safety or welfare, or to domestic, commercial, industrial, agricultural, recreational or other legitimate uses of water, or to livestock, wild animals, fish or other aquatic life. It also includes changes in temperature due to the discharge of hot water (thermal pollution).

Sources of Water Pollution and Types of Pollutant

Pollution may be accidental — and sometimes with grave consequences — but is most often caused by the uncontrolled disposal of sewage and other liquid wastes resulting from domestic uses of water, industrial wastes containing a variety of pollutants, agricultural effluents from animal husbandry and drainage of irrigation water, and urban run-off. The deliberate spreading of chemicals on the land to increase crop yields or the addition of chemicals to water to control undesirable organisms is another cause of pollution. Examples are the applications of chemical fertilizers, and of pesticides for the control of aquatic weeds, insects and molluscs.

In addition to the increased production of sewage due to the growth of population, the *per caput* production of waste water is also growing, so that in many cities it may amount to 600 litres per day per person. At the same time its content of organic and mineral pollutants is also large and may amount to 10 litres of wet sludge per person daily, or about 50 kg of dry solids per person per year (WHO Scientific Group on the Treatment and Disposal of Wastes, 1967). Domestic and municipal sewage contains decomposable organic matter that exerts a demand on the oxygen resources of the receiving waters. This biochemical oxygen demand (BOD) is a measure of the weight (per unit volume of water or waste water) of dissolved oxygen consumed in the biological processes that degrade organic matter; it is determined by means of a standard test procedure. BOD values range from around 1 mg/litre (for natural waters) to 300–500 mg/litre (for untreated domestic sewage). The organic matter consists primarily of carbohydrates, proteins from animal matter and miscellaneous fats and oils. The specific classes of organic compounds found in sewage include amino-acids, fatty acids, soaps, esters, anionic detergents, amino-sugars, amines, amides, and many others. Much of the impurity in municipal wastes is settleable material that may be deposited at the bottom of receiving waters to form deep layers of organic sludge. Dissolved salts in the form of ions such as sodium, potassium, calcium, manganese, ammonium, chloride, nitrate, nitrite, bicarbonate, sulfate and phosphate are the main inorganic constituents of sewage and other waste-waters. Domestic and municipal sewage invariably contains a variety of micro-organisms, some of which may be pathogenic. Although most human intestinal pathogens do not survive for extended periods outside the body of the host, there is evidence that they may remain sufficiently viable in different types of aquatic environment to infect man. The presence of indicator organisms, especially the faecal *Escherichia coli*, affords presumptive, though not conclusive, evidence of pollution by sewage and thus of the possibility of a public health hazard.

Industrial pollutants are even more difficult to characterize, and detailed inventories of industrial wastes on a national scale are practically non-existent. Industrial wastes usually contain traces or larger quantities of the raw materials, intermediate products, final products, co-products and by-products and of any ancillary or processing chemicals used. The composition and amounts of pollutants discharged by a specific industry can usually be determined only by detailed analysis of its effluents. The complete enumeration of the substances present in industrial waste waters as a whole would run into thousands. They include detergents, solvents, cyanides, heavy metals, mineral and organic acids, nitrogenous substances, fats, salts, bleaching agents, dyes and pigments, phenolic compounds, tanning agents, sulfides and ammonia; of the compounds mentioned, many are biocidal and toxic. In spite of this variety, many industrial wastes can be measured by the same parameters as those applicable to municipal wastes, such as BOD and chemical oxygen demand (COD), turbidity, and suspended solids; however, the lack of information on the composition of industrial discharges has caused the greatest difficulties in water quality management.

Pollution from agricultural practices is due to animal wastes, material eroded from land, plant nutrients, inorganic salts and minerals resulting from irrigation, herbicides and pesticides; to these may be added various infectious agents contained in wastes. The total quantity of such wastes is large. In the USA, for instance, the production of animal wastes exceeds that of human wastes by a factor of at least five on a BOD basis, seven on a total nitrogen basis, and 10 on a total solids basis (Loehr, 1970).

Although the variety of dissolved and suspended materials in natural waters and aqueous liquid wastes is large, their total concentration is comparatively small. Thus the water content of sea-water is 96.5 % of the total, of domestic sewage 99.9 % and of rivers 99.95 %. The concentrations of pollutants may range from around 1 g/litre (total dissolved and suspended matter in sewage) down to microgram quantities per litre (e.g., carcinogenic hydrocarbons) or even less.

The concentration of pollutants present in original waste waters is normally altered when the water is treated before discharge. The fate of pollutants after release to a natural water will in general depend on their nature (solubility, biodegradability) and on that of the body of water concerned. They will normally be subject to physical processes of dispersion and dilution, and may be affected by chemical or biological reactions. Prediction of the variations in their concentration with time and distance from the point of discharge is often easiest where physical processes are alone involved, as is the case when the pollutant is non-degradable. Methods of prediction for these circumstances are, however, more advanced for soluble substances, which travel with the water in which they are dissolved, than for suspended matter with a tendency either to float or settle under gravity. The situation can be even more complicated when chemical or biological mechanisms are involved, though good progress has been made in developing techniques of forecasting. Prediction of the fate and effects of substances that undergo biochemical oxidation and thereby influence the level of dissolved oxygen presents particular difficulties because of the large number of factors that can affect reaction rates, including temperature, concentration of dissolved oxygen, and presence or absence of inhibiting or accelerating materials. The oxygen depletion may proceed to the point where anaerobic conditions prevail. The variation in concentration of dissolved oxygen with distance often follows a so-called "oxygen-sag" curve showing a minimum below the point of discharge, usually followed by a zone of recovery. Knowledge of all these processes is of great importance in water pollution control. Calculations, however, are often made on the basis of one-point discharge and do not necessarily give a true picture of the situation.

Specific problems: groundwater and coastal waters

Untreated non-saline *groundwater* is normally much safer to drink than any untreated surface water, since the ground itself provides an effective purifying medium; such water constitutes a major source of drinking-water supplies. Nevertheless, many cases are known where groundwater has been polluted by domestic and industrial waste waters, by soluble materials leached out of tips for municipal refuse or industrial waste, by accidental spillage of other liquids, especially oil, and by intrusion of highly saline water (Buchan & Key, 1956; Baars, 1957).

Pollution of *coastal waters* may arise from various sources, such as the discharge of sewage and industrial waste from coastal outfalls, the dumping of wastes at sea, and the discharge of sewage and rubbish from ships; the handling of cargo, and the exploration and exploitation of the sea bed and ocean floor; accidental pollution by oil and other substances; and conveyance by air and other routes of pollutants from the land. If wastes contain persistent pollutants, discharge into rivers even at considerable distances upstream from the mouth can result in substantial quantities reaching the sea. Undoubtedly the most frequent cause of coastal pollution problems is the discharge of municipal sewage and industrial wastes into coastal waters or into estuaries through unsatisfactory disposal facilities. Nevertheless, considerable quantities of waste waters are disposed of without causing a nuisance or problems of other kinds. The major classes of pollutant reaching coastal waters are decomposable organic materials, heavy metals and other toxic matter, dissolved and suspended non-toxic inorganic substances, and pathogenic organisms (IMCO/FAO/UNESCO/ WMO/WHO/IAEA/UN Joint Group of Experts on Scientific Aspects of Marine Pollution, 1971).

Many factors, such as dilution, temperature, adsorption, sedimentation and nutrient deficiencies, influence self-purification of the sea. The marine environment is generally unfavourable to the survival of most pathogenic organisms. However, under special circumstances, particularly in temperate and warm coastal waters near large cities, pathogenic agents may be found in marine waters in the proximity of the coast-line and in estuaries (Brisou, 1968; Mallman, 1970).

Health Hazards of Water Pollution and Water-Related Diseases

Water, as a part of the human environment, occurs in four main forms—as groundwater, in freshwater surface masses, in the sea, and as vapour in the atmosphere. Human health may be affected by ingesting water directly or in food, by using it in personal hygiene or for agriculture, industry or recreation, and by living near it. Two main categories of water-associated health hazards are considered here: (1) hazards from biological agents that may affect man following ingestion of water or other forms of water contact, or through insect vectors; and (2) hazards from chemical and radioactive pollutants, usually resulting from discharges of industrial wastes.

Biological hazards

Water-associated hazards from ingestion of biological agents

The principal biological agents transmitted in this way can be grouped into the following categories: pathogenic bacteria; viruses; parasites; and other organisms.

The contamination of water by pathogenic bacteria, viruses and parasites can be attributed either to the pollution of the water source itself or to the pollution of the water during its conveyance from source to consumer. The pollutants may include the excretions, faecal and urinary, of man and animals, sewage and sewage effluents, and washings from the soil. Infections are spread both by patients and by carriers who shed the pathogen in faeces or urine. Carriers may be patients who have recovered but still harbour the infective agent without suffering any further ill-health themselves, or patients with mild or asymptomatic disease that has neither been discovered nor diagnosed. The prevention of pollution and the purification of water are largely concerned with, and were developed to bring about, the eradication of water-borne infections.

(1) Pathogenic bacteria

Pathogenic bacteria transmitted directly by water or indirectly through water to food, constitute one of the principal sources of morbidity and mortality in many developing countries. They include the causative agents of the great epidemic diseases—cholera and typhoid—and of the less spectacular but far more numerous cases of infantile diarrhoea, dysenteries and other enteric infections that occur continuously, and often with fatal results, among rural and urban populations, particularly in the developing countries.

Bacterial infections, especially those caused by the *Salmonella* group, may also be transmitted by shellfish grown in contaminated waters, unless a sufficient period is allowed for self-cleansing in tanks containing pathogen-free water treated with chlorine or by ultraviolet light.

Table 1 shows the principal diseases attributable to the ingestion of water-borne bacteria.

TABLE 1

BACTERIAL DISEASES CAPABLE OF BEING TRANSMITTED
THROUGH CONTAMINATED WATER OR FOOD PREPARED WITH SUCH WATER

Disease	Causative organism
Cholera	*Vibrio cholerae*, including biotype El Tor
Bacillary dysentery	*Shigella* spp.
Typhoid fever	*Salmonella typhi*
Paratyphoid fever	*Salmonella paratyphi* A, B & C
Gastoenteritis	Other *Salmonella* types, *Shigella*, *Proteus* spp., etc.
Infantile diarrhoea	Enteropathogenic types of *Escherichia coli*
Leptospirosis	*Leptospira* spp.
Tularaemia (rarely)	*Pasteurella (Brucella* or *Francisella) tularensis*

During the last decade, classical cholera caused by *Vibrio cholerae* has receded remarkably, even in such areas as Calcutta. However, cholera "El Tor", which emerged in 1961 from its endemic foci in Indonesia, has spread to many countries in the Western Pacific and in South-East and Central Asia. During 1970, a series of outbreaks of cholera "El Tor" occurred in areas not normally affected, e.g., the Eastern Mediterranean region and the USSR, as well as a number of African countries (*Off. Rec. Wld Hlth Org.*, 1971). In 1971, cholera spread to nine more African countries, and small outbreaks or individual cases of cholera occurred in six European countries. Person-to-person transmission of cholera does occur, but by far the most important mode of dissemination is through the environment, especially water (Barua et al., 1970). Typhoid and paratyphoid fevers are still widely disseminated throughout the world; in Europe, the explosive outbreak of typhoid fever in Zermatt in 1963 was a salutary warning (Bernard, 1965). Outbreaks of salmonellosis, although usually food-borne, may occasionally be spread by water (Greenberg & Ongerth, 1966).

(2) *Viruses*

Certain viruses that multiply in the alimentary tract (including the oropharynx) of man, and may be excreted in considerable amounts in faeces, can be found in sewage and polluted waters but their mere presence is not necessarily evidence of significant risk to man. The viruses most commonly present in polluted waters and sewage are the enteroviruses (poliovirus, coxsackieviruses and echoviruses), adenoviruses, reoviruses and the virus (not yet identified) of infectious hepatitis (Chang, 1968). Of the enteroviruses, the spread of poliovirus by water has rarely if ever been demonstrated, because of the extremely high dilution of the virus and the consequent difficulty of isolating it, whilst the more direct faecal-oral route is the most likely mode of spread of the echoviruses and coxsackieviruses; adenoviruses and reoviruses are usually transmitted to other persons from the oropharynx (respiratory route).

Although the virus of infectious hepatitis has not yet been isolated and identified, there is ample epidemiological evidence that outbreaks of this infection, which has a global distribution, are caused by polluted waters (Mosley, 1967; Taylor et al., 1966; Koff, 1970). A striking example was the epidemic of infectious hepatitis in Delhi (1955–56), in which more than 28 000 cases were identified, with a case fatality rate of 0.9 per 1000 and an estimated total case incidence of 97 600 (Viswanathan, 1957).

Infectious hepatitis can also be spread·by shellfish contaminated with sewage effluent (WHO Expert Committee on Hepatitis, 1964).

(3)   Parasites

Of the parasites that may be ingested, Entamoeba histolytica is the causal agent of both intestinal amoebiasis (e.g., amoebic dysentery and its complications) and extra-intestinal forms of the disease, such as amoebic liver abscess. It is widespread throughout the warm countries of the world and wherever sanitary conditions are poor. Fine filtration, as practised for the removal of bacteria, is both effective and essential against vegetative and encysted amoebae, since amoebic cysts are resistant to chlorine in the doses normally applied in water treatment (WHO Expert Committee on Amoebiasis, 1969). The guinea-worm, which causes dracontiasis, is common among the rural populations of many developing countries. This parasite is transmitted principally through open village wells and ponds infested with the copepod intermediate host.

Some intestinal helminths, such as Ascaris lumbricoides and Trichuris trichiura, may also be water-borne, although ingestion of contaminated soil is the normal means of transmission. Distomatosis is another parasitic disease that may be contracted by swallowing contaminated water containing, in this case, cysts of species of Fasciola or Dicrocoelium.

Hydatid disease (hydatidosis), a zoonosis that usually involves a dog-sheep-dog cycle in maintaining the reservoir of infection (cattle, pigs and other animals, including wildlife, may act as intermediate hosts), is occasionally transmitted to man through drinking-water or foods contaminated with the excreta of the primary hosts.

Hazards from biological agents transmitted through water contact other than ingestion

In economically advanced countries, direct contact with water, other than in personal hygiene, occurs mostly in recreational activities—swimming, waterskiing, etc.—and ordinarily involves only minimal hazards. In many developing countries, on the other hand, water in rivers, ponds, canals, etc., is used for a variety of purposes—ablutions, washing of clothes, disposal of human excreta, domestic uses—so that these waters become highly polluted and serve as an important vehicle for the transmission of enteric infections, such as cholera, typhoid fever and the dysenteries, and of certain parasitic infections.

Of the communicable diseases spread by the penetration, by parasites, of the skin and certain mucous membranes, the most widespread is schistosomiasis. Certain bacteria also cause disease in this way.

(1) *Schistosomiasis and other communicable diseases*

Schistosomiasis is a chronic, insidious, debilitating disease that may cause serious pathological lesions, saps energy, lowers resistance and reduces output of work. In certain endemic areas, it may be classed not only as an important health problem, but as a major social and economic one as well. Accurate figures for morbidity and mortality are lacking, but a conservative estimate is that the number of people infected with the parasite at any given time amounts to some 200 million. In some endemic areas, the prevalence may exceed 50 % (WHO Expert Committee on Bilharziasis, 1965; WHO Expert Committee on the Epidemiology and Control of Schistosomiasis, 1967). The accelerated construction of artificial lakes, reservoirs and water impoundments to meet the needs of agriculture and industry in developing countries must inevitably lead to an increase in freshwater snail populations and a corresponding increase in schistosomiasis if preventive measures are not taken.

The disease in man is chiefly due to three species of trematodes, namely *Schistosoma mansoni*, *S. japonicum* and *S. haematobium*.

Of these, the first two give rise to intestinal manifestations, and the third is the causative agent of genito-urinary or vesical schistosomiasis. The eggs, released in faeces or urine, hatch as miracidia on reaching a free body of water, where they penetrate snails (such as *Biomphalaria*, *Bulinus* and *Oncomelania*). They emerge from the snails in the form of cercariae ready to infect man. Penetration is through the skin, while wading, bathing, etc. Water flowing with only a very gentle current, as in slow-moving canals, is preferred by all species of aquatic snail hosts.

In many parts of the world, bathers in lakes may be affected by "swimmer's itch". This dermatitis is caused by the penetration of the skin by cercariae of schistosomes from animals, such as birds and rodents.

Other parasitic diseases where entry is through the skin are ancylosto-miasis and strongyloidiasis. *Necator americanus* and *Ancylostoma duode-nale* are the hookworms (roundworms) responsible for most cases of ancylostomiasis. The eggs, passed in the faeces of the infected person, hatch and larvae emerge that develop into a filariform stage infective to man. Strongyloidiasis is caused by the nematode *Strongyloides stercoralis*, which inhabits the submucous tissue of the small intestine. The mode of transmission is identical to that of ancylostomiasis. While water may serve as the medium whereby these infective agents are swallowed, infection is usually acquired by skin penetration from soil, or by auto-infection in the case of *Strongyloides*.

Leptospirosis is the principal bacterial infection transmissible from vertebrate animals to man through direct contact with water. The natural hosts are wild and domestic animals that excrete leptospires in urine, and man is infected through the skin and mucous membranes from contact with the water of contaminated ponds, canals, rivers, etc.

(2) *Health hazards from bathing beaches and coastal waters*

With the increased use by large groups of people of beaches for recrea-tional purposes and because of the possible consumption of marine fish and shellfish from polluted waters, it is understandable that coastal pollution has received increased attention in many countries.

Epidemiological studies on coastal pollution have given equivocal findings and no definite conclusions have yet been reached (Brisou, 1968, 1971; Moore, 1954, 1970).

In a large-scale survey of over 40 bathing beaches around the English coast that were known to be contaminated with sewage, only four cases of paratyphoid fever probably due to bathing were recorded; these were from two beaches with median coliform counts of more than 1000 per 10 ml; both beaches also showed gross macroscopic faecal pollution. There was no evidence that bathing in polluted coastal waters played any part in the occurrence of 150 cases of poliomyelitis among children living near the sea (Committee on Bathing Beach Contamination of the Public Health Laboratory Service, 1959). More information is needed about the possibility of young children acquiring superficial mycotic diseases, such as thrush, or becoming infected with enteroviruses other than poliovirus, as a result of bathing in such waters.

There is no agreed basis for establishing a limiting bacteriological quality for coastal water, above which there is a danger of infection from bathing. Maximum acceptable counts in different countries for coliforms may be as high as 10 000 per litre of water; for *Streptococcus faecalis* the corresponding figure is 200 per litre (Brisou, 1968). There are no inter-nationally accepted criteria for the quality of coastal water, with respect either to microbial contamination or chemical pollution.

Hazards of diseases transmitted by water-associated insect vectors

Of diseases caused by water-associated vectors, the most widespread is malaria, transmitted by the anopheline mosquito. The habitats of different vector species of anophelines, their ecology and bionomics are well known (see Chapter 5, Insects and rodents).

Onchocerciasis, or river blindness, is associated, under natural conditions, with clear springs running over rocky beds. In artificial works of water resources development, the same conditions may arise on dam spillways or concrete lined channels if suitable precautions are not taken. The disease, transmitted by blackflies (*Simulium* spp.), is of considerable health, social and economic importance in the vicinity of breeding grounds for the vector, where a large proportion of the resident population may become partially or completely blind. The creation of new breeding areas, as a result of water resources development, may outweigh in significance any potential benefits of the works concerned (WHO Expert Committee on Onchocerciasis, 1966). An indirect effect of onchocerciasis on the environment may follow the application of control measures against the vector if persistent insecticides, such as DDT, are used for this purpose. However, it is now recommended that these insecticides should be replaced in onchocerciasis vector control by newly developed biodegradable larvicides.

Other diseases of a similar nature include yellow fever (transmitted by a water-breeding mosquito); trypanosomiasis, or sleeping sickness, which is widespread in Africa and is transmitted by the tsetse fly (the form of the disease caused by *Trypanosoma gambiense* is particularly associated with waterside vegetation); and filariasis.

Filariasis, which affects more than 250 million people throughout the world, continues to be one of the major parasitic infections. The public health importance of the causative organisms, *Wuchereria bancrofti* and *Brugia malayi*, is widely recognized, but control programmes, although successful to some extent, have not succeeded in containing the infection significantly on a world basis. Indeed, in many of the developing countries the amount of infection and disease may in fact be increasing. This trend is due primarily to the rapid urbanization now taking place in many of the new countries of Africa and Asia, a phenomenon characterized by vast population movements and the growth of urban ghettos in which breeding sites for the major vector, *Culex pipiens fatigans*, have been greatly increased (WHO Expert Committee on Filariasis (*Wuchereria* and *Brugia* infections), 1967).

C. p. fatigans may occupy the first place as the mosquito that has profited most by increasing urbanization and industrialization. In Kaduna, Nigeria, for instance, a survey carried out in 1942 failed to detect the presence of this species at all. However, in 1958, another survey found as many as 760 per room (Mattingly, 1963). The significance of this rather spectacular development is that it occurred unrecognized. There seems little doubt that similar rapid increases in numbers are taking place in other areas. In addition to its well developed ability to shelter in houses, *C. p. fatigans* possesses a remarkable genetic adaptability in developing resistance to insecticides; it was noted in Malaya that the urban strain of this species was about 20 times as efficient a vector of *W. bancrofti* as a rural strain.

Nuisance organisms

Other organisms constitute, so far as is known at present, only indirect health hazards in that they may make a safe water unpalatable or unattractive, or interfere with treatment and distribution processes. Such organisms include the biological slimes that accumulate on the interior surfaces of mains and upon which methane-utilizing bacteria may grow; algae and bryozoal growths, such as *Plumatella*, which may interfere with the operation of filters; molluscs, such as *Dreissena*, which may choke mains; crustacea, such as *Asellus* ("water louse" or "sow bug"), and nematodes, which while not in themselves pathogenic, may harbour bacteria or viruses in their intestines, thus protecting possible pathogens from destruction by chlorine; and certain algae, which may impart bad tastes and odours to water. Table 2 lists the nuisance organisms normally found in drinking-water.

TABLE 2

NUISANCE ORGANISMS NORMALLY FOUND IN DRINKING-WATER

Organism	Effects
Biological slimes	Choking of treatment plants and distribution systems. Support for methane-utilizing bacteria. Risk of rendering water unacceptable
Molluscs (Dreissena)	Choking of water mains
Plumatella, algae	Interference with filtration
Asellus	Risk of rendering water unacceptable
Nematodes	Possible concentration of pathogens

Nuisance organisms, which, once they have entered a distribution system, may multiply there, can be kept to insignificant levels by regular cleansing of mains and storage tanks, and by the use of harmless pesticides, such as pyrethrin, to which some of these organisms (e.g., *Asellus*) are particularly sensitive. Research is needed on the influence of organic matter in treated water on bacterial growths, leading to the production of bad tastes and odours.

Hazards from chemical and radioactive pollution

Types of hazard

If present above a certain level, some chemical pollutants (e.g., nitrates, arsenic and lead) may constitute a direct toxic hazard when ingested in water. Other water constituents, such as fluorides, are beneficial, and may be essential to health, if present in small concentrations, though toxic if taken in larger amounts. Certain other substances or chemical characteristics may affect the acceptability of water for drinking purposes. They include substances causing odours or tastes; acidity or alkalinity; anionic detergents; mineral oil; phenolic compounds; and naturally occurring salts of magnesium and iron, as well as sulfate and chloride ions, if present in excessive concentrations. Both international and national criteria and standards have been established to provide a basis for the control of human exposure to many of these substances through ingestion of polluted water (World Health Organization, 1970, 1971b) (see also pp. 65-68).

Ingestion is, however, only one possible pathway to exposure. Man can be exposed to water pollutants through other types of direct contact, e.g., in recreation or the use of water for personal hygiene. The possible health implications of these non-drinking uses of water (including agricultural and industrial uses) are less well understood, and no international criteria or guidelines exist for the control of such exposure.

In addition to the possible effects of ingestion and other direct water contacts, chemical water pollutants may influence man's health indirectly by disturbing the aquatic ecosystems or by accumulating in aquatic organisms used in human food. For some pollutants, at the levels now existing in water bodies, these effects may be the most important public health aspects of water pollution, and should be considered particularly in respect of such substances as compounds of toxic metals and organo-chlorine pesticides.

The various chemical and biochemical transformations that pollutants may undergo in the aquatic environment also deserve attention. Chemical change may affect their biological availability or toxicity, which may be either enhanced or reduced. Degradation or transformation products may appear that are more toxic than the original pollutant. Little is known of these physical, chemical and biological processes and their mechanisms, yet they are essential to the understanding of the health implications of chemical water pollution.

Many water pollutants also appear in air and food, which are often more important sources of intake than water. Such pollutants include metals, organic substances resistant to biodegradation, and radionuclides. The assessment of pollutant levels in water should always be made in relation to the actual intake of drinking water and to the body burden resulting from other sources in a given locality (World Health Organization, 1971b).

Specific pollutants

A few specific pollutants will be discussed as examples of toxic substances that may be transmitted from the source to man by water. For details of the toxicology of some of these substances, the reader is referred to Chapters 12 and 13.

(1) Nitrates

The concentration of nitrate in surface waters is usually below 5 mg/litre. Much higher concentrations are sometimes found in groundwater. For example, a survey of 2000 wells in Canada (Robertson & Riddel, 1949) showed that 25.5 % of wells examined contained over 20 mg/litre of nitrate nitrogen, 18.8 % over 50 mg/litre, and 5.3 % over 300 mg/litre. The consumption of water (or baby food preparations) with a high nitrate concentration may result in infant methaemoglobinaemia. The mean nitrate content of water consumed by affected children, for example, in Czechoslovakia (Schmidt & Knotek, 1970) ranged from 18 to 257 mg/litre, but about three-quarters of them had consumed water containing more than 100 mg/litre of nitrate.

(2) Fluorides

Fluorides occur naturally in many public water supplies and are regarded as essential constituents of drinking-water, particularly with regard to the prevention of dental caries in children (McClure, 1970). If the concentration of fluorides in drinking-water is less than 0.5 mg/litre, the incidence of dental caries is likely to be high. When present in much greater concentrations, they can cause endemic cumulative fluorosis with resulting skeletal damage (Adler et al., 1970). It has therefore been recommended that the fluoride content of water should be kept within well-defined limits (World Health Organization, 1971b), which vary with water temperature (see also Chapter 12). Areas exist where the natural fluoride content of the water is high, e.g., the Kurnool district of Andhra Pradesh, India (up to 6 mg/litre, with 23 % of samples exceeding 1.5 mg/litre) (Ramamohana Rao & Bhaskaran, 1964), New Mexico (up to 12 mg/litre) (Cholak, 1959), and elsewhere (Adler et al., 1970).

(3) Arsenic and selenium

Concentrations of *arsenic* in surface water bodies are usually low. Rather high concentrations have been reported in some drinking-water supplies in Latin America (0.6–0.8 mg/litre) and the Western Pacific (0.24–0.96 mg/litre), and are associated with endemic arsenic poisoning

(Astolfi, 1971; Bruning, 1971) and the so-called "blackfoot" disease (I-Cheng Chi' & Blackwell, 1968). Arsenic is also known to accumulate in some marine organisms, such as clams and shrimps, which were found in certain areas to contain up to 50–100 mg/kg and more of this element (Angino et al., 1970). Selenium seems to counteract arsenic toxicity (Stokinger, 1969). The specific protective action of selenium against the toxic effects of cadmium and mercury seems well established (Muth, 1967; WHO Scientific Group on the Biochemistry and Microbiology of the Female and Male Genital Tracts, 1965).

Selenium levels in water appear to be subject to natural control by adsorption by sediments and precipitation. The levels found are of the order of a few μg/litre, but in some seleniferous areas may reach 50–300 μg/litre (Smith & Westfall, 1937). In trace amounts selenium is a micronutrient; at higher levels (over 2000 μg/litre), it may have adverse effects on mammals. In only one instance, that of an Indian family who, by chance, used well water in an isolated location where the selenium content was as high as 9000 μg/litre (cited in Rosenfeld & Beath, 1964), has drinking-water been associated with typical selenosis. Some recent studies have indicated that selenium increased the susceptibility to dental caries in early life (Hadjimarkos, 1965), but this view is not generally accepted (Schwarz, 1967).

(4)   *Mercury, lead, cadmium and other toxic metals*

Reported concentrations of *mercury* in tap water range from 0.01 to 0.3 μg/litre (Stock & Cucuel, 1934; Cerkez & Goldwater, 1969, unpublished data). Surveys of mercury in natural waters have been made, e.g., in Sweden (Wiklander, 1968), in Italy (Dall'Aglio, 1968), and in the USSR (Aidinjan, 1962); the levels found were generally below 0.1 μg/litre. The average concentration of mercury (mainly of natural origin) in sea-water is of the order of 0.03 μg/litre (Goldberg, 1963), but in contaminated areas, such as Minamata Bay in Japan, levels as high as 1–10 μg/litre were observed (Kiyoura, 1963). High contents (up to 30–40 mg/kg) were found in the mud of Minamata Bay (Kitamura, 1968).

In both marine and fresh water environments (bottom sediments), most organic mercury compounds, except alkylmercury, decompose to give the inorganic form, which then gradually changes into the simplest alkylmercury, namely methylmercury, $(CH_3)_2Hg$, a very toxic compound having a high tendency to accumulate throughout the aquatic food chain (Jensen & Jernelöv, 1969); it appears that these transformations take place only if the mercury concentration is above 1–10 mg/litre.

The well-known outbreak of methylmercury poisoning in Japan following the consumption of polluted fish and shellfish (Study Group on Minamata Disease, 1968; Tsuchiya, 1969) is referred to in Chapters 3 and 12.

In addition to other sources, the *lead* content of drinking-water may be due to the use of lead pipes or of plastic pipes stabilized with lead compounds. Natural and untreated water supplies contain about 0.01–0.03 mg/litre of lead. A recent survey of trace metal concentrations in rivers and lakes in the USA found only 2 % of samples with a lead concentration in excess of 0.05 mg/litre (Kopp & Kroner, 1970). The estimated average daily intake of lead from water (0.01–0.1 mg) (Working Group on Lead Contamination, 1965) is small, however, as compared with the total average daily intake from all sources, including urban air (0.33–0.44 mg; Joint FAO/WHO Expert Committee on Food Additives, 1967). Lead accumulates in oysters and other shellfish. Little is known of the possible chemical transformations of lead in the aquatic environment.

Cadmium levels ranging from less than 1 µg/litre (in areas not known to be polluted) up to more than 10 µg/litre have been reported both in natural waters and in water for human consumption (Friberg et al., 1971). In addition to industrial discharges, metal or plastic pipes constitute a possible source of cadmium in water (Schroeder et al., 1967). Like other metals in solution, cadmium tends to be adsorbed by suspended particles and in bottom sediments. For this reason, even in polluted rivers, the cadmium levels in the water phase may be below the detection limit. Irrigation water containing suspended solids was implicated in the pollution of rice paddy soils surrounding the Jintsu River, Japan, the area where "itai-itai" disease had occurred (Yamagata & Shigematsu, 1970).

The concentration of *nickel* in water, as reported by the National Water Quality Network in the USA (Lutz et al., 1967), ranges from 1–70 µg/litre. Our knowledge of the possible chronic effects of small quantities of nickel in environmental samples, including food and water, is very limited and much more research is needed.

Other toxic elements and their compounds are found in natural and polluted water, usually in very small concentrations. They include barium, beryllium, cobalt, molybdenum, tin, uranium, vanadium and many others. Insufficient information is available to assess the health significance of the presence of these substances in water and to enable safety levels to be determined.

(5) *Water hardness and cardiovascular disease*

Reports from several countries have shown an inverse statistical association between the hardness[1] of drinking-water and the death rate from cardiovascular diseases. Areas supplied with soft drinking-water almost consistently experience a significantly higher prevalence of either arterioscle-

---

[1] The "hardness" of water is defined as the sum of the concentrations of the metallic ions (with the exception of those of the alkaline metals) present in it. In most cases, the hardness is due to the content of calcium and magnesium (and sometimes aluminium and iron).

rotic heart disease, or degenerative heart disease, hypertension, sudden deaths of cardiovascular origin, or a combination of these.

There are also indications from one study that, in certain cities, where the water had become softer during the past few decades, the mortality from cardiovascular diseases increased, while the opposite was true for cities where the water had become harder. A few animal experiments tend to confirm the view that soft water may be one of the factors responsible for the development of atherosclerosis. Further details and references to these studies can be found in WHO publications (*WHO Chronicle*, 1972; Masironi, 1970; Miesch et al., 1972).

However, the conclusion that soft water has harmful effects in human cardiovascular diseases is based solely on circumstantial evidence and statistical associations; there is still no definite information as to which water components may be "protective" or "harmful", whether these are major constituents or trace elements, and whether it is their presence or absence that is responsible for the effects. The evidence for a possible connexion between certain water characteristics and the development of cardiovascular diseases is nevertheless suggestive enough to justify deeper studies.

(6) *Organochlorine compounds*

Several groups of organochlorine compounds are of interest in water pollution. They include insecticides, such as DDT, aldrin, and endosulfan; chlorinated phenoxyacetic acids used as herbicides (e.g., 2,4,5-T); and fungicides, such as hexachlorobenzene and pentachlorophenol. Chlorinated aromatics are used mainly in industry and include chlorinated naphthalenes and biphenyls.

There are two main sources of *organochlorine pesticides* in water: run-off from agricultural land and discharge of industrial wastes (from the manufacture and formulation of pesticides or their use as mothproofing chemicals). Because of their low solubility in water and tendency to be adsorbed on solid surfaces, only traces of these compounds are found in raw and treated water. Residues reported in water surveys are mainly of insecticides carried on particulate matter suspended in water. Much larger quantities may be found in mud and bottom sediments. Major river basins in the USA were found to contain the following mean concentrations of pesticides (in nanograms per litre or parts per 10^{-12}) (Edwards, 1970):

> DDT and related compounds: 8.2–10.3
> lindane: 2.8–28
> aldrin: 0.2–5
> dieldrin: 2.3–10
> heptachlor and heptachlor epoxides: 0.1–6.3
> endrin: 1.4–541

Similar studies in the United Kingdom gave values of 1.6–64.6 ng/litre for DDT and related compounds; 18.7–38.6 for lindane; and 3.3–114 for dieldrin (Lowden et al., 1969).

The presence of *polychlorinated biphenyls* (PCB) in the environment has been detected only since 1966, because of the complexity of the analytical techniques needed to identify them in mixtures with other organochlorine compounds. In the effluents of municipal sewage plants and in receiving waters, PCB concentrations typically range from a few nanograms per litre to microgram/litre levels (Duke et al., 1970). They precipitate with sludge, and are adsorbed by clays to such an extent that only barely detectable traces should appear in drinking-water. Like some other organochlorine compounds, they are soluble in fat and tend to accumulate in aquatic animals.

Biochemical breakdown of some organochlorine compounds is slow, the time required for 50 % degradation being of the order of 0.05–2 years, The rate of chemical degradation in water may be much slower (Robinson. 1971).

(7) *Polynuclear aromatic hydrocarbons*

Many polynuclear aromatic hydrocarbons (PAH), particularly benzo [a] pyrene (BP), have been found in water and other environmental media (cf. Andelman & Suess, 1970). Their solubility in pure water is very low, but can be increased by the presence of fairly high concentrations of anionic detergents. The adsorption of PAH on surfaces is an important characteristic, both in relation to their presence in water and their removal in water-treatment processes. The stability of PAH is affected by light and oxygen. The concentration of carcinogenic PAH in fresh waters has been estimated as follows (Borneff & Kunte, 1964):

groundwater: 0.001–0.010 µg/litre

treated river and lake water: 0.010–0.025 µg/litre

surface water: 0.025–0 100 µg/litre

strongly contaminated surface water: > 0.100 µg/litre

The health significance of traces of carcinogenic PAH in fresh waters is not known. PAH are also present in the marine environment. BP contents of up to 400 µg/kg of dry sample have been detected in marine plankton.

(8) *Anionic detergents*

Residues of alkyl benzene sulfonate (ABS), used as the surface-active component in synthetic detergent mixtures, cause foaming, particularly in turbulent reaches of rivers, and interfere with sewage-treatment processes and the self-purification of streams. The introduction in the 1960s of more easily biodegradable linear alkyl sulfonates (LAS) helped greatly to reduce these effects (Brenner, 1969).

Detergent "builders" are chelating agents that produce a marked improvement in detergent properties. The most effective and the most widely used compound today is sodium tripolyphosphate (STP). Ordinary sewage-treatment processes do not remove phosphates and nitrates, and increased levels of such substances in many lakes and rivers of industrially advanced countries have been associated with the process of eutrophication. Various proposals have been made to replace phosphates in detergents by other substances, including the sodium salt of nitrilotriacetic acid (NTA). Although toxicological data for NTA are incomplete (US Senate Committee on Public Works, 1970), they indicate a potential human hazard in that NTA alters the toxicity of metals by affecting their entry into the body, as well as their distribution and concentration in the tissues. Pending further toxicological evaluation, the US Government has recommended that NTA detergents should not be used.

(9) Radionuclides

The radioactivity of water from natural causes is usually low and of no immediate health significance, except where water is drawn from deposits of highly radioactive minerals. Pollution by radioactive wastes, however, may be highly dangerous and should be dealt with at the point of discharge rather than by attempting to treat contaminated water after it has been withdrawn for supply purposes. Radioactive material may be ingested directly through water supplies, but may also be present in more concentrated form in fish, in shellfish (^{65}Zn), in edible seaweeds (^{108}Ru) or in plants irrigated with contaminated water (World Health Organization, 1968; Straub, 1970).

The most common naturally-occurring radionuclides in drinking-water sources are ^{226}Ra and ^{222}Rn, ^{232}Th and its decay products, and to a lesser extent ^{238}U. Concentrations of ^{226}Ra (in picocuries per litre—pCi/litre) in river waters amount to 0.01–0.08 and in groundwater from 0.07 to 139 pCi/litre (some springs in France). For ^{222}Rn, the concentrations in pCi/litre vary from 0.2 (river water, United Kingdom) to 3×10^5 (some springs in the USA) (UNSCEAR, 1962).

The radioactivity of public water supplies is affected by the treatment that they undergo. Thus up to 98 % of ^{226}Ra in water can be removed by precipitation processes and filtration. The concentrations of natural radioactive substances in water available for public water supplies differ greatly. In Bad Gastein, Austria, for example, the ^{226}Ra concentration was 0.6 pCi/litre, in certain areas of the Federal Republic of Germany only 0.03-0.3 pCi/litre and in tap water in the USA on average 0.04 pCi/litre

(UNSCEAR, 1962). About 10 % of ^{226}Ra present in bone is assumed to originate from the water supply.

Artificial radioactive substances in water are derived from the fallout from nuclear testing, discharges from nuclear power reactors and reprocessing plants, and the disposal of radioactive wastes. The radionuclides of importance are ^{90}Sr, ^{137}Cs and to some extent ^{131}I, but the concentrations of these radionuclides in drinking-water are normally very low. More detailed information on this topic can be found in the UNSCEAR reports (e.g., UNSCEAR, 1966, 1969).

Water Quality Criteria and Standards

Internationally recommended water quality requirements exist only for drinking-water, and are discussed in some detail in this section. There is also an urgent need for internationally agreed water quality criteria for recreational uses of water, for water used for irrigation and fisheries, and for water used in the food industry.

Drinking-water standards

International standards for drinking-water (World Health Organization, 1971b) contains proposed minimum standards considered to be within the reach of all countries throughout the world at the present time. In view of the different economic and technological capabilities of various countries, however, areas will exist in which higher standards than those proposed for the world as a whole will be attainable, and these areas should be encouraged to attain such high standards. It is for this reason that WHO has also proposed *European standards for drinking-water* (World Health Organization, 1970).

The international standards are referred to in the *International Health Regulations* (World Health Organization, 1971a) as requirements to be satisfied by water supplied at international ports and airports. Apart from this, they have no legal force in any country unless and until legislative action is taken to adopt them as national standards.

International standards for drinking-water distinguishes five classes of quality parameters: biological pollutants, radioactive pollutants, toxic substances, specific chemical substances that may affect health, and characteristics affecting the acceptability of water.

Standards for bacteriological water quality are based on an organism that is not itself pathogenic but merely an indicator of possible contamination. For chlorinated or otherwise disinfected supplies, it should not be possible to demonstrate the presence of coliform organisms in any 100-ml sample of water entering the distribution system; in established non-disinfected supplies, there should be no (faecal) *E. coli* in 100 ml;

if (faecal) *E. coli* is absent, the presence of not more than three coliform organisms per 100 ml may be tolerated in occasional samples.[1] If more than three coliform organisms per 100 ml are found, the supply is not suitable without disinfection.

In principle, all samples taken from the distribution system (including consumers' premises) should be free from coliform organisms. In practice, these requirements cannot always be satisfied.

In small community supplies, such as individual wells, bore wells or springs, it should be possible to reduce the coliform count of even shallow water to less than 10 per 100 ml. If this cannot be achieved, the water should not be used for drinking purposes.

As regards the possible contamination of drinking-water by enteroviruses, 0.5 mg/litre of free chlorine for one hour following normal water treatment processes should be sufficient to inactivate viruses even in water that was originally polluted. The same effect would be achieved by 0.4 mg/litre of free ozone for four minutes. "If not even one plaque-forming unit (PFU) of virus can be found in one litre of water it can be reasonably assumed that the water is safe to drink. It would, however, be necessary to examine a sample of the order of 10 litres to obtain a proper estimation of the PFU at this level" (World Health Organization, 1971b).

International standards for drinking-water also gives guidelines for the biological examination of water that may be useful in determining the causes of objectionable tastes and odours and for controlling remedial treatments.

The recommended limits for levels of radioactivity are derived from the recommendations of the International Commission on Radiological Protection (1959, 1964, 1966) and the IAEA *Basic safety standards for radiation protection* (International Atomic Energy Agency, 1967) and are summarized in Table 3.

TABLE 3

RECOMMENDED LEVELS OF RADIOACTIVITY IN DRINKING-WATER *

Type of activity	Proposed levels [1]	Remarks
Gross alpha	3 pCi/litre	Before the analysis, the activity of ^{222}Rn and ^{220}Rn should be eliminated by aeration of the sample. Short-lived daughtei products can be excluded by allowing them to decay. Concentration of 3 pCi/litre or less is acceptable even if all is due to ^{226}Ra. If 3 pCi/litre is exceeded, radiochemical analysis is required.
Gross beta	30 pCi/litre	Concentration of 30 pCi/litre or less is acceptable even if all is due to ^{90}Sr. If this is exceeded, radiochemical analysis is required. If presence of ^{3}H is suspected, special examination is needed.

* Data from: World Health Organization (1971b), pp. 29-30.
[1] Applicable to the mean activity of all measurements obtained during a 3-month period.

[1] This applies to supplies that are regularly and frequently tested.

For toxic substances, *International standards for drinking-water* proposes the tentative limits set out in Table 4, together with upper limits of concentration for some specific substances that may affect health, such as nitrates and polynuclear aromatic hydrocarbons (PAH). The recommended limits (lower and upper) for fluorides in drinking water depend on the temperature and vary from 0.9 to 0.6 mg/litre (lower limit) and from 1.7 to 0.8 mg/litre (upper limit).

TABLE 4

TENTATIVE LIMITS FOR TOXIC SUBSTANCES AND
SOME SPECIFIC SUBSTANCES THAT MAY AFFECT HEALTH *

Substance		Upper limit of concentration (mg/litre)
Toxic substances [1]		
Arsenic	(as As)	0.05
Cadmium	(as Cd)	0.01
Cyanide	(as CN)	0.05
Lead	(as Pb)	0.1
Mercury (total)	(as Hg)	0.001
Selenium	(as Se)	0.01
Specific chemical substances that may affect health		
Nitrates	(as NO₃)	45
Polynuclear aromatic hydrocarbons (PAH) [2]		0.0002
Pesticides		
Insecticides		No limit specified. The concept
Herbicides		of acceptable daily intake (ADI)
Fungicides		serves as a guideline for toxicological evaluation

* Data from: World Health Organization (1971b), pp. 31-37.
[1] Based on an assumed daily intake of 2.5 litres by a man weighing 70 kg.
[2] This refers to the six representative PAH compounds: benzo[*a*]pyrene, benzo[*g,h,i*]perylene, fluoranthene, benz[*e*]acephenanthrylene, benzo[*k*]fluoranthene, and indeno[1,2,3-*cd*]pyrene.

The highest desirable levels for characteristics or substances affecting the acceptability of water (such as substances causing odours, substances causing tastes, suspended matter, pH range, anionic detergents, mineral oil, phenolic compounds, iron and magnesium) are also specified in *International standards for drinking-water*.

Quality criteria for recreational uses of water

In much of the available literature on quality criteria for water used for recreational purposes, the need for the protection of the health and safety of the user is emphasized. Recreational uses may involve "primary" and "secondary" contact. Primary contact includes those activities in which there is prolonged and intimate contact with water (swimming, diving, waterskiing and surfing). Secondary contact refers to sports in which contact with water is either incidental or accidental and the probability of ingesting appreciable amounts of water is small.

Since contamination with pathogenic microbes is a possible health hazard in the recreational use of water, e.g., in swimming pools, regular microbiological examination of such waters is recommended. Other parameters deserving consideration are acidity and chlorine concentration, because of their possible relation to eye irritation. Additional desirable criteria include clarity and suitable temperature. Secondary contact criteria might include microbiological standards, in addition to aesthetic requirements.

REFERENCES

Adler, P. et al. (1970) *Fluorides and human health*, Geneva, World Health Organization, (*Monograph Series*, No. 59)

Aidinjan, N. K. (1962) *Trudy Inst. Geol. rudn. Mestorož.*, No. 70, pp. 9-14

Andelman, J. B. & Suess, M. J. (1970) *Bull. Wld Hlth Org.*, **43**, 479-508

Angino, E. E., Magnuson, L. M., Waugh, T. C., Galle, O. K. & Bredfeldt, J. (1970) *Science*, **168**, 389-390

Astolfi, E. (1971) *Pren. méd. argent.*, **58**, 1342-1343

Baars, J. K. (1957), *Bull. Wld Hlth Org.*, **16**, 727-747

Barua, D., Burrows, W. & Gallut, J.C. (1970). In: *Principles and practice of cholera control*, Geneva, World Health Organization (*Publ. Hlth Pap.*, No. 40)

Bernard, R. P. (1965) *J. Hyg. (Lond.)*, **63**, 537-563

Borneff, J. & Kunte, H. (1964) *Arch. Hyg. (Berl.)*, **148**, 585-597

Brenner, T. E. (1969) *Biodegradable detergents in water pollution*. In: Pitts, J. N. & Metcalf, R. L., eds, *Advances in environmental sciences and technology*, Vol. 1, New York, Wiley Interscience

Brisou, J. (1968) *Bull. Wld Hlth Org.*, **38**, 79-118

Brisou, J. (1971) *La pollution des mers par les microorganismes*, Geneva, World Health Organization (Unpublished document WHO/EP/71.1)

Bruning, W. (1968) *Rev. chil. Pediat.*, **39**, 49-51

Buchan, S. & Key, A. (1956) *Bull. Wld Hlth Org.*, **14**, 949-1006

Chang, S. L. (1968) *Bull. Wld Hlth Org.*, **28**, 410-414

Cholak, J. (1959) *J. occup. Med.*, **1**, 501-511

Committee on Bathing Beach Contamination of the Public Health Laboratory Service (1959) *J. Hyg. (Lond.)*, **57**, 435-472

Dall'Aglio, N. (1968) *The abundance of mercury in 300 natural water samples from Tuscany and Latium (Central Italy)*. In: Abrams, L. H., ed., *Origin and distribution of the elements*, Oxford, Pergamon Press, pp. 1056-1081

Duke, T. W., Lowe, J. I. & Wilson, A. J. (1970) *Bull. environm. Contam.*, **5**, 171-180

Edwards, C. A. (1970) *CRC Crit. Rev. environm. Control*, **1**, 7-67

Friberg, L., Piscator, M. & Nordberg, G. (1971) *Cadmium in the environment*, Stockholm, Karolinska Institute

Goldberg, E. D. (1963) *The ocean as a chemical system*. In: Hill, N. N., ed., *The sea*, Vol. 2, New York, Interscience Publishers, pp. 3-25

Greenberg, A. E. & Ongerth, J. H. (1966) *J. Amer. Wat. Wks Ass.*, **58**, 1145-1150

Hadjimarkos, D. M. (1965) *Arch. environm. Hlth*, **10**, 893-899

I-Cheng Ch'i & Blackwell, R. Q. (1968) *Amer. J. Epidem.*, **88**, 7-24

IMCO/FAO/UNESCO/WMO/WHO/IAEA/UN Joint Group of Experts on the Scientific Aspects of Marine Pollution (GESAMP) (1971) *Report of the Third Session, Rome 22-27 February* 1970, Geneva, World Health Organization (Unpublished document WHO/W.POLL/71.8; GESAMP 111/19)

International Atomic Energy Agency (1967) *Basic standards for radiation protection*, Vienna (*Safety Series* No. 9)

International Commission on Radiological Protection (1959) *Recommendations...* Oxford, Pergamon Press (*ICRP Publication* No. 2)

International Commission on Radiological Protection (1964) *Recommendations...* Oxford, Pergamon Press (*ICRP Publication* No. 6)

International Commission on Radiological Protection (1966) *Recommendations...* Oxford, Pergamon Press (*ICRP Publication* No. 9)

Jensen, S. & Jernelöv, A. (1969) *Nature (Lond.)*, **223**, 753-754

Joint FAO/WHO Expert Committee on Food Additives (1967) *Specifications for the identity and purity of food additives and their toxicological evaluation: some emulsifiers and stabilizers and certain other substances, Tenth report*, Geneva (*Wld Hlth Org. techn. Rep. Ser.*, No. 373)

Kitamura, S. (1968) *Determination of mercury content in bodies of inhabitants, cats, fishes and shells in Minamata district and the mud of Minamata Bay.* In: *Minamata Disease*, Kukamoto University, pp. 257-266

Kiyoura, R. (1963) *Int. J. Air Wat. Pollut.*, **7**, 459-470

Koff, R. S. (1970) *CRC Crit. Rev. environm. Control*, **1**, 383-442

Kopp, J. F. & Kroner, R. C. (1970) *Trace metals in waters of the United States: A 5-year summary of trace metals in rivers and lakes of the U.S. (October 1, 1962-September 30, 1967)*, Cincinnati, Ohio, US Department of the Interior, FWPCA, Division of Pollution Surveillance

Loehr, R. C. (1970) *CRC Crit. Rev. environm. Control*, **1**, 69-99

Lowden, G. F., Saunders, C. L. & Edwards, R. W. (1969) *Wat. Treat. Exam.*, **19**, 275-294

Lutz, C. A. et al. (1967) *Design of an overview system for evaluating the public health hazards of chemicals in the environment, Vol. 1, Test case studies*, Columbus, Ohio, Battelle Memorial Institute

Mallman, W. L. (1970) *CRC Crit. Rev. environm. Control*, **1**, 221-255

Masironi, R. (1970) *Bull. Wld Hlth Org.*, **43**, 687-697

Mattingly, P. F. (1963) *Bull. Wld Hlth Org.*, **29**, Suppl., 135-139

McClure, F. J. (1970) *Water fluoridation*, Bethesda, Md, US Department of Health, Education, and Welfare, National Institute of Health

Miesch, A. T., Crawford, M. D., Masironi, R. & Hamilton, E. L. (1972) *Bull. Wld Hlth Org.* (in press)

Moore, B. (1954) *Bull. Hyg.*, **29**, 689-704

Moore, B. (1970) *Rev. int. Océanogr. Méd.*, **18-19**, 1-26

Mosley, J. W. (1967) *Transmission of viral diseases by drinking water.* In: Berg. G., ed., *Transmission of viruses by the water route*, New York, Interscience

Muth, O. H., ed. (1967) *Selenium in biomedicine*, Westport, Conn., Avi Publishing Co.

Off. Rec. Wld Hlth Org., 1971, No. 193, p. 144

Ramanohana Rao, N. V. & Bhaskaran, C. S. (1964) *Indian J. Med. Res.*, **52**, 180-186

Robertson, H. E. & Riddel, W. A. (1949) *Canad. J. publ. Hlth*, **40**, 72-77

Robinson, J (1971) *Chem. Brit.*, **7**, 472-475

Rosenfeld, I. & Beath, O. A. (1964) *Selenium: geobotany, biochemistry, toxicity and nutrition*, New York, Academic Press

Schmidt, P. & Knotek, Z. (1970) *Epidemiological evaluation of nitrates as ground water contaminants in Czechoslovakia* (Paper presented to the Sixth International Water Pollution Research Conference, San Francisco)

Schroeder, H. A., Nason, A. P., Tipton, I. H. & Balasser, J. J. (1967) *J. chron. Dis.*, **20**, 179-210

Schwartz, K. (1967). In: Muth, O. H., Oldfield, J. E. & Weswig, P. H., eds, *Selenium in biomedicine*, Westport, Conn., Avi Publishing Co.

Smith, M. I. & Westfall, B. B. (1937) *Publ. Hlth Rep. (Wash.)*, **53**, 1375-1384

Stock, A. & Cucuel, F. (1934) *Naturwissenschaften*, **22-24**, 390-393

Stokinger, H. E. (1969) *Amer. industr. Hyg. Ass. J.*, **30**, 195-217

Straub, C. P. (1970) *Public health implications of radioactive waste releases*, Geneva, World Health Organization

Study Group on Minamata Disease (1968) *Minamata disease*, Kumamoto University

Taylor, F. B. et al. (1966) *Amer. J. publ. Hlth*, **56**, 2093-2105

Tsuchiya, K. (1969) *Keio J. Med.*, **18**, 213-227

United Nations Scientific Committee on the Effects of Atomic Radiation (UNSCEAR) (1962) *Report...*, New York United Nations (Official Records of the General Assembly, Seventeenth session, Supplement No. 16 (A/5216))

United Nations Scientific Committee on the Effects of Atomic Radiation (UNSCEAR) (1966) *Report...*, New York, United Nations (Official Records of the General Assembly, Twenty-first session, Supplement No. 14 (A/6314))

United Nations Scientific Committee on the Effects of Atomic Radiation (UNSCEAR) (1969) *Report...*, New York, United Nations (Official Records of the General Assembly, Twenty-fourth session, Supplement No. 13 (A/7613))

United States Senate Committee on Public Works (1970) *Toxicological and environmental implications of the use of nitrilotriacetic acid as a detergent builder*, Washington, D.C., US Government Printing Office

Viswanathan, R. (1957) *Indian J. med. Res.*, **45**, Suppl. No. 1

WHO Chronicle, 1972, **26**, 51

WHO Expert Committee on Amoebiasis (1969) *Report*, Geneva (*Wld Hlth Org. techn. Rep. Ser.*, No. 421)

WHO Expert Committee on Bilharziasis (1965), *Third report*, Geneva (*Wld Hlth Org. techn. Rep, Ser.*, No. 299)

WHO Expert Committee on the Epidemiology and Control of Schistosomiasis (1967) *Report*, Geneva (*Wld Hlth Org. techn. Rep. Ser.*, No. 372)

WHO Expert Committee on Filariasis (*Wuchereria* and *Brugia* infections) (1967) *Report*, Geneva (*Wld Hlth Org. techn. Rep. Ser.*, No. 359)

WHO Expert Committee on Hepatitis (1964) *Second report*, Geneva (*Wld Hlth Org. techn. Rep. Ser.*, No. 285)

WHO Expert Committee on Onchocerciasis (1966), *Second report*, Geneva (*Wld Hlth Org. techn. Rep. Ser.*, No. 335)

WHO Scientific Group on the Biochemistry and Microbiology of the Female and Male Genital Tracts (1965) *Report*, Geneva (*Wld Hlth Org. techn. Rep. Ser.*, No. 313), pp. 11-12

WHO Scientific Group on the Treatment and Disposal of Wastes (1967) *Report*, Geneva (*Wld Hlth Org. techn. Rep. Ser.*, No. 367)

Wiklander, L. (1968) *Grundförbättring*, **21**, 151-155

Working Group on Lead Contamination (1965) *Survey of lead in the atmosphere of three urban communities*, Cincinnati, Ohio, US Department of Health, Education, and Welfare, Public Health Service, Division of Air Pollution

World Health Organization (1968) *Routine surveillance for radionuclides in air and water*, Geneva

World Health Organization (1970) *European standards for drinking-water*, 2nd ed., Geneva

World Health Organization (1971a) *International Health Regulations (1969)*, 1st annotated ed., Geneva

World Health Organization (1971b) *International standards for drinking-water*, 3rd ed., Geneva

Yamagata, N. & Shigematsu, I. (1970) *Bull. Inst. publ. Hlth*, **19** (1), 1-27

CHAPTER 3

FOOD

Biological Contamination

Food may serve as a vehicle for the distribution of two major groups of organisms pathogenic to man: (1) those associated with endogenous animal infections transmissible to man (zoonoses), including bacterial, viral, fungal, helminthic, and protozoan species (Joint FAO/WHO Expert Committee on Zoonoses, 1967); and (2) micro-organisms from the environment that contaminate food and may cause infection or intoxication in man. We shall be concerned mainly with the latter.

Food may become contaminated with microbes at many points during its production, processing, transportation, storage, distribution, and preparation for consumption. The degree of hazard and points of maximum danger vary, depending on the types of contamination, and the food and its method of production, including handling and processing procedures.

Principal types and sources of contamination

General surveys of the question of the principal types and sources of microbiological contamination of food can be found in a number of publications (Frazier, 1967; Thatcher & Clark, 1968; US National Academy of Sciences, 1964; WHO Expert Committee on Enteric Infections, 1964; WHO Expert Committee on the Microbiological Aspects of Food Hygiene, 1968).

Initial contamination

Animals may themselves be diseased (Joint FAO/WHO Expert Committee on Zoonoses, 1967) or may be merely the passive carriers of organisms infectious to man, as in the case of some *Salmonella* infections (Dräger, 1971). Sewage bacteria and viruses (e.g., the virus of infectious hepatitis) may be concentrated in shellfish, such as oysters and clams, and fish may carry *Vibrio parahaemolyticus*, *Salmonella* spp., *Clostridium botulinum* type E, and other organisms. Vegetables may become contaminated by contact with field soils (e.g., with *Cl. botulinum*) and with polluted water carrying typhoid bacilli, *Shigella*, and other micro-organisms (see Chapter 2).

— 72 —

Contamination during food processing

The many potential routes of contamination during processing include contamination from human sources, vermin, or the ingredient materials.

Foods may be contaminated by each other and by pieces of equipment with which they come into contact. Contaminants may build up in numbers on such equipment and constantly transmit seed organisms into the foods. Disease outbreaks due to commercially processed foods are not uncommon (Cockburn et al., 1962; Riemann, 1969).

Hazards during transportation

Proliferation of organisms in food is related mainly to the temperature at which it is kept during transit, and is most hazardous when products are improperly refrigerated. Secondary contamination may occur, however, through contact with vermin and other carriers.

Handling in retail markets and houses

The handling of food contaminated with food-borne pathogens, particularly *Salmonella*, can easily lead to cross-contamination and create a health hazard in butchers' shops, bakeries, retail dairy shops and similar establishments, and in the home. Common sources of such contamination include the cutting of both raw and cooked meat on the same board; dirty kitchen utensils, particularly those in bad repair; storage of raw and processed foods in the same place; and unwashed hands.

Contamination from water

Food may be contaminated by water used as an ingredient, for washing foods, and for cooling heated foods, and from ice used for preserving foods (Frazier, 1967). Gas-forming bacteria may enter milk from cooling-tank water and cause difficulties in cheese made from that milk. Anaerobic gas formers may enter foods from soil-laden water. Cannery cooling water may contain pathogenic micro-organisms that enter canned foods during cooling through minute defects in the seams or seals of the cans (Scottish Home and Health Department, 1964).

Contamination of various kinds of foods

A list of the principal microbiological contaminants of foods, showing the diseases caused and the foods involved, is provided in the accompanying table (pp. 74-77).

Meat and meat products

The inner flesh of meats of poultry and fish from healthy animals contain few or no micro-organisms, although they may be present in other parts of the carcase.   Contamination can occur, however, during slaughtering, handling and processing (Albertsen et al., 1957; Joint FAO/WHO Expert Committee on Meat Hygiene, 1962; Matyáš et al., 1965).

PRINCIPAL BIOLOGICAL CONTAMINANTS OF FOODS [1]

Disease	Causative agent	Source	Principal foods involved
Bacterial diseases			
Salmonelloses (including typhoid and paratyphoid fever)	Salmonella spp.	Faeces and urine of infected domestic or wild animals and man.	Meat, poultry, shellfish, raw vegetables, eggs, and their products.
Staphylococcal intoxication	Enterotoxin A, B, C, D, or E of *Staphylococcus aureus*	Nose and throat discharges; hands and skin; infected cuts, wounds, burns; boils; pimples, acne; faeces.	Cooked ham, meat products; cream-filled pastry; potato, ham, poultry, and fish salads; milk, cheese.
Botulism	Toxin A, B, E, or F of *Clostridium botulinum* or *Cl. parabotulinum*	Soil, mud, water, and intestinal tract of animals.	Improperly canned low-acid foods, smoked vacuum-packed fish, fermented foods.
Clostridium perfringens food-borne illness	*Clostridium perfringens (welchii)* type A	Faeces of infected persons and animals. Soil, dust, sewage.	Cooked meat and poultry.
Bacillus cereus food infection	*Bacillus cereus*	Soil and dust.	Custards, cereal products, puddings, sauces, and meat loaf.
Arizona infection	*Arizona arizonae*	Faeces of infected persons and animals.	Turkey, cream-filled pastry, ice cream.
Enteropathogenic *Escherichia coli* infection	*Escherichia coli*	Human faeces.	Coffee substitute, salmon (?).
Vibrio parahaemolyticus infection	*Vibrio parahaemolyticus*	Sea-water and marine life.	Raw foods of marine origin. Fish, shellfish, and fish products.
Shigellosis (bacillary dysentery)	*Shigella sonnei, S. flexneri, S. dysenteriae, S. boydii*	Faeces of infected human beings.	Moist, mixed foods. Milk, beans, potato, tuna, shrimp, poultry.
Scarlet fever, septic sore throat (beta hemolytic streptococcal infections)	*Streptococcus pyogenes*	Infected persons; nose, throat, and lesion discharges. Main mode of transmission: airborne.	Milk, eggs, and their products.
Cholera	*Vibrio cholerae* and *V. cholerae* biotype El Tor	Faeces and vomitus of infected human cases.	Raw vegetables; mixed and moist foods.
Diphtheria	*Corynebacterium diphtheriae*	Discharges and secretion from mucous surfaces of nasopharynx.	Milk.

[1] Sources: Bryan, 1971; Ingram et al., 1967; Joint FAO/WHO Expert Committee on Zoonoses, 1967; Riemann, 1969; Sedlák & Rische, 1961; WHO Expert Committee on the Microbiological Aspects of Food Hygiene, 1968; Wogan, 1964.

Disease	Causative agent	Source	Principal foods involved

Viral and rickettsial diseases

Disease	Causative agent	Source	Principal foods involved
Infectious hepatitis	Virus of infectious hepatitis (virus A)	Faeces, urine, blood of infected human cases and persons incubating or convalescing from the disease.	Shellfish, milk, unheated foods.
Bolivian haemorrhagic fever	Machupo virus	Urine of infected rodent (*Calomys callosus*).	Cereals. Possibly any food contaminated with rodent urine. (?)
Russian spring-summer encephalitis (diphasic milk fever)	Russian tick-borne virus complex. Russian spring-summer louping-ill group viruses.	Ruminants infected by ticks.	Raw milk from goats or sheep.
Q fever	*Coxiella* (*Rickettsia*) *burnetti*	Cattle, sheep, and goats.	Milk.

Parasitic diseases: [1]

Disease	Causative agent	Source	Principal foods involved
Trichinosis (trichinelliasis)	*Trichinella spiralis*	Meat of infected animals.	Pork, bear meat, walrus flesh.
Taeniasis	*Taenia saginata* (beef tapeworm)	Human faeces.	Beef.
	Taenia solium (pork tapeworm)	Human faeces.	Pork.
Cysticercosis	*Taenia solium* larva, *Cysticercus cellulosae*.	Human faeces.	Any food or water contaminated by human faeces containing eggs of the parasite.
Diphyllobothriasis	*Diphyllobothrium latum* (broad or fish tapeworm)	Faeces of human beings, dogs, and other fish-eating mammals.	Raw or partly cooked or inadequately pickled fresh-water fish (pike, pickerel).
Sparganosis	Sparganum of *Diphyllobothrium latum* and *Spirometra* spp.	Cat and dog faeces.	Tadpoles, snakes, frogs.
Angiostrongyliasis (eosinophilic meningo-encephalitis)	*Angiostrongylus cantonensis* (rat lung worm)	Rat faeces.	Raw crabs, prawns. shrimps, snails,
Anisakiasis	*Anisakis* spp.	Fish-eating mammals, birds, predatory fish (shark and rays).	Herring (raw, partially cooked, pickled, smoked).
Fasciolopsiasis	*Fasciolopsis buski*	Human, dog, or hog faeces.	Water chestnuts, water bamboos, water hyacinths, water caltrop, lotus plant root.
Echinostomiasis	*Echinostoma ilocanum* and other species	Infective faeces of man, dog, rats.	Raw snails and clams. Also limpets, fresh-water fish, or tadpoles.
Clonorchiasis	*Clonorchis sinensis* (Chinese liver fluke)	Faeces of man, cats, dogs, hogs.	Raw or partly cooked, fresh, dried, salted, or pickled fish (carp and 80 other species).
Opisthorchiasis	*Opisthorchis felineus* and *O. viverrini*.	Faeces from man and fish-eating mammals.	Fresh-water fish.

[1] These are mainly endogenous infections of animals for which polluted water or soil serves as a vehicle of one of the stages in the life cycle of the parasite.

Disease	Causative agent	Source	Principal foods involved
Fascioliasis (liver fluke infection)	Fasciola hepatica and F. gigantica	Faeces from man, sheep, cattle, or other herbivorous and omnivorous animals.	Aquatic vegetation, watercress.
Heterophyid infection	Heterophyes heterophyes	Faeces of fish-eating birds and mammals.	Raw, partially cooked, salted, or dried fresh-water or brackish-water fish (mullet).
Metagonimiasis	Metagonimus yokogawai	Faeces of fish-eating birds and mammals.	Raw, partially cooked, salted or dried fresh-water or brackish-water fish (trout).
Paragonimiasis	Paragonimus westermani (oriental lung fluke) P. skrjabini P. heterotremus	Sputum and faeces from man and other carnivores.	Raw or partly cooked crabs or crayfish.
Hymenolepiasis diminuta	Hymenolepis diminuta (rat tapeworm)	Faeces of rats, mice, man.	Grains and cereals.
Gnathostomiasis (creeping eruption, larva migrans)	Gnathostoma spinigerum	Dogs and cats.	Raw, fermented, or partially cooked fresh-water fish; snakes, birds, mammals.
Intestinal myiasis and pseudomyiasis	Diptera. Piophila casei (cheese skipper), Musca domestica (common housefly), and other diptera.	Flies.	Meat, fruit, water-cress, cheese, or other contaminated food or water.
Amoebiasis (amoebic dysentery)	Entamoeba histolytica	Human faeces containing cysts.	Raw vegetables and fruits.
Ascariasis	Ascaris lumbricoides	Infective eggs from human faeces.	Raw vegetables and fruits.
Trichuriasis	Trichuris trichiura	Human faeces.	Any soil-contaminated food.
Enterobiasis	Enterobius vermicularis (pinworm)	Human faeces.	Any contaminated raw foods.
Echinococcosis, hydatidosis	Echinococcus granulosus (dog tapeworm)	Faeces of carnivores (dog and wolf).	Any contaminated raw foods.
Balantidiasis (balantidial dysentery)	Balantidium coli	Swine or human faeces.	Pork, raw foods.
Giardiasis	Giardia lamblia	Human faeces.	Raw foods.
Isospora infection	Isospora hominis and I. belli	Human faeces.	Raw foods.
Dientamoeba infection	Dientamoeba fragilis	Human faeces.	Raw foods.
Toxoplasmosis	Toxoplasma gondii	Cat faeces.	Raw foods.

Fungal diseases:

Disease	Causative agent	Source	Principal foods involved
Alimentary toxic aleukia (ATA) (epidemic panmyelo-toxicosis)	Sporofusariogrenin glycoside and other toxins from Fusarium sporotri-chioides (F. poae,, Cladosporium, Alter-naria, Penicillium,, and Mucor spp.)	Soil, air.	Grains (millet, wheat, oats, barley, rye, buckwheat).

Disease	Causative agent	Source	Principal foods involved
Urov disease (Kaschin-Beck disease)	Toxins from *Fusarium sporotrichiella*	Soil, air.	Moist grains.
"Drunken bread" poisoning	Toxins from *Fusarium graminearum (roseum)*	Soil, air.	Grain, bread.
Ergotism (St Anthony's fire)	Ergot alkaloids from *Claviceps purpurea.* Toxic alkaloids: ergotamine, ergotoxine, and ergometrine groups.	Soil, air.	Rye meal or bread.
Epidemic polyuria	Toxins from *Rhizopus nigricans*	Soil, air.	Millet grains.
Toxic mouldy rice disease	Toxins from *Penicillium islandicum, P. atrinum, P. citreoviride, Fusarium, Rhizopus, Aspergillus*	Soil, air.	Yellow rice.

Milk and milk products

A number of reviews of the subject of milk hygiene are available (Abdussalam et al., 1962; Arhangel'skij & Kartasova, 1966; Joint FAO/WHO Expert Committee on Milk Hygiene, 1970; Lerche, 1966; Manzari, 1965; Schönherr, 1967; Zahariev, 1964).

Milk contains few bacteria when it leaves the udder of the healthy cow, but is liable to contamination from the exterior of the animal, especially the exterior of the udder and adjacent parts. Micro-organisms of manure, soil and water may enter from this source.

Automatic milking apparatus and various milk utensils may add contaminants after the milk leaves the udder. Contamination can also occur from the tanker truck and various utensils and equipment at the market milk plant, cheese factory, condensery or other processing plant.

Other possible sources of contamination are the hands of the milker or other dairy workers, and flies, which may add spoilage organisms or pathogens.

Fish and shellfish

Fish do not naturally carry a wide variety of pathogens, and those that may contaminate the marketed product are normally derived from the environment—e.g., from pollution of the water in which they live, and improper handling after they are removed from the water (Borgstrom et al., 1961-65; WHO Expert Committee on the Microbiological Aspects of Food Hygiene, 1968).

Various species of bacteria, and particularly *Proteus spp.*, if present in the flesh of scombroid fishes may, under conditions favourable to their growth, break down histidine in flesh into saurine, a histamine-like substance, which has caused disease in human beings on numerous occasions (Halstead, 1967) (see also p. 88).

Many outbreaks of infectious hepatitis and typhoid have been attributed to shellfish as vehicles (Riemann, 1969). Bivalve molluscs, such as oysters, clams and mussels, are the usual offenders.

Eggs

Although the majority of freshly laid eggs are sterile inside, the shells become contaminated by faecal matter from the hen, by washing water if the eggs are washed, and by handling. Micro-organisms, including pathogenic *Salmonella*, can penetrate a cracked shell and enter the egg (WHO Expert Committee on the Microbiological Aspects of Food Hygiene, 1968).

Cereals, fruits and vegetables

The exterior of these foods can become contaminated from air, soil, water, handling, vermin and other sources (see Chapters 2 and 12).

Chemical Contamination

Chemical contamination of food has recently become cause for concern, particularly in the more developed and industrialized countries. The specific toxic effects of the chemical substances described in this chapter are covered in Chapters 12 and 13.

Metal contaminants

Lead

Lead is sometimes found in foods and beverages. The use of lead arsenate sprays, once a common source of contamination, has decreased as the use of alternative pesticides has increased. In North America it is estimated that over 90 % of the total lead ingested results from non-agricultural uses (FAO/WHO, 1969a). Lead contamination of illicitly distilled alcoholic beverages has been a source of poisoning (Standstead et al., 1970).

Although the total lead intake through food and water is usually several times that inhaled in air (Goldsmith, 1969), only 5 % is absorbed by the oral route compared to 30–40 % via inhalation (Kehoe, 1959).

Arsenic

Arsenic occurs naturally in foods and beverages and is normally present in relatively high concentrations in crustacea and other shellfish. The naturally occurring form found in marine animals is probably not very toxic (Coulson et al., 1936; Pattison et al., 1970). Arsenic can occur as a contaminant if employed as a pesticide; its use for this purpose is declining

Mercury

In recent years there has been increasing concern over the presence of mercury in food, and particularly in fish, in which it accumulates. High levels have been found in fish caught in polluted bays and estuaries, because fish appear to be able to concentrate mercury from water several thousand-fold; they are thus the major source of food contamination by mercury. In addition, mercury is most frequently encountered in fish as methyl-mercury (Westöö, 1969), which is the most dangerous form. This compound was responsible for 200 cases of poisoning in Japan (Minamata disease) with scores of deaths and many cases of irreversible brain damage (Tokuomi et al., 1961). Approximately 25 cases of "congenital Minamata disease" have been attributed to the consumption of contaminated fish and shellfish by pregnant women who themselves were usually asymptomatic (Matsumoto et al., 1965).

The presence of mercury in fish has also been recognized in studies in the Nordic countries, in Canada and in the USA, and it is probably present in fish in other industrialized countries. The presence of mercury in deep sea fish (e.g., tuna and swordfish) at levels often above 0.5 mg/kg (Edwards, unpublished data) cannot be explained entirely on the basis of industrial pollution; it is likely that such fish take up mercury naturally present in the environment.

In certain predominantly fish-eating populations, the body burden of organic mercury increases. Raised levels of mercury in eggs and bird tissues have resulted from feeding on mercury-contaminated fish and on organo-mercury-treated seed (Kazantzis, 1971). Mercury, when present in fish, cannot be removed by cooking or processing and appears to be firmly bound as methylmercury to the sulfhydryl groups of proteins (Westöö, 1969).

Methylmercury compounds have been used as seed dressings, and this has resulted in residues in the plant, though at an insignificant level (0.01 mg/kg) (FAO/WHO, 1968). Its use as a direct fungicidal spray has resulted in higher levels (up to 0.1 mg/kg) in cereals (Smart, 1961; Novick, 1969).

Cases of poisoning by alkylmercury compounds have resulted from the illegal use of seed grain treated with these compounds in the preparation and consumption of food (Jalili & Abbasi, 1961; *New York Times*, 1972).

The consumption of meat from pigs fed on treated seed grain has led to alkylmercury poisoning in man (Pierce et al., 1972).

A correlation has been found between the number of chromosome breaks in the lymphocytes and the mercury levels in the blood cells of persons who have eaten fish contaminated with mercury but who do not display the neurological symptoms of methylmercury poisoning (Skerfving et al., 1970). The significance of this finding is not yet known.

Cadmium

Levels of cadmium in food have been determined for a number of crops. Levels as high as 0.07 mg/kg in wheat flour and 0.004 mg/kg in milk seem typical for non-polluted areas (Schroeder & Balassa, 1961). Uptake of cadmium from the soil by a number of plants has been demonstrated by deliberately increasing its cadmium content. Thus, in a typical soil in Japan under normal conditions, rice contained 0.16 mg/kg, but after the addition of an excessively large amount (to bring the level up to 0.01 %) of cadmium oxide to the soil, the level in the rice rose to 0.78 mg/kg. Even greater increases in cadmium content were found with wheat (Yamagata & Shigematsu, 1970). Some marine animals are reported to be capable of concentrating cadmium more than 4500-fold from water (Noddack & Noddack, 1940). In non-polluted areas, shellfish have been reported to contain 0.05 mg/kg (Schroeder & Balassa, 1961), whereas in polluted waters values up to 420 mg/kg have been reported in the livers of shellfish and cuttlefish (Ishizaki et al., 1970). Oysters from the East coast of the USA have had levels from 0.2 to 2.1 mg/kg (Pringle et al., 1968).

Cobalt

In Quebec in 1965, 48 people developed symptoms of cardiac insufficiency and there were 20 deaths from cobalt poisoning. A similar outbreak with 16 deaths developed in Omaha, and another in Minneapolis (one death). The disease was characterized by severe myocardial failure appearing usually 3–4 weeks after the first appareance of cardiac symptoms. All the patients drank 3–7 litres of beer daily, had poor dietary habits, and displayed thiamine deficiency (*J. Amer. med. Ass.*, 1966). The outbreaks were traced to the use of cobalt in beer in amounts not exceeding 1.5 mg/kg to improve foam stability and to prevent gushing. This use has since been prohibited. Although the average amount of cobalt consumed in the beer was 8 mg per day, high concentrations were found in the cardiac muscle (Sullivan et al., 1968). Intake of cobalt at this level would not normally be toxic but evidence has been presented suggesting that a low protein diet and high consumption of alcohol potentiated its cardiomyopathological effect (Alexander, 1969).

It was reported from Belgium that 16 cases of a syndrome typical of "beri-beri" heart disease were due to the effects of high alcoholic intake (Kesteloot et al., 1966). This disease has since been attributed to the use of cobalt in local breweries (Lafontaine, personal communication, 1967).

Tin

Tin may be encountered as a contaminant in tinned food products; the presence of nitrate in such products may contribute to increased amounts of tin being dissolved from the container (Horio et al., 1967; Cheftal, personal communication, 1971).

A number of acute poisoning incidents have resulted from ingestion of fruit juices containing tin. The symptoms observed were vomiting, diarrhoea, fatigue and headache. The levels of tin that produced symptoms are uncertain but appear to be around 300–500 mg/kg (Horio et al., 1967; Kojima, personal communication). In human test subjects, nausea and diarrhoea occurred at 1370 mg/kg of tin, but not at lower levels and not when the test was repeated one month later (Benoy et al., 1971).

Manganese

Certain marine animals tend to concentrate this element, and levels in the range 0.1–30 mg/kg have been reported (Pringle et al., 1968).

Although an essential ingredient of the human diet in trace amounts, manganese is toxic in higher concentrations. Chronic exposure is characterized by neurological lesions involving the basal ganglia, the frontal cortex and occasionally the extra-pyramidal system, resulting in a Parkinsonianlike syndrome (Stokinger, 1963).

Other chemical contaminants

Selenium

Certain plants are known to accumulate selenium when grown in soils containing a high natural content of this element or where selenium has entered the soil from industrial waste. Cereals such as wheat can accumulate up to 30 mg/kg without impairment of growth (Miller & Byers, 1937). It is thus possible for food crops to be contaminated by selenium. In certain areas (e.g., parts of the mid-Western USA) some plants (e.g., loco weed) accumulate selenium to such an extent that grazing animals display toxic symptoms (Moxon & Rhian, 1943).

There is some evidence that selenium compounds may be teratogenic to certain species. Of four pregnant women exposed to selenites, only one went to term and the infant had a bilateral clubfoot. No other incidents of this type have been recorded (Clegg, 1971).

N-*Nitroso compounds*

Nitrosodimethylamine, which has been shown to be carcinogenic in experimental animals (see Chapter 12), has been found as a contaminant in certain foodstuffs treated with sodium nitrate, such as herring meal (Ender et al., 1964). Levels of 30–100 mg/kg of nitrosodimethylamine were reported in some batches of Norwegian herring meal.

Polychlorinated biphenyls (PCBs)

These compounds enter the marine environment through the discharge of industrial wastes into estuaries and bays, and are found in fish. In fish-eating birds, levels as high as 100 mg/kg have been detected (Jensen et al., 1969), but there is virtually no evidence as to their presence or absence in human tissues as a result of natural exposure (see, however, Chapter 12).

PCBs may also enter foodstuffs directly as a result of contamination from packaging (Bailey et al., 1970).

Oil and petroleum

High levels of polycyclic aromatic hydrocarbons have been detected in oysters in contact with oil pollution (Callaghan, 1961), and there is thus a potential carcinogenic hazard if these shellfish are used as food. In addition, it has been suggested that emulsifier formulations used for dispersing oil spillage may facilitate the penetration of water-insoluble carcinogens into marine organisms (Hueper, 1963). As a result of the pollution of the Caspian Sea by petroleum, a marked decline both in quantities of phytoplankton and fish stocks occurred; nearly all the sea pike were killed (Kasymov, 1970).

Organochlorine insecticides (see also Chapter 12)

The major importance of this group of compounds arises from their stability and persistence in the environment.

A serious incident of poisoning by endrin, with several deaths, occurred in Saudi Arabia when bread prepared from wheat that had been contaminated with this insecticide was consumed (Weeks, 1967).

The presence of DDT in mothers' milk has given rise to particular concern (Quinby et al., 1965; Curley & Kimbrough, 1969; Egan et al., 1965; Komarova, 1970), especially in view of the low levels of detoxifying enzymes present in the infant. Levels of DDT found as a contaminant in food would lead to intakes far below that necessary to induce tumours in rodent species (Duggan & Weatherwax, 1967; Campbell et al., 1965).

Hexachlorocyclohexane (HCH) is easily manufactured and is used as a crude mixture of isomers in a number of developing countries. The 99 % pure isomer is called lindane, and most of the information on residue levels in food refers to this isomer. Lindane has been widely used for protecting harvested cereals, pulses and nuts and for treating storage areas. In certain countries, it is mixed at about 3 mg/kg with cereals in store, while in some tropical countries maize, millet, guinea corn and rice paddy have been treated at doses up to 11 mg/kg. It is destroyed to some extent by cooking. Application of lindane directly to animals to control insects has led to the occurrence of lindane in meat, and its use is usually not permitted on lactating animals (FAO/WHO, 1967). Information on the use pattern of the mixture of isomers and its level in food is very limited (FAO/WHO, 1969a), although it does appear to be widely used in many parts of the world. Information is available on the levels of lindane and its isomers encountered in various countries of the world and on many crops (FAO Working Party of Experts on Pesticide Residues and WHO Expert Committee on Pesticide Residues, 1971).

Total diet studies in at least two countries have confirmed the presence of significant residues of organochlorine insecticides in the diet of man (Duggan, 1968; Duggan & Weatherwax, 1967; Abbott et al., 1969). Thus a daily intake of 0.05 mg of DDT and its metabolites has been reported to arise from man's consumption of meat, fish and poultry (Duggan & Weatherwax, 1967). This intake can be expected to decrease in many countries with the decline in use of DDT.

Organophosphorus insecticides

Evidence from total diet studies indicates that levels of parathion in food are very low, namely 0–0.001 mg/kg in food as consumed (Duggan & Weatherwax, 1967). High residue levels of unchanged parathion may, however, occur in some crops (e.g., in carrots) (Maier-Bode, 1965).

Although parathion can be used safely if the necessary precautions are taken, it is associated with many incidents of poisoning and death. An outbreak in Tijuana, Mexico, in 1967 with 16 deaths was attributed to the contamination of bread as a result of the shipment of flour together with parathion (*The Times*, 1967; Weeks, 1968).

Some widely used organophosphorus insecticides, e.g., dichlorvos, are rapidly broken down and leave little or no toxic residues in food (Casida et al., 1962).

Carbamate insecticides

Probably the most commonly used carbamate insecticide in agriculture today is carbaryl. This compound is only partly broken down in plants to non-toxic compounds, and metabolites with anticholinesterase properties can become translocated to a certain extent into plant tissues (Kuhr & Casida, 1967). Total diet studies indicate a daily intake of 0.02 mg of carbaryl from meat, fish and poultry (Duggan & Weatherwax, 1967).

Other pesticides

A number of other classes of pesticides are used on food crops. Examples are the phenoxy herbicides and the dithiocarbamate fungicides. Total diet studies have demonstrated that these compounds are found only in very low levels in foodstuffs. For example, it has been calculated that the five-year daily average level of total herbicides ingested in the diet is 0.0001 mg/kg (Duggan et al., 1971).

Hazards from the use of fungicides appear to arise largely because of the application of high levels to treat seed grain. Occasionally such grain has mistakenly been used as food with serious toxic effects. The outbreak of porphyria in Turkey following the consumption of hexachlorobenzene-treated seed (Schmid, 1960) is such an example. Reference has already been made to cases where poisoning and death have resulted from eating mercury-treated grain (Jalili & Abbasi, 1961; *New York Times*, 1972).

Food additives

These substances, widely used in the more industrialized countries, are normally defined as "non-nutritive substances which are added intentionally to food, generally in small quantities, to improve its appearance, flavour, texture or storage properties" (Joint FAO/WHO Expert Committee on Nutrition, 1955). Although not contaminants in the strict sense, they are dealt with briefly here because of the harmful chemical changes that may occur. Food additives should be regarded as potentially toxic materials and should be properly tested and evaluated toxicologically. For example, nitrates or nitrites have been widely used as preservatives, but have been found to cause methaemoglobinaemia, especially in young children, and may give rise to carcinogenic nitrosamines (see Chapter 12).

Certain non-nutritive sweetening agents, e.g., cyclamates, have been widely used in recent years, but it has now been found that bladder tumours develop in animals to which they are fed in relatively high doses (Price et al., 1969). As a result, the use of these agents has been restricted or completely prohibited in a number of countries.

Certain methods of processing foods may lead to the formation of toxic contaminants. Thus smoking of foods has been shown to produce significant levels of the carcinogen benzo[a]pyrene (Dobes et al., 1954). The incidence of neoplasms seems to be increased in areas where the consumption of smoked fish reaches a high level (Bailey & Dungal, 1958; Kaufman et al., 1959; Voitelovič et al., 1957). Trace amounts of similar polycyclic hydrocarbons occur in extraction solvents; as a result, concentrated residues of such carcinogens may be present in processed food when the solvent has been evaporated.

The problem of antibiotics used as food additives, and of antibiotics and other chemotherapeutic agents that might under certain conditions leave residues in foods of animal origin (see next section), was reviewed by the Joint FAO/WHO Expert Committee on Food Additives (1969). Most countries have strict regulations against the intentional addition of antibiotics to food for preservative purposes. There are rare exceptions to this, such as the use of antibiotics in ice used to preserve fish in trawlers.

Animal feed additives and growth promoters

A widespread practice in animal husbandry in recent years has been to add substances to animal feeds, or to inject hormone-like agents, in order to promote the growth of animals. These substances include a wide variety of antibiotics and other chemotherapeutic agents (e.g., antiprotozoal and antibacterial compounds). They are presumed to act mainly as suppressors of disease agents, although they may also exert as yet ill-defined non-specific effects that promote animal growth. Undesirable effects of these substances include the emergence of antibiotic-resistant strains of micro-organisms that, when transferred to man, may cause considerable medical and public health problems. Allergic reactions and toxic effects in man may also occur, but knowledge of the toxicology of many of these substances is only rudimentary. This has led to a considerable tightening up of regulations for the use of these chemical compounds in many countries (Joint FAO/WHO Expert Committee on Food Additives, 1969; United Kingdom, Joint Committee on the Use of Antibiotics in Animal Husbandry and Veterinary Medicine, 1969).

Naturally occurring poisonous substances

Mycotoxins

If a plant crop is grown or stored under certain conditions, it may become infested with a fungus. Often these fungi are toxic only to the plant itself and control is necessary only to prevent loss of the crop. In some cases, however, the fungi produce highly toxic chemicals, e.g., aflatoxin in groundnuts, that present a hazard to the consumer. Often normal processing and cooking do not destroy the toxins and their presence is not immediately apparent. Many are of uncertain composition.

(1)   *Aflatoxin*

In 1960 an unusual fatal disease involving hepatoxicity became prevalent in turkeys in the United Kingdom, and after severe losses of turkey poults the disease was traced to certain lots of groundnuts in the ration (Allcroft & Carnaghan, 1963a). The groundnuts were contaminated by a toxin-producing strain of *Aspergillus flavus* (Sargeant et al., 1963). The toxic factor was termed "aflatoxin", and is now known to consist of a number of compounds of similar chemical structure. Aflatoxin B_1 and G_1 are highly hepatoxic to animals (van der Merwe et al., 1963).

The presence of aflatoxin-related compounds has been demonstrated in the milk of animals, following the use of feeds containing aflatoxin (Allcroft & Carnaghan, 1963b; de Iongh et al., 1964). Animal species vary widely in their response to aflatoxin. All species display acute liver damage and cell death following a dose near the LD_{50}. Hepatocarcinomas may be observed in the survivors, notably in the rat and some other species. Non-human primates appear to be fairly sensitive to the acute toxic effects, but liver tumours have not been induced in them (Barnes, 1970). The acute oral LD_{50} of aflatoxin in male vervet monkeys is 3.7 mg/kg. Aflatoxin causes bile duct proliferation and a central and mid-zonal necrosis of the liver, accompanied by haemorrhage. It also causes degenerative necrotic changes in the kidneys and extensive damage of the adrenals (van der Watt & Purchase, 1970).

A human death in circumstances strongly suggesting that aflatoxin was the cause has recently been reported (Serck-Hanssen, 1970). The case concerned a 15-year-old boy who died 6 days after eating cassava containing a high level (1.7 mg/kg) of aflatoxin. Histological examination of the liver showed centrilobular degeneration and necrosis with loss of stainable cytoplasm and mild fatty changes in the mid-zonal cells. Similar effects have been found in many animals fed aflatoxin and the histological changes strikingly resemble those found in the livers of 5 monkeys fed 0.01–1.0 mg aflatoxin per day until death (Elpert, 1970). As the boy's diet had consisted principally of cassava, his daily intake of aflatoxin could easily have been comparable to the lower level fed to the monkeys (*Food Cosmet. Toxicol.*, 1971).

Studies conducted in Kenya appear to show a correlation between the incidence of human liver cancer in one district and the levels of aflatoxin in food samples. Other similar studies are said to be in progress, in particular in Mozambique, where the world's highest incidence of liver cancer has been reported (International Agency for Research on Cancer, 1971).

(2) *Ergot*

The toxic effect of certain cereals contaminated with ergot has been documented over several centuries. The contaminant is produced by the fungus *Claviceps purpurea*, which infects seed grain, particularly rye (Barger, 1931). The adrenergic blocking activity of ergot results in vaso-constriction of the capillaries in the extremities, giving rise to a burning sensation known as "St Anthony's fire". If consumption of the conta-minated food is continued, progressive restriction of the blood supply to the limbs results in severance of the distal portions. Convulsive seizures and hallucinogenic manifestations also develop; the dancing mania of medieval Europe has been attributed to ergotism. Reports of human ergotism due to contaminated food are very rare today.

(3) "Yellow rice"

Liver tumours in rats and mice have been reported following contamination of rice with a strain of *Penicillum islandicum* (Kobayashi et al., 1959). Two compounds have been isolated. There is no evidence that the contaminants have been responsible for human cancer.

Marine biotoxins

With the rapid expansion of fisheries as a means of providing a source of protein, particularly in tropical developing countries, there is increasing concern over the presence of toxins in fish. The hazard of marine biotoxins is particularly insidious because species of fish that have been eaten for many years without danger often suddenly become poisonous and many deaths and harmful effects have resulted. In this section, only those fish having poisonous edible flesh will be considered. In many cases ordinary cooking procedures do not destroy the toxins. An extensive review has recently been published (Bagnis et al., 1970).

(1) Paralytic shellfish poisoning

This form of poisoning is caused by eating certain shellfish, particularly mussels, oysters and clams, that have been feeding on toxic dinoflagellates. Numerous outbreaks in both temperate and tropical areas of the world have been reported. The specific toxin, saxitoxin, has been partially identified chemically (Schuett & Rapoport, 1962). Symptoms usually develop within 30 minutes of ingestion, the initial paraesthesias being followed by more severe central nervous system involvement. The case fatality rate is said to be as high as 10 %; death is usually attributed to respiratory paralysis (Russell, 1965).

(2) Venerupin shellfish poisoning

Species of shellfish, particularly the clam *Venerupis semidecussata*, caught in Japan during certain months of the year, have been involved in this form of poisoning. Symptoms appear about 48 hours after ingestion, the liver being particularly affected. Death occurs in about one-third of cases (Halstead, 1965).

(3) Cephalopod poisoning

This intoxication results from the ingestion of squid and octopus from certain areas of Japan. From 1952 to 1955 there were 779 outbreaks involving 2874 persons and resulting in 10 deaths. Symptoms included gastrointestinal upset, abdominal pain, headache, weakness, paralysis and convulsions (Kawabata et al., 1957).

(4) *Ciguatera fish poisoning*

Ciguatera poisoning is one of the most serious and widespread forms of ichthyosarcotoxism. So far about 400 species have been implicated and in many cases useful food fishes suddenly became toxic without warning, possibly because they had been feeding on various forms of toxic marine life. Symptoms consist of paraesthesias of the lips, tongue and limbs with profound muscular weakness. Further neurological symptoms may develop, leading to convulsions. The case fatality rate is about 7 %. The poison has been isolated but its chemical structure is unclear (Mosher, 1966; Bagnis et al., 1970).

(5) *Puffer-fish poisoning (tetraodontoxism)*

Tetraodon poisoning is one of the most violent forms. There are at least 40 toxic species. Both central and peripheral nervous systems are involved and death may result from respiratory distress and convulsions. The case fatality rate is about 60 %. The compound responsible has been isolated and a probable chemical structure has been elucidated (Woodward, 1964; Bagnis et al., 1970).

(6) *Clupeotoxism*

This form of poisoning is caused by fish of the order *Clupeiformes*, which includes several well-known species, such as herrings, anchovies, tarpons, etc. The symptoms are usually violent, sometimes commencing immediately after the fish has been eaten. Vascular collapse and a variety of neurological symptoms may lead to death in less than 15 minutes. The case fatality rate is said to be very high, but there are no accurate statistics (Bagnis et al., 1970).

(7) *Scombrotoxism*

This form of poisoning is caused by the consumption of fish belonging to the family *Scombridae*, which includes tuna and related species. It is generally the consequence of improper preservation, whereby bacteria convert the histidine of the muscle into saurine, a histamine-like substance. The symptoms of scombrotoxism therefore resemble those of histamine intoxication. In extreme cases, death from anaphylactic shock has been reported. On a world-wide basis, scombrotoxism accounts for the greatest incidence of morbidity from ichthyosarcotoxism (Bagnis et al., 1970).

Radiological Contamination

Natural background radiation is high in certain parts of the world, so that there is a risk of food contamination from this source. Certain fish can concentrate heavy metals, and will concentrate radioisotopes of these metals in the same way. Thus ^{65}Zn has been accumulated by oysters at levels sufficient to present a hazard from their consumption as food (Fitzgerald et al., 1962). Fish, such as salmon, tuna, and saury, accumulate ^{55}Fe and high levels of consumption of these fish may increase the body-burden of radioactivity (Palmer et al., 1966). Certain marine animals e.g., molluscs, have concentrated the especially dangerous ^{90}Sr and high levels have been found largely in the shells or bones of the animals and also in the edible portions (Mauchline & Templeton, 1966).

Food Standards

The need for international food standards has been recognized. As a result, FAO and WHO have established the Joint FAO/WHO Food Standards Programme, with the Codex Alimentarius Commission as the principal organ of implementation of the Programme. Various subsidiary bodies have undertaken to establish levels or standards for contaminants that can be agreed upon at the international level; such levels or standards have already been established for some pesticide residues, food additives and food contaminants. Thus two series of recommended international tolerances for pesticide residues have been issued (FAO/WHO, 1969b, 1970), and maximum levels of many food contaminants and food additives have been included in many standards on food commodities. These standards are circulated to Member States for their acceptance. In addition, a publication entitled *General principles of food hygiene* (FAO/WHO, 1969b) has been prepared. As these standards become generally accepted they will be published in the *Codex Alimentarius* as world-wide Codex standards.

REFERENCES

Abbott, D. C., Holmes, D. C. & Tatton, J. D. G. (1969) *J. Sci. Fd Agric.*, **20**, 245

Abdussalam, M. et al. (1962) *Milk hygiene*, Geneva, World Health Organization (*Monograph Series*, No. 48)

Albertsen, V. E. et al. (1957) *Meat hygiene*, Geneva, World Health Organization (*Monograph Series*, No. 33)

Alexander, C. S. (1969) *Ann. intern. Med.*, **70**, 411

Allcroft, R. & Carnaghan, R. B. A. (1963a) *Chem. Industr.*, p. 50

Allcroft, R. & Carnaghan, R. B. A. (1963b) *Vet. Rec.*, **75**, 259

Arhangel'skij, I. I. & Kartasova, V. M. (1966) *Gigiena moloka i kontrol' jego sanitarnogo kačestva [Milk hygiene and control of the hygienic quality of milk]*, Moscow, Izdatel'stvo Kolos

Bagnis, R., Berglund, F., Elias, P. S., van Esch, G. J., Halstead, B. W. & Kojima, K. (1970) *Bull. Wld Hlth Org.*, **42,** 69

Bailey, E. J. & Dungal, N. (1958) *Brit. J. Cancer*, **12,** 348

Bailey, S., Bunyan, P. J. & Fishwick, F. B. (1970) *Chem. Industr.*, p. 705

Barger, G. (1931) *Ergot and ergotism*, London, Gurney & Jackson

Barnes, J. M. (1970) *J. appl. Bact.*, **33,** 285

Benoy, C. J., Hooper, P. A. & Schneider, R. (1971) *Fd Cosmet. Toxicol.*, **9,** No. 5

Borgstrom, G. et al. (1961-1965) *Fish as food*, Vols 1-4, London and New York, Academic Press

Bryan, F. L. (1971) *Diseases transmitted by foods (a classification and summary)*, Atlanta, Ga., US Public Health Service, Center for Disease Control

Callagan, J. (1961) *Trans. N. Amer. Wildl. Conf.*, **26,** 328

Campbell, J., Richardson, L. & Schafer, M. (1965) *Arch. environm. Hlth*, **10,** 831

Casida, J. E., McBride, L. & Niedermeier, P. R. (1962) *J. Agric. Fd Chem.*, **10,** 370

Clegg, D. J. (1971) *Fd Cosmet. Toxicol.*, **9,** 195

Cockburn, W. C., Taylor, J., Anderson, E. S. & Hobbs, B. C. (1962) *Food poisoning*, London, Royal Society

Coulson, E. J., Remington, R. E. & Lynch, K. M. (1936) *J. Nutr.*, **10,** 225

Curley, A. & Kimbrough, R. (1969) *Arch. environm. Hlth*, **18,** 156

Dobes, M., Hopp, K. & Šula, J. (1954) *Čs. Onkol.*, **1,** 254

Dräger, H. (1971) *Salmonellosen (ihre Entstehung und Verhütung)*, Berlin, Akademie-Verlag

Duggan, R. E. (1968) *Pestic. Monit. J.*, **1** (4), 2

Duggan, R. E., Lipscomb, G. D., Cox, E. L., Heatwole, R. E. & Kling, R. C. (1971) *Pestic. Monit. J.*, **5** (2), 73

Duggan, R. E. & Weatherwax, J. R. (1967) *Science*, **157,** 1006

Egan, H., Goulding, R., Roburn, J. & Tatton, J. O'G. (1965) *Brit. med. J.*, **2,** 66

Elpert, A. R. (1970) *Arch. environm. Hlth*, **20,** 723

Ender, F., Havre, G., Helgebostad, A., Koppang, N., Madsen, R., & Čeh, L. (1964) *Naturwissenschaften*, **225,** 554

FAO/WHO (1967) *Evaluations of some pesticide residues in food* (Unpublished document FAO PL:CP/15; WHO/Food Add./67.32)

FAO/WHO (1968) *1967 evaluations of some pesticide residues in food*, Rome (Unpublished document FAO/PL: 1967/M/11/1; WHO/Food Add./68.30)

FAO/WHO (1969a) *1968 evaluations of some pesticide residues in food*, Geneva (Unpublished document FAO/PL: 1968/M/9/1; WHO/Food Add./69.35)

FAO/WHO (1969b) *Recommended International Code of Practice. General principles of food hygiene. Joint FAO/WHO Food Standards Programme*, Rome (Unpublished document No. CAC/RCP 1-1969)

FAO/WHO (1970) *Recommended International Tolerances for Pesticide Residues, Second Series, Joint FAO/WHO Food Standards Programme*, Rome (Unpublished document No. CAC/RS 35-1970)

FAO Working Party of Experts on Pesticide Residues and WHO Expert Committee on Pesticide Residues (1971) *Pesticide residues in food*, Geneva, World Health Organization (*Wld Hlth Org. techn. Rep. Ser.*, No. 474)

Fitzgerald, B. W., Rankin, J. S. & Skarien, D. M. (1962) *Science*, **135,** 926

Food Cosmet. Toxicol., 1971, **9,** 575

Frazier, W. C. (1967) *Food microbiology*, 2nd ed., New York, McGraw-Hill

Goldsmith, J. R. (1969) *J. Air Pollut. Control Ass.*, **19**, 714

Halstead, B. W. (1965) *Poisonous and venomous marine animals of the world*, vol. 1, *Invertebrates*, Washington, D. C., US Government Printing Office

Halstead, B. W. (1967) *Poisonous and venomous marine animals of the world*, vol. 2, *Vertebrates*, Washington, D.C., US Government Printing Office.

Horio, T., Iwamoto, Y. & Shiga, I. (1967) *Communications of the 5th International Congress on Canning, Vienna*

Hueper, W. C. (1963) *Ann. N.Y. Acad. Sci.*, **108**, 961

Ingram, M. & Roberts, T. A., eds (1967) *Botulism 1966: Proceedings of the Fifth International Symposium on Food Microbiology, Moscow, 1966*, London, Chapman & Hall

International Agency for Research on Cancer (1971) *Annual Report 1970*, Lyon, p. 86

de Iongh, H., Vles, R. O. & van Pelt, J. G. (1964) *Nature*, **202**, 466

Ishizaki, A., Fukushima, M. & Sakamonto, M. (1970) *Jap. J. Hyg.*, **25**, 207

Jalili, M. A. & Abbasi, A. H. (1961) *Brit. J. industr. Med.*, **18**, 303

J. Amer. med. Ass., 1966, **197**, 25 July, p. 27

Jensen, S., Johnels, A. G., Olsson, M. & Otterland, G. (1969) *Nature (Lond.)*, **224**, 247

Joint FAO/WHO Expert Committee on Food Additives (1969) *Twelfth report*, Geneva (*Wld Hlth Org. techn. Rep. Ser.*, No. 430)

Joint FAO/WHO Expert Committee on Meat Hygiene (1962) *Second report*, Geneva (*Wld Hlth Org. techn. Rep. Ser.*, No. 241)

Joint FAO/WHO Expert Committee on Milk Hygiene (1970) *Third report*, Geneva (*Wld Hlth Org. techn. Rep. Ser.*, No. 453)

Joint FAO/WHO Expert Committee on Nutrition (1955) *Fourth report*, Geneva (*Wld Hlth Org. techn. Rep. Ser.*, No. 97)

Joint FAO/WHO Expert Committee on Zoonoses (1967) *Third report*, Geneva (*Wld Hlth Org. techn. Rep. Ser.*, No. 378)

Kasymov, A. G. (1970) *Mar. Pollut. Bull.*, **11**, 100-103

Kaufman, B. D., Moronova, A. I. & Šabad, L. M. (1959) *Vop. Onkol.*, **5** (9), 314

Kawabata, T., Halstead, B. W. & Judefind, T. F. (1957) *Amer. J. trop. Med. Hyg.*, **6**, 935

Kazantzis, G. (1971) *Int. J. environm. Stud.*, **1**, 301-306

Kehoe, R. A. (1959) *Industr. Med. Surg.*, **28**, 156

Kesteloot, H., Terryn, R., Bosmans, P. & Joosens, J. V. (1966) *Acta Cardiol. (Brux.)*, **21**, 341

Kobayashi, Y., Uraguchi, K., Sakai, F., Tatsuno, T., Tsukioka, Y., Noguchi, Y., Tsunoda, H., Miyake, M., Saito, M., Enomoto, M., Shikata, T. & Ishiko, T. (1959) *Proc. Japan Acad.*, **35**, 501

Komarova, L. I. (1970) *Pediat. Akush. Ginec.*, **35** (1), 19

Kuhr, R. J. & Casida, J. E. (1967) *J. Agric. Fd Chem.*, **15**, 814

Lerche, M. (1966) *Lehrbuch der tierärztlichen Milchüberwachung*, Berlin, Parey

Maier-Bode, H. (1965) *Pflanzenschutzmittel-Rückstände*, Stuttgart, Ulmer, p. 455

Manzari, P. (1965) *Manuale di microbiologia del latte*, Rome, Pozzi

Matsumoto, H., Koya, G. & Takeuchi, T. (1965) *J. Neuropath. exp. Neurol.*, **24**, 563

Matyáš, Z. et al. (1965) *Hygiena potravin I Maso a masné výrobky* [*Food hygiene I. Meat and meat products*], Prague, Státni zemĕdĕlské nakladatelstvi

Mauchline, J. & Templeton, W. L. (1966) *J. Cons. perm. int. Explor. Mer*, **30,** 2

Miller, J. T. & Byers, H. G. (1937) *J. agric. Res.*, **55,** 59

Mosher, H. S. (1966) *Science*, **51,** 860

Moxon, A. L. & Rhian, M. (1943) *Physiol. Rev.*, **23,** 305

New York Times (1972) 9 March

Noddack, I. & Noddack, W. (1940) *Arch. Zool.*, **32A** (4), 1

Novick, S. (1969) *Environment*, **11** (4), 2

Palmer, H. E., Beasley, T. M. & Folson, T. R. (1966) *Nature (Lond.)*, **211,** 1253

Pattison, E. S., Collins, I. V. & Argino, E. E. (1970) *Science*, **170,** 870

Pierce, P. E., Thompson, J. F., Likosky, W. H., Nickey, L. N., Barthel, W. F. & Hinman, A. R. (1972) *J. Amer. med. Ass.*, **220,** 1439-1442

Price, J. M., Bravia, C. G., Oser, B. C., Vogin, E. E., Steinfield, J. & Saffiotti, U. (1969) *BIBRA Bull.*, **8,** 456

Pringle, B. H., Hissong, D. E., Katz, E. W. & Mulawaka, S. T. (1968) *J. sanit. Engng Div. Amer. Soc. civ. Engrs*, **94,** 455

Quinby, G. E., Armstrong, J. F. & Durham, W. F. (1965) *Nature (Lond.)*, **207,** 726

Riemann, H., ed. (1969) *Food-borne infections and intoxications*, New York and London, Academic Press

Russell, F. E. (1965) *Adv. marine Biol.*, **3,** 255

Sargeant, K., Carnaghan, R. B. A. & Allcroft, R. (1963) *Chem. Industr.*, p. 53

Schmid, R. (1960) *New Engl. J. Med.*, **263,** 397

Schönherr, W., ed. (1967) *Tierärztliche Milchhygiene*, Leipzig, Hirzel

Schroeder, H. A. & Balassa, J. J. (1961) *J. chron. Dis.*, **14,** 236

Schuett, W. & Rapoport, N. (1962) *J. Amer. chem. Soc.*, **84,** 2266

Scottish Home and Health Department (1964) *The Aberdeen typhoid outbreak 1964. Report of the Departmental Committee of Enquiry*, Edinburgh, HM Stationery Office

Sedlák, J. & Rische, H. (1961) *Enterobacteriaceae-Infektionen: Epidemiologie und Laboratoriumsdiagnostik*, Leipzig, Thieme

Serck-Hanssen, A. (1970) *Arch. environm. Hlth*, **20,** 729

Skerfving, S., Hausson, A. & Lindsten, J. (1970) *Arch. environm. Hlth*, **21,** 133

Smart, N. A. (1961) *Pl. Path.*, **10,** 150

Stanstead, H. H., Michelakes, A. M. & Temple, T. E. (1970) *Arch. environm. Hlth*, **20,** 356

Stokinger, H. E. (1963). In: Patty, F. A., Fassett, D. W. & Irish, D. D., eds, *Industrial hygiene and toxicology*, 2nd ed., New York, Interscience

Sullivan, J., Parker, M. & Carson, S. B. (1968) *J. Lab. clin. Med.*, **71,** 893

Thatcher, F. S. & Clark, D. S., eds (1968) *Micro-organisms in foods: their significance and methods of enumeration*, Toronto, University of Toronto Press

The Times, 29 September 1967

Tokuomi, H., Okajima, T., Kanai, J., Tsunoda, M., Ichiyasu, Y., Misumi, H., Shimomura, K. & Tokaha, M. (1961) *Wld Neurol.*, **2,** 536; *Kumamoto med. J.*, **14,** 47

United Kingdom, Joint Committee on the Use of Antibiotics in Animal Husbandry and Veterinary Medicine (1969) *Report*, London, H.M. Stationery Office

US National Academy of Sciences (1964) *An evaluation of public health hazards from microbiological contamination of foods*, Washington, D.C.

van der Merwe, K. J., Fourie, L. & de Scott, B. (1963) *Chem. Industr.*, p. 1660

van der Watt, K. J. & Purchase, I. F. H. (1970) *Brit. J. exp. Path.*, **51**, 183

Voitelovič, F. A., Dikun, P. P., Dymarskii, L. U. & Šabad, L. M. (1957) *Vop. Onkol.*, **3** (3), 351

Weeks, D. E. (1967) *Bull. Wld Hlth Org.*, **37**, 499

Weeks, D. E. (1968) Geneva, World Health Organization (Unpublished document WHO/VBC/68.98)

Westöö, G. (1969) In: Miller, M. W. & Berg, G. G., eds, *Chemical fallout*, Springfield, Thomas, pp. 75-93

WHO Expert Committee on Enteric Infections (1964) *Report*, Geneva (*Wld Hlth Org. techn. Rep. Ser.*, No. 288)

WHO Expert Committee on the Microbiological Aspects of Food Hygiene (1968) *Report*, Geneva (*Wld Hlth Org. techn. Rep. Ser.*, No. 399)

Wogan, G. N., ed. (1964) *Mycotoxins in foodstuffs: Proceedings of a Symposium held at the Massachusetts Institute of Technology...*, Cambridge, Mass., Massachusetts Institute of Technology

Woodward, R. B. (1964) *Pure appl. Chem.*, **9**, 49

Yamagata, N. & Shigematsu, I. (1970) *Bull. Inst. publ. Hlth*, **19** (1), 1

Zahariev, C. (1964) *Higiena: veterinarno-sanitarna ekspertiza na mljakoto i mlečnite produkti s osnovami na tehnologijata*, [*Hygiene: veterinary sanitary assessment of milk and milk products on a technological basis*], Sofia, Zemizdat

CHAPTER 4

SOIL AND LAND

Soil pollution is usually a consequence of insanitary habits, various agricultural practices, and incorrect methods of disposal of solid and liquid wastes, but can also result from fallout from atmospheric pollution. It is closely linked with the ultimate fate of those substances that are unlikely to undergo the natural recycling processes to which putrescible matter is subject.

In industrialized countries, soil pollution is associated mainly with:

(1) the use of chemicals, such as fertilizers and growth-regulating agents, in agriculture;

(2) the dumping on land of large masses of waste materials from the mining of coal and minerals and the smelting of metals. Toxic or harmful substances can be leached out of such materials and enter the soil;

(3) the dumping on land of domestic refuse and solids resulting from the treatment of sewage and industrial wastes (WHO Scientific Group on the Treatment and Disposal of Wastes, 1967; WHO Expert Committee on Solid Wastes Disposal and Control, 1971).

The soil is thus becoming increasingly polluted with chemicals, including heavy metals and products of the petroleum industry, which can reach the food chain, surface water, or ground water, and ultimately be ingested by man.

In many countries of the world, and particularly in the developing ones, soil pollution with pathogenic micro-organisms is still of major importance. In such countries, intestinal parasites constitute the most important soil pollution problem, as a result both of the improper disposal of human excreta, waste water, and solid wastes, and of incorrect agricultural practices. Thus it is estimated that about one-third of the world's population is infected by hookworm (CCTA/WHO African Conference on Ancylostomiasis, 1963), while one out of every four people in the world may be infected with *Ascaris lumbricoides* (WHO Expert Committee on the Control of Ascariasis, 1967).

Soil Pollution by Biological Disease Agents

Biological agents that can pollute the soil and cause disease in man can be divided into three groups:

(1) pathogenic organisms excreted by man and transmitted to man by direct contact with contaminated soil or by the consumption of fruit or vegetables grown in contaminated soil (man-soil-man);

(2) pathogenic organisms of animals, transmitted to man by direct contact with soil contaminated by the wastes of infected animals (animal-soil-man); and

(3) pathogenic organisms found naturally in soil and transmitted to man by contact with contaminated soil (soil-man).

Man-soil-man

Enteric bacteria and protozoa

Enteric bacteria and protozoa can contaminate the soil as a result of: (a) insanitary excreta disposal practices; or (b) the use of night soil or sewage sludge as a fertilizer, or the direct irrigation of agricultural crops with sewage. Soil and crops can become contaminated with the bacterial agents of cholera, salmonellosis, bacillary dysentery (shigellosis) and typhoid and paratyphoid fever, or with the protozoan agent of amoebiasis. However, these diseases are most often water-borne, and transmitted by direct person-to-person contact, or by the contamination of food (see Chapters 2 and 3). Flies that breed in, or come into contact with, faecal-contaminated soil can serve as mechanical carriers of disease organisms.

Parasitic worms (helminths)

Soil-transmitted parasitic worms or geo-helminths are characterized by the fact that their eggs or larvae become infective after a period of incubation in the soil.

Infections with such helminths on the whole provide, by their prevalence and intensity, an index of a community's progress towards a desirable level of sanitation. From the standpoint of the prevalence and severity of such infections, the most important soil-transmitted helminths are *Ascaris lumbricoides* (roundworm), *Trichuris trichiura* (whipworm), *Necator americanus*, and *Ancylostoma duodenale*, the last two being the causative agents of hookworm disease. An additional species that is less widely distributed and less restricted to soil transmission is *Strongyloides stercoralis*.

The free-living stages of soil-transmitted helminths have to face many natural hazards. Because of its particular requirements, each species tends to occur in broad ecological zones, determined by the climatic conditions. The range of conditions permitting maximum survival and development is narrow, however, and depends more on the micro-environment than on the macro-environment. The optimum conditions for each species are related to rainfall, atmospheric temperature, vegetation, sunlight, and air movement, as well as to the texture, moisture, and structure of the soil. It is for this reason that eggs of *Ascaris lumbricoides* have been found to survive at extremely low air temperatures under a thick cover of snow, and that hookworm disease does not occur everywhere in moist tropical regions and is also found outside the tropics.

There appears to be little doubt that infections, whether heavy or moderate, with intestinal geo-helminths constitute a continuing drain on the host's supply of nutrients, particularly protein and certain vitamins. Malnutrition may also be induced or aggravated by the resulting impairment of the digestion and absorption of essential nutritional substances. It was recently shown, for instance, that *Ascaris* infection in children produces marked nutritional deficiencies when a high parasite load is associated with a low protein intake (Tripathy et al., 1971). The sucking motions of hookworms lead to the loss of large quantities of blood and iron; in subjects who receive an inadequate supply of food iron, as is the case in many rural populations, such blood loss is of great importance in the causation of anaemia in the tropics (Roche & Layrisse, 1966). The amount of nutrients lost to human beings throughout the tropical world as a result of intestinal geo-helminths is of formidable proportions. If diverted from the parasites to their human hosts, it could not fail to bring considerable benefits to their health (WHO Expert Committee on the Control of Ascariasis, 1967).

Contamination of soil and crops

Despite the enormous progress made by mankind over the past 50 years, there still remain, even relatively close to the largest modern cities, a vast number of human beings whose standards of living, level of education, and economic and social status have changed little, and whose habits, particularly with regard to micturition and defecation, are still such as to maintain the cycle of infection with soil-transmitted pathogens.

Human faeces are nevertheless a valuable fertilizer when chemical fertilizers are in short supply, as is the case in most parts of the world. The contents of latrines, septic tanks, and sewage systems are therefore frequently used for the fertilization of crops. In areas subject to water shortages, the reclamation of waste water often provides a valuable additional source of water for irrigation, but unless certain precautions are taken this practice is dangerous to health. Soil and crops may thus be contaminated by pathogenic enteric bacteria, protozoan parasites, such as *Entamoeba histolytica*, and the larvae of intestinal helminths, leading to direct transmission either by contact or by the ingestion of uncooked vegetables.

Untreated domestic sewage or night soil usually contains the complete spectrum of pathogenic micro-organisms harboured by the community. Conventional sewage treatment processes cannot remove all these pathogenic organisms, but it is generally accepted that the extent of removal of coliform organisms serves as an indication of the efficiency of such processes from a bacteriological point of view. It has been found that, in primary sedimentation, a 30–40 % reduction in the numbers of coliform organisms can be achieved, while in most full biological treatment processes the reduction is about 90 %. Stabilization ponds with a 30-day detention period have generally shown more than 99 % reduction of coliform organisms (Shuval, 1963). A number of studies have been carried out to determine the efficiency of sewage treatment processes in the removal of specific pathogens. In general, the data closely parallel those for the removal rates for coliform organisms. For practical purposes, it cannot be assumed that even a well-run biological sewage treatment plant can consistently remove more than 90 % of the pathogenic organisms present in the sewage, unless heavy chlorination is applied. In the case of primary sedimentation, a considerably lower rate of removal of pathogenic organisms must be expected.

Various control methods have been devised on the basis of studies made on the viability of pathogenic organisms and their resistance to detrimental environmental factors and to chemicals. Research has shown, for instance, that *Salmonella* organisms persist for up to 70 days in soil irrigated with sewage under moist winter conditions and for about half that length of time under drier summer conditions (Bergner-Rabinovitz, 1956). *Ascaris* eggs can withstand more than two years' exposure on fields in temperate regions, and it has been reported that even dried, digested sludge from some sewage plants contains viable eggs of this parasite (WHO Expert Committee on Helminthiases, 1964). Methods adapted to the particular characteristics of each species of soil-transmitted pathogen are therefore required for the effective treatment of sewage effluents used for irrigation purposes.

The problem of the unsupervised scattering of fresh, untreated night-soil and raw sewage still remains. In the recent spread of cholera throughout the Middle East, vegetable crops irrigated with raw sewage were implicated in one instance as the major pathway for the dissemination of the disease. In a few cases the suspected contaminated vegetables were consumed cooked, but it may be assumed that kitchen surfaces and utensils became contaminated in the process of preparing these vegetables, thus leading to the contamination of other foods eaten uncooked (Cohen et al., 1971).

Animal-soil-man

In a number of zoonoses (diseases of animals transmissible to man), the soil may play a major part in transmitting the infective agent from animal to man.

Leptospirosis

This disease affects both animals and man in all parts of the world. The epidemiology of the disease follows a characteristic pattern similar to that of other zoonoses, namely animal to animal, and animal to man. Leptospirosis now constitutes a major problem in cattle and a problem of undetermined size in swine. In some areas, sheep, goats, and horses become infected. Rodent carriers include rats, mice, and voles. The dispersion of leptospires is associated with specific environmental conditions, particularly those that bring animal carriers, water, mud, and man together. Animal carriers often excrete a profusion of leptospires—up to 100 million per ml—in the urine. If this is excreted into water or mud that is neutral or slightly alkaline, the leptospires may survive for weeks. Susceptible animals and man entering this environment are exposed to the agent and may develop infection varying from an inapparent reaction to an acute fulminating fatal disease. Leptospires usually enter the body through the mucous membranes or broken or macerated skin. Agricultural workers in irrigated fields, and in rice and cane fields in particular, often become infected (Joint ILO/WHO Committee on Occupational Health, 1962; Joint FAO/WHO Expert Committee on Zoonoses, 1967).

Anthrax

The number of reported cases of anthrax in man is relatively small compared with the figures for other zoonoses; nevertheless, anthrax is still of importance both as a human disease and because of its economic impact on animal husbandry. The spores of *Bacillus anthracis* are very resistant to chemical and environmental influences and can survive for years in certain soils as well as in animal products, such as hides, hair, and wool. When anthrax infections in livestock become established in a district, a relatively permanent enzootic focus of infection is created because of the long period for which the spores can remain viable in the soil (Joint FAO/WHO Expert Committee on Zoonoses, 1967).

Q fever

Q fever, caused by the rickettsia *Coxiella burnetii*, is an important public health problem affecting almost all the countries of the world. Rickettsiae may be present in soil and dust, where they can survive for long periods, since they are highly resistant to drying. This is particularly important in those countries where ewes are brought into yards to lamb. Very high concentrations of rickettsiae may then be present in the dust of such yards, which is therefore highly infective when sheltered from direct sunlight (Joint FAO/WHO Expert Committee on Zoonoses, 1967).

Cutaneous larva migrans

Cutaneous larva migrans, or creeping eruption, is a common infection of man in warm climates where dog and cat hookworms *(Ancylostoma braziliense)* are widespread. Man becomes infected by the entry of the hookworm larvae into the skin, where they migrate causing a dermatitis of varying intensity. Infection is usually found among those exposed to animal faeces, especially children on beaches, lawns, or playgrounds where larvae are present. Soil disinfection can be practised in selected areas (Joint FAO/WHO Expert Committee on Zoonoses, 1967).

Other diseases

Among other diseases that follow the sequence animal-soil-man, mention should be made of the following: visceral larva migrans, due mainly to *Toxocara canis*, listeriosis, *Clostridium perfringens* infections, lymphocytic choriomeningitis, South American types of haemorrhagic fever, tuberculosis, salmonellosis, and tularaemia. Although most of these diseases and infections are transmitted predominantly by direct animal-man contact, or through the contamination of food by animal droppings and wastes, soil pollution may also play an important part (Joint FAO/WHO Expert Committee on Zoonoses, 1967).

Soil-man

Mycoses

Most of the serious subcutaneous, deep-seated and systemic mycoses are caused by fungi and actinomycetes that grow normally as saprophytes in soil or vegetation. Under certain circumstances, however, they become pathogenic and invade specific tissues or entire systems.

The usual modes of transmission are by inhalation of spores or by penetration of the skin following an injury. Thus mycetomas are produced when various mycetes penetrate the skin through puncture wounds, such as those caused by thorns. As with chromomycosis and other fungal diseases, they are commonest among those who walk barefooted or are inadequately protected by shoes or clothing; they are the cause of long periods of disability ending, if left untreated, in the amputation of the affected limbs. Coccidioidomycosis is due to the fungus *Coccidioides immitis*, which is found in arid and semi-arid regions in the top few inches of soil and in the vicinity of rodent burrows. In the heat of early summer, the little ground cover that exists withers and dies; wind then disturbs the surface dust and lifts the spores into the air. The same process is involved in infections with many other fungi that grow in soil (geotrichosis), on leaf mould or decaying fruit (phycomycosis), on soil enriched by excreta from chickens, other birds, or bats (histoplasmosis), in the nests and manure of pigeons (cryptococcosis), in vegetable compost (aspergillosis), or on timber or water seepage (sporotrichosis).

The ecology of most of these free-living organisms potentially pathogenic to man and the pathogenesis of the diseases they produce are still far from being elucidated. Such mycoses have up to now been a neglected field of medicine, but nevertheless constitute world-wide or regional problems of great magnitude affecting, in particular, workers engaged in digging operations or agriculture.

Tetanus

Tetanus is an acute disease of man induced by the toxin of the tetanus bacillus growing anaerobically at the site of an injury. The organism has a world-wide distribution, though cases of the disease are comparatively infrequent today. It is an occasional disease among farmers, especially following the contamination of wounds with manured soil (Joint ILO/WHO Committee on Occupational Health, 1962). The infectious agent, *Clostridium tetani*, is excreted by infected animals, especially horses. The immediate source of infection may be soil, dust, or animal and human faeces.

Botulism

This is a frequently fatal type of poisoning caused by bacterial toxins produced by *Clostridium botulinum*. The reservoir of the organism is soil and the intestinal tract of animals. The toxin is formed by the anaerobic growth of spores in food, which is the immediate source of poisoning. The disease is usually transmitted by the ingestion, without previous cooking, of food from jars or cans imperfectly sterilized during canning, the canned or preserved food having been infected with soil contaminated b *Cl. botulinum* (see Chapter 3, p. 74).

Soil Pollution and Solid Wastes Disposal

Urban areas

The land serves as a major repository for the solid wastes of urban and industrial areas. Solid wastes disposal in metropolitan areas has a number of public health implications (Hanks, 1967).

The problem of greatest concern stems from the fact that, with increasing urbanization and the consequent increase in the area occupied by buildings, the land available for depositing wastes is correspondingly reduced.

In highly industrialized countries, even the solid wastes from agriculture can become a problem, particularly when livestock and poultry wastes near urban centres become a breeding ground for flies and cause a serious odour nuisance on decomposition.

Production per head of solid wastes varies considerably from country to country, but with rising living standards the amount of refuse produced is everywhere on the increase. In the USA and some European countries this increase is estimated at about 3 % per year by volume, and 2 % per year by weight (Ellis, 1969).

The problems of land pollution by wastes differ in a number of important respects from those of water or air pollution, since the polluting material remains in place for relatively long periods of time unless removed, burned, washed away, or otherwise destroyed.

In many of the more developed countries, aesthetic considerations have become important in wastes disposal and there is less readiness to accept unsightly, open refuse dumps and junk heaps as an inevitable blot on the landscape. Insects and rodents, which breed in such dumps, and odours from decomposing organic matter or from slow smouldering fires, can cause severe nuisance and public health problems.

With the increasing utilization of land for urban development, pressure to dispose of solid wastes by methods other than land disposal has led to new pollution problems. Improper incineration can lead to severe air pollution, while discharge into water leads to overloading of treatment facilities and to increased pollution in already heavily burdened watercourses.

Agricultural land pollution

In the past, nutrient materials in the agricultural economy followed a clearly defined cycle: from the land to plants, from plants to animals, and then back to the land again. In some of the more highly industrialized countries, the use of chemical fertilizers has short-circuited this cycle, and many agricultural areas now have large surpluses of plant and animal wastes that, unless properly disposed of, can cause soil pollution. The problem becomes particularly severe where urban areas border on agricultural land. In these fringe areas, agricultural solid wastes may ultimately have to be handled in the same way as urban wastes.

As agriculture becomes more intensive, so that increasing quantities of synthetic materials, such as pesticides, nutrients, and control agents, are used, chemical soil pollution coupled with increasing amounts of excess organic waste materials leads ultimately to severe land pollution problems in agricultural areas (Shuval, 1962).

Contamination of the Soil by Toxic Chemicals

Agricultural chemicals

Fertilizers are intended to fortify the soil for the raising of crops, but incidentally may contaminate the soil with their impurities. Irrigation of farmlands and orchards may do this if the source of water is polluted by industrial wastes that contain synthetic organic chemicals. During the last few decades, herbicides, insecticides, fungicides, soil conditioners, and fumigants have produced intentional alterations of agricultural, horticultural, and silvicultural soils. The chemicals used may pollute the soil water.

Fumigants and soil conditioners are unstable and are metabolized by the micro-organisms of the soil. For example, even the chlorinated phenol derivatives, such as polychlorophenoxyacyl acids, used as herbicides, are metabolized by special strains of bacteria that adapt themselves to use them as nutrients. This holds true also for dinitro-*o*-cresol and allied compounds. The bacterial and fungal flora of the soil are much richer in numbers than the flora of watercourses, even when these are contaminated by organic matter. It is therefore possible for chemicals that can remain unchanged for a long time in water to be rapidly degraded by microbial activity in the soil. For example, if a soil is "fed" with chemicals such as phenols, bacteria that thrive on naturally occurring phenols will multiply.

Experience with new antibacterial drugs shows how effective some bacteria are in developing resistance to new substances. The metabolic enzymes undergo the necessary alteration so as to detoxify the compounds (adaptive enzyme formation). By such mechanisms chemicals disappear from the soil, and farmlands must be sprayed every year with herbicides if weeds are to be kept in check.

Ideally, only such chemicals should be employed as have been proved to be readily attacked and degraded by the common soil micro-organisms. Compounds of lead and mercury—the mercurials being mostly organic compounds—and salts of arsenious acids are likely to accumulate as persistent soil contaminants and to introduce lead, mercury, and arsenic into plant products.

The present trend in the manufacture of pesticides for use in agriculture is to synthesize short-lived degradable compounds because this minimizes the persistence of residues of pesticides and their degradation products on food and forage crops.

Little is known, however, about the breakdown products of many of these chemicals. In some cases new toxic breakdown products can be formed in the soil although little of the original toxic compound can be detected.

Among the organic pesticides now in use that resist bacterial degradation and have no inert end-products, by far the most important are the chlorinated hydrocarbons, e.g., DDT, lindane, aldrin, and dieldrin. Remnants of these stable pesticides appear to be bound to or adsorbed on soil particles, which are made up of inorganic minerals coated with organic compounds. These chemicals may contaminate root crops grown in soils of this kind; for example, lindane can taint carrots or beets. The behaviour of chemicals that do not affect the quality or reduce the yield of crops can escape notice, but true absorption and incorporation of these pollutants by plants is unlikely to occur in normal practice (World Health Organization, 1968). Five years after the last insecticide treatment, 4 to 5 % of the quantity applied remains in the soil.   Some of the breakdown products are more toxic to insects than the original insecticides themselves, while others may be completely non-toxic.

Thousands of soil samples have been analysed in the USA and other countries during the last five years.   In some orchard soils the concentrations of DDT and other chlorinated hydrocarbons reached 120 ppm, but most frequently were in the range 0.1–5 ppm (World Health Organization, 1971).   (For a recent comprehensive discussion of the persistence of pesticides in the soil flora and fauna, see Edwards, 1970.)

Solid wastes from industry

Leachate from industrial solid wastes may contain poisonous chemicals in solution; these may be concentrated in nature by various organisms in the human food chain.

A recent study (United Kingdom, 1970) has shown that the disposal of industrial solid wastes constitutes a major source of land pollution by toxic chemicals.   It has been estimated that some 50 % or more of the raw materials used by industry ultimately become waste products, and that about 15 % can be considered deleterious or toxic.   In the United Kingdom, close to one million tons of materials classified as flammable, acid, caustic, or indisputably toxic are dumped annually by industry.   This amounts to about 20 kg per person per year.   A major portion of these wastes is dumped on the land either by private contractors or by arrangement with local authorities.   Some wastes are dumped at sea or incinerated.

These wastes have, in certain instances, given rise to severe problems of soil pollution, either by poisoning the soil or crops, or by eventual entry into ground-water and surface-water sources.

Observation of the contamination of farmland in the neighbourhood of chemical factories has indicated that there is a potential danger of fallout from the plume emitted by the smoke-stacks of chemical works.   This applies mainly to inorganic contaminants, e.g., fluorine (Macúch et al., 1963).   Synthetic organic chemicals can be destroyed in properly operated stacks.

Radioactive materials

Radioactive materials can reach the soil and accumulate there, either from atmospheric fallout from nuclear explosions, or from the release of liquid or solid radioactive wastes produced by industrial or research establishments. The two most important radionuclides with long half-lives produced by nuclear fission are ^{90}Sr (half-life 28 years) and ^{137}Cs (half-life 30 years). Fallout of relatively recent origin and discharges from nuclear reactors also contain a number of other radionuclides of importance from the ecological point of view, e.g., ^{131}I, ^{140}Ba + ^{140}La, ^{106}Ru + ^{106}Rh, ^{144}Ce + ^{144}Pr, etc. These radionuclides contribute primarily to the gamma radiation emitted by the radioactive material accumulated in the soil. ^{14}C has also to be taken into account; this is produced from nitrogen in the air by neutron-proton processes, e.g., during the explosion of a hydrogen weapon, and also by cosmic radiation. It participates in the carbon metabolism of plants, and is thus also introduced into animals and the soil. Levels are not expected to become high enough, however, for adverse effects to occur.

Concentrations of radioactive strontium in the soil are generally a function of the amount of precipitation, since this element is brought to the soil primarily by rain. Within the soil, the deposited ^{90}Sr is held firmly by electrostatic forces in the upper few inches. If soil is eroded, the deposited radionuclides are carried away with the silt and clay.

Radioactive cesium is held even more tightly by the soil than strontium; however, certain plants, e.g., mushrooms and lichens, accumulate cesium, and high concentrations of this element can be reached in animals that feed on these plants. It is known that, during the period 1962-1963, cesium levels in the bodies of Lapps, who live mainly on reindeer meat, were about ten times as great as those for other population groups in northern countries.

Levels of radiation from fission products deposited in the soil by fallout in the northern hemisphere are about 10–30 % of those due to natural radioactive substances in the soil. Many authorities feel that there is very little evidence to date to show that this increase in radiation levels could affect soil fauna or their predators, but increased radioactive fallout could in time result in levels of soil contamination high enough to cause concern.

Conclusion

Pollution of the land by the biological agents of disease remains one of the major causes of debilitating infections in the rural and semi-rural areas inhabited by the majority of the world's population. Land pollution by toxic chemicals from agriculture and industry, leading to the contamination of soil, food, and water, may prove to be a significant hazard to health in the more industrialized areas of the world. The problems arising from the dumping on land of the ever-increasing amounts of domestic and industrial solid wastes will become more acute as world population and the degree of urbanization increase.

REFERENCES

Bergner-Rabinovitz, S. (1956) *Appl. Microbiol.*, **4**, 101

CCTA/WHO African Conference on Ancylostomiasis (1963) *Report*, Geneva, World Health Organization (*Wld Hlth Org. techn. Rep. Ser.*, No. 255) p. 5

Cohen, J. et al. (1971), *Lancet*, **2**, 86-89

Edwards, C. A. (1970) *Persistent pesticides in the environment*, London, Butterworths

Ellis, H. M. (1969) *A new appraisal of the solid-waste problem.* In: *Problems in community wastes management*, Geneva, World Health Organization (*Publ. Hlth Pap.*, No. 38) p. 22

Emmons, C. W. (1950) *The natural occurrence in animals and soils of fungi which cause disease in man.* In: *Proc. Seventh Int. Bot. Congr.*, Stockholm, pp. 416-421

Hanks, T. G. (1967) *Solid waste/disease relationships: a literature survey*, Cincinnati, US Public Health Service, Solid Wastes Program (*US Public Health Service Publication* No. 999-UIH-6)

Joint FAO/WHO Expert Committee on Zoonoses (1967) *Third report*, Geneva, World Health Organization (*Wld Hlth Org. techn. Rep. Ser.*, No. 378)

Joint ILO/WHO Committee on Occupational Health (1962) *Occupational health problems in agriculture. Fourth report of the Joint ILO/WHO Committee on Occupational Health*, Geneva, World Health Organization (*Wld Hlth Org. techn. Rep. Ser.*, No. 246)

Macúch, P. et al. (1963) *J. Hyg. Epidem. (Praha)*, **7**, 389-403

Roche, M. & Layrisse, M. (1966) *Amer. J. trop. Med. Hyg.*, **15**, 1032-1102

Schmelzer, L. L. & Tabershaw, I. R. (1968) *Amer. J. publ. Hlth*, **58**, 107-113

Shuval, H. I. (1962) *Bull. Wld Hlth Org.*, **27**, 791

Tripathy, K. et al. (1971) *Amer. J. trop. Med. Hyg.*, **20**, 212-218

United Kingdom, Ministry of Housing and Local Government/Scottish Development Department (1970) *Disposal of solid toxic wastes. Report of the Technical Committee on the Disposal of Toxic Solid Wastes*, London, HM Stationery Office

WHO Expert Committee on the Control of Ascariasis (1967) *Report*, Geneva (*Wld Hlth Org. techn. Rep. Ser.*, No. 379) p. 6

WHO Expert Committee on Helminthiases (1964) *Soil-transmitted helminths. Report*, Geneva (*Wld Hlth Org. techn. Rep. Ser.*, No. 277)

WHO Expert Committee on Solid Wastes Disposal and Control (1971) *Report*, Geneva (*Wld Hlth Org. techn. Rep. Ser.*, No. 484)

WHO Scientific Group on the Treatment and Disposal of Wastes (1967) *Report*, Geneva (*Wld Hlth Org. techn. Rep. Ser.*, No. 367)

World Health Organization (1968) *Research into environmental pollution: report of five WHO scientific groups*, Geneva (*Wld Hlth Org. techn. Rep. Ser.*, No. 406) pp. 63-65

World Health Organization (1969) *The medical research programme of the World Health Organization. Report by the Director-General*, Geneva, pp. 319-320

World Health Organization (1971) *Contamination through water contact: Criteria, standards and guides for permissible levels of human exposure*, Geneva (unpublished document WHO/EH/71.3) p. 24

CHAPTER 5

INSECTS AND RODENTS

Virtually all human communities are affected by insects, other arthropods, and rodents, in several important ways, the most obvious of which stems from their role as vectors and reservoirs of human disease. Throughout most of the tropical world, vector-borne diseases constitute many of the main public health problems, since they are responsible for a great deal of mortality and morbidity. Information on the various vectors and reservoirs and the diseases they carry is voluminous; the accompanying table lists briefly some of the more important of the latter, together with their vectors and geographical distribution.

Insects, ticks, mites, and rodents can also be severe pests of man and his domestic animals even in areas where they are not vectors of disease; this question will also be dealt with briefly below.

Finally, these groups consume and destroy large quantities of foodstuffs. In so doing, they pollute them with substantial amounts of their excreta, thus increasing the risk of infection during handling or consumption.

SOME MAJOR INSECT-BORNE AND RODENT-BORNE DISEASES OF MAN

Disease	Vectors	Organism	Distribution
Viruses			
Yellow fever	Aedes mosquitos of subgenus *Stegomyia* and *Haemagogus* mosquitos	Arbovirus group B	Tropics and sub-tropics of Africa and Central and South America
Viral encephalitides: (a) Mosquito-borne (Eastern and Western equine, California, Japanese B, West Nile, Murray Valley, and St Louis encephalitis)	Mosquitos: *Culex* and *Aedes* species	Arbovirus specific to each form	Many temperate and tropical or sub-tropical areas
(b) Tick-borne (Russian spring-summer encephalitis, diphasic meningoencephalitis, louping ill, Powassan encephalitis, etc.)	Ticks: *Ixodes* species	Closely related arboviruses of group B	Temperate areas of Eurasia and America
Dengue	*Aedes aegypti* and *Ae. albopictus*	Arbovirus group B	Western and South Pacific, South East Asia, Caribbean and tropical South America

Disease	Vectors	Organism	Distribution
Rickettsiae			
Typhus and other rickettsial fevers:			
(a) Louse-borne typhus fever (epidemic)	Body louse, *Pediculus humanus*	*R. prowazeki*	Certain cold areas of Africa, Asia and Central America; also the Balkans
(b) Murine (endemic) typhus	Rat fleas, usually *Xenopsylla cheopis*	*R. typhi (R. mooseri)*	Cosmopolitan
(c) Tick-borne (several forms of tick-borne fever)	Several species of Ixodid tick	*R. rickettsii, R. australis, R. sibirica, R. conori,* etc.	Widespread
(d) Mite-borne scrub typhus	Trombiculid mites *Leptotrombidium akamushi* and *L. deliensis*	*R. tsutsugamushi*	Eastern Mediterranean and South East Asia regions
Bacteria			
Plague	Rodent fleas *(Xenopsylla sp.)*	*Pasteurella pestis*	Endemic in many cosmopolitan foci
Relapsing fever			
(a) Louse-borne	*Pediculus humanus humanus*	A spirochete, *Borrelia recurrentis*	Parts of Africa (mainly Ethiopia), South America, Middle East, Europe, Asia
(b) Tick-borne	*Ornithodoros* ticks	See above	Parts of Africa, North and South America, Middle East, India, Spain, Asia
Leptospirosis	Rodents and other mammals are reservoirs	Many serotypes of *Leptospira*	Worldwide
Rat bite fevers	House rats, rarely other rats	1) *Streptobacillus moniliformis* 2) *Spirillum minus*	World wide, but local differences in frequency of the two forms
Protozoa			
Malaria	*Anopheles* mosquitos	*Plasmodium* spp.	Broadly tropical and sub-tropical
Leishmaniasis	Sandflies, *Phlebotomus*	*Leishmania* spp.	Near East, India, China, Southern Europe, North and Equatorial Africa, South and Central America, Central Asia
Chagas' disease	*Triatominae* (kissing bugs)	*Trypanosoma cruzi*	Central and South America
African trypanosomiasis	Tsetse flies, genus *Glossina*	*Trypanosoma gambiense* and *rhodesiense* (sleeping sickness); *T. brucei, T. congolense, T. simiae, T. vivax* (animal trypanosomiasis)	Inter-tropical Africa
Helminths			
Onchocerciasis	Black flies, genus *Simulium*	*Onchocerca volvulus*	Tropical Africa, Central America, North-eastern South America
Filariasis	Many mosquito species	*Wuchereria bancrofti Brugia malayi*	Western and South Pacific, South East Asia, Africa, West Indies, North-eastern South America
Loaiasis	Mangrove flies, genus *Chrysops*	Loa loa	Equatorial rain belt in Africa

Insects and Disease

Insects or rodents can be so numerous that, once transmission of a disease has been established in a particular area, especially in the tropics and where sanitation is poor, many or most of the members of the human communities in that area can be affected at one time or another in their lives. Perhaps the best example is provided by malaria in areas where eradication of the disease has not as yet been achieved or is in its early stages. In many parts of West Africa, there is probably no child who has not been infected once maternal immunity has been lost. Consequently, there are areas where as much as 10 % of the mortality and a major part of the morbidity occurring among young children may be due to malaria (Bruce-Chwatt, 1952). Such a high incidence of disease can be accounted for when it is realized that many anopheline mosquitos may feed on a person every night, thus making it almost certain that at least one of them will carry the malaria infection.

Epidemics of arboviruses may involve large numbers of individuals at one time and may affect almost the entire community, not only in rural areas but also in large cities. Recent examples of such outbreaks are the estimated 200 000 cases of dengue over a period of some 2–3 months in and around Kanpur, India, in 1968 (Chaturvedi et al., 1970); the 1000 cases of dengue haemorrhagic fever in children hospitalized in Manila in 1956 (Dizon, 1967); the outbreak of yellow fever in Ethiopia where, in the 18 months preceding April 1962, as many as 100 000 cases and 30 000 deaths may have occurred (Sérié et al., 1968); and the recent dengue outbreaks in the Caribbean region involving some tens of thousands of cases (*Wkly epidem. Rec.*, 1969).

Examples of outbreaks of many other diseases can be given, ranging from those of the past when the Black Death pandemic of plague transmitted by rat fleas killed a quarter of the population of Europe in the 14th century, to the present time when all the efforts being made in many countries to improve living conditions and productive capacity are frustrated by endemic diseases, such as onchocerciasis, the cause of river blindness and a major factor in the desertion of large fertile river valleys (Waddy, 1969), or African trypanosomiasis, the control of which would make it possible to more than double the cattle population of the African continent (Wilson et al., 1963).

Unfortunately, the multiplication of many of the important vectors and reservoirs of disease is often the result of man's own actions. Community sanitation in many of the cities in the tropical and semitropical areas of the world depends on the conveyance of sewage in open channels that permit the breeding of enormous numbers of *Culex pipiens fatigans*, the main urban vector of Bancroftian filariasis. As human populations increase beyond the capacity of municipal services to dispose of wastes, more and more bodies of water become suitable for the breeding of *C.p. fatigans*, with a consequent increase in filariasis transmission.[1] Flies and rodents multiply in accumulating solid wastes, setting the stage for the transmission of enteric diseases and other rat-borne infections. Much of the transmission of arboviruses in the USA, the Western Pacific and South East Asia is due to species of mosquitos that breed in irrigated pastures or rice fields.

In South East Asia, the extensive epidemics of dengue and dengue haemorrhagic fever that have occurred are transmitted by *Aedes aegypti*, which in that part of the world breeds in man-made containers, such as the large clay jars used for the storage of drinking water, discarded tin cans and bottles, old tyres, and other receptacles. In Africa, where this species is one of the important vectors of yellow fever, its main larval habitat in urban areas is now artificial containers. As the food habits of the human population change and more containers are used and carelessly discarded, the problem of *Ae. aegypti* in cities grows, as does the threat of disease transmission.

Leishmaniasis, transmitted by sandflies, is still well entrenched in many parts of the world and has recently caused epidemics of alarming proportions. Because this disease has animal reservoirs, both the cutaneous and visceral forms are liable to increase with urbanization and with the reclamation of vast expanses of forest or desert, where human habitation encroaches on the habitats of reservoir animals.

Insects and Rodents as Pests of Man and Animals

Although the harm done by insects and rodents as annoying pests is hardly comparable to the loss and illness they cause as vectors of disease, it is by no means negligible. Certain pests can seriously affect human well-being. Thus in many areas the persistent bites of mosquitos, blackflies, and other blood-sucking insects can seriously impair the working capacity of exposed persons and may even bring work to a stop. Infestations of bedbugs, scabies, mites, head lice, and crab lice cause great discomfort. Furthermore, many of them transmit important diseases (see table on pp. 106-107).

Among the non-bloodsucking insects, flies and cockroaches are annoying pests and may transmit agents of disease mechanically on their legs and body hairs.

Apart from their importance as reservoirs of disease and destroyers of food, rats can attack human beings direct. In New York City more than 600 cases of rat bite are reported each year, and throughout the USA some 14 000 cases occur in a year (Clinton, 1969). One hospital in Bombay,

---

[1] Some diseases transmitted by vectors associated with water, such as onchocerciasis and filariasis, are also discussed in Chapter 2.

India, reported having treated 20 000 cases of rat bite in a single year (Deoras, 1966). Most cases of rat bite are among children, and the bites frequently cause secondary infection and disfigurement.

Insects, Rodents, and Man's Food

Insects and rodents consume and contaminate great quantities of stored food products. On a worldwide basis, 33 million tons of bread grains and rice in storage are estimated to be lost to rodents each year, and the loss to insects is at least as great, if not greater. Such enormous losses, especially in tropical countries where nutrition is often already inadequate, cannot help but adversely affect the wellbeing of the community.

The numbers in which most of the urban insect vectors and rodent reservoirs of disease are present in cities and towns are in most cases directly related to the level of sanitation; the poorer the methods of disposal of solid and liquid wastes, the greater the numbers of mosquitos, flies, and rats. While many pesticides are available for the control of these insects and rodents, the most fundamental and effective approach is to improve sanitary conditions and practices to the extent that conditions no longer exist that encourage the multiplication of insects and rodents. Control of vector-borne diseases in rural regions where insect breeding places or reservoir habitats are spread over large areas raises far greater problems, calling for the mobilization of resources beyond the capabilities of the local community.

REFERENCES

Bruce-Chwatt, L. J. (1952) *Ann. trop. Med. Parasit.*, **46**, 173-200

Chaturvedi, U. C. et al. (1970) *Bull. Wld Hlth Org.*, **43**, 281-287

Clinton, J. M. (1969) *Publ. Hlth Rep. (Wash.)*, **14**, 1-7

Deoras, P. J. (1966) *Indian J. Ent.*, **28**, 543-547

Dizon, J. J. (1967) *J. Philipp. med. Ass.*, **43**, 346-365

Série, C. et al. (1968) *Bull. Wld Hlth Org.*, **38**, 879-884

Waddy, B. B. (1969) *Bull. Wld Hlth Org.*, **40**, 843

Wilson, S. G. et al. (1963) *Bull. Wld Hlth Org.*, **28**, 595

Wkly epidem. Rec., 1969, **44**, 497-505

CHAPTER 6

THE HOME ENVIRONMENT

In most countries, particularly in the developing areas, the problem of housing, including living space, calls for urgent solutions. This is mainly due to the great increase in world population, and its influx into urban areas. In many regions, particularly in Africa, Latin America, and Asia, the urban population has doubled in the past ten years and this trend is expected to continue. Rapid and uncontrolled urbanization generates a whole series of complex problems, ranging from housing, basic sanitation, and environmental pollution to such little studied and poorly understood phenomena as the effects of life in urban environments on moral and social attitudes and values, and the morbidity associated with urban life.

The two most striking features of poor housing are overcrowding and a lack of basic sanitation. The action required seems obvious, but the economic implications are such that no adequate solution has been found in any country to deal effectively with, and to eliminate, these basic deficiencies of human settlements. More than one thousand million people throughout the world live in substandard housing conditions, and this situation is likely to worsen in the years to come (United Nations Conference on the Problems of the Human Environment, 1972).

Poverty and filth are often closely associated with poor housing. Without a water supply, it is very difficult to maintain personal cleanliness, and wastes accumulate where there is no public service of refuse collection. Even when the occupants attempt, within the limits of their meagre resources, to improve the hygiene of their dwellings, the results are seldom lasting. This is mainly because the physical condition of the house, with leaking roof, cracked walls, and earth floors, facilitates the admission and accumulation of dirt, dust, and soot, and gives rise to dampness. Filth attracts lice, fleas, bugs, and mites that may transmit disease. Poor housing permits the harbouring of mice and rats, which can also be carriers and transmitters of disease, and the entrance of flies and mosquitos, with the resultant spread of such diseases as trachoma, malaria, yellow fever, filariasis, and dengue (see Chapter 5).

Housing and Health

The history of studies on the influence of poor housing on health has recently been reviewed by Martin (1967) and Cassel (unpublished observations, 1971). In spite of the advances in epidemiological techniques there are still difficulties in methodology, and the evidence produced is by no means conclusive. A few examples will illustrate the uncertainty that exists in this field.

A positive association between infant mortality and socioeconomic conditions, including overcrowding, was reported by Ellis (1956) but not confirmed by Willie (1959). Stockwell (1962) examined five specific indices (occupation, education, income, rent, and crowding) but the only significant association found was between neonatal mortality and income. Halliday (1928) and Wright & Wright (1942) showed that measles and whooping cough tended to occur at earlier ages in overcrowded homes, and higher mortality rates would therefore be expected in overcrowded conditions. Many studies have been made to assess the importance of housing conditions in relation to tuberculosis, but the results are conflicting. According to Stein (1950, 1954), Britten (1942), and Laidlaw (1946), higher mortality and incidence rates were associated with poor housing and overcrowding. Benjamin (1953) could not distinguish satisfactorily the respective roles of income, housing, nutrition, and occupation. McKinley (1947), Lockhart (1949), Holmes (1956), McMillan (1957), and Brett & Benjamin (1957) could find no relationship between overcrowding and tuberculosis. A number of investigators pointed out the relationship between overcrowding and the incidence of acute rheumatic fever or rheumatic heart conditions (cf. Ryle, 1946), but it is doubtful how far the findings are still applicable (Martin, 1967). Fisher & Pierce (1967) and Kent et al. (1958) suggested that crowding and isolation may be contributory factors in intellectual deterioration in old age and in increased mortality from arteriosclerotic heart disease. Other studies reported that poor housing was associated with meningococcal disease (Blum, 1949), anaemia (Britten & Altman, 1941), digestive diseases (Britten, 1942), and higher admission rates to hospitals for communicable and nutritional disease (Worth, 1963). No effect of housing on the incidence and spread of common respiratory diseases was found by Bernstein (1957), and rheumatic fever and streptococcal illness were found to be equally frequent in two communities in New York State with different housing conditions (Coulter, 1952).

It has often been stated that the design and construction of the house may help to produce mental unrest and thus exacerbate mental disorders already afflicting the occupants; that sensory annoyance and dissatisfaction may make an important contribution to mental unrest; that noise and unpleasant smells easily lead to nervous irritability and bad temper; and that gloomy, bleak, and unattractive rooms and surroundings may accentuate mental depression. The effects of such adverse conditions are thought to be particularly serious where individuals are already exposed to other mental tensions and preoccupations in their work and outside their homes. Lack of privacy and freedom of movement in the house as a consequence of overcrowding is also considered a cause of mental unrest. Shared and interconnected bedrooms, bathrooms without direct access, a family room where it is impossible to find a quiet place if so desired, windows and doors that do not permit visual privacy, are typical of the deficiencies that may generate feelings of irritation, resentment, and frustration as a result of intrusions, interruptions, and general interference (WHO Expert Committee on the Public Health Aspects of Housing, 1961; Lemkau, 1970).

The difficulty of establishing a relationship between behavioural disorders and housing, however, is considerable. Neuroses, which may be considered as etiologically related to psychological and physical stress, are perhaps easier to relate to the frustrations inherent in living in an inconvenient, uncleanable, noisy, drab house with too many people in too little space (Lemkau, 1970; Carlestam & Levi, 1971; Schorr, 1970) (see also Chapter 10). Recent studies by de Groot et al. (1970) indicate that only in the totality of man's behaviour, in all its interactional and transactional aspects, can spatial characteristics of housing be evaluated meaningfully.

The effects of rehousing have been considered in several studies. Ferguson & Pettigrew (1954) found that the proportion of surviving children was higher in the rehoused group. Lunn's study (1961) showed little difference in the incidence of illness in spite of a very marked improvement as regards overcrowding and home management. Similar results were obtained by Wilner (1962) for persons in the 35–39-year age group; under the age of 35 an improvement was noticed, particularly in persons under 20. Finally, certain studies have indicated that the morale and general adjustment of slum dwellers did not improve on rehousing, and that neuroses and death rates increased after slum populations were moved to better housing (Martin et al., 1957; Wilner, 1962; Loring, 1964).

These conflicting findings on the relationship between the quality of housing and health show the inadequacy of available means of measurement and the need to develop standardized methods of data collection and appraisal, as well as for prolonged observation to take account of delayed effects. At the same time an increasing number of investigators (cf. Loring, 1964; Foster, 1970) are beginning to stress the need to examine the mechanisms through which housing quality may be linked to health. According to Cassel (unpublished observations, 1971), such an approach suggests that the link between housing and health may be quite indirect, and that changes in the physical structure of the housing alone may have no effect on health unless the intervening processes are understood and changed simultaneously.

Housing Standards

In the past, the housing standards adopted in many countries were based mainly on the local climate, geography, social practices, customs and tradition. At best, such standards were the expression of the judgement of some authority as to the goals to be aimed at, or were based on limited observations made under the conditions with which that authority was concerned. It is now recognized that a thorough knowledge of human requirements is essential for the establishment of standards, in order to ensure that full provision is made for the health, safety, and general well-being of the people (Goromosov, 1968). Until more knowledge is acquired about the physiological and psychological responses of the human body to the physical and social environment, standards of housing will be applicable only for the region in which they are adopted and to the physical, social, and economic conditions of the time (Cassel, unpublished observations, 1971).

Another difficulty with currently proposed standards for the design and utilization of indoor and outdoor space is that they are not generally attainable, even in highly developed countries; moreover, they do not take sufficiently into account the variation in housing requirements resulting from such variables as the demographic characteristics of the population (age, sex, family, and household), social values, and socio-cultural heterogeneity (Task Force on Research Planning in Environmental Health Science, 1970).

Home Accidents

An inter-country study in Europe, initiated by WHO in 1964 (WHO Regional Office for Europe, 1969), showed that home accidents accounted for 1–2 % of all deaths, for 20 % of all accidental deaths among men, and about 50 % of accidental deaths among females. However, mortality statistics should not be used as the only measure of the importance of home accidents. For each fatal accident, there are probably 150 non-fatal home accidents, many of which require hospitalization or prolonged home care (Backett, 1965).

In the United States, for example, approximately 16 million persons are injured each year in or around the home (United States Department of Health, Education and Welfare, 1969). About 700 thousand to one million of these accidents are estimated to result from toys and other children's products (Hart, 1971).

Mortality and morbidity statistics reveal three highly accident-prone population groups: children, elderly people, and persons who are physically, mentally, or socially handicapped. Patterns of domestic accidents change with time, and there are marked differences within and between countries, depending on age and sex and on social, economic, cultural, geographic, and climatic conditions. In addition to environmental factors, the liability to accidents is influenced by such factors as marital status, mental health, handicaps in sight, hearing, and smell, skeletal deformation, and chronic diseases (WHO Regional Office for Europe, 1969). Irrespective of local, national, or regional differences, the major causes of accidental injuries at home include falls, fires, burns and scalds, electrocution, suffocation, and poisoning (including gassing).

In many countries, falls are the most important cause of accidental deaths. They cause up to two-thirds of accidental deaths in the home among males and up to four-fifths among women—the bulk of fatal cases occurring in persons over 65 years of age (WHO Regional Office for Europe, 1969). Young children have the highest rate of fall injuries requiring medical treatment, but the fatality rate is low except for infants (Iskrant & Joliet, 1968).

Fires also rank very high as causes of accidental deaths in residential environments. The study by Brose (1967) in Pittsburgh is a rare example of the application of epidemiological methods to such problems. He found, for example, that smoking caused a quarter of fires, a finding also noted by the Advisory Committee to the Surgeon General of the US Public Health Service (1964). Matches started only 7 % of fires, and of these over 80 % resulted from the play of children. Other frequent causes of fires are faulty house wiring, electrical appliances, and heating equipment. There is a strong association between the incidence of fires and poor housing. The very young and the very old face the highest risk of fire death. Common causes of domestic accidents are the burning of clothes and flammable liquids (solvents). In Japan, burns and scalds taken together are the most important external cause of domestic accidental death. In Western countries, burning is also of considerable importance, particularly as a cause of accidental death among children (Backett, 1965). Among old people, relatively small areas of burnt skin are fatal.

Electrocution is a form of domestic accident that often follows rural electrification schemes. With the present proliferation of electrical domestic gadgets, this hazard is likely to increase. The lowering of voltages and standardization of wiring systems could help to reduce the number and severity of such accidents.

The vast majority of "mechanical suffocation" deaths occur in children under 5 years of age, and particularly in infancy.

Consumer products

In addition to the conventional causes of accidental injuries, such as falls, fires, flammable liquids, and hot and corrosive liquids, modern technology has introduced a variety of consumer products that present new chemical, electrical, mechanical, and radiation hazards (see, for example, Chapter 14). The proliferation of consumer chemicals since the Second World War makes the task of protecting the population from such hazards increasingly difficult. The first annual list of toxic substances prepared in compliance with the US Occupational Safety and Health Act, 1970, contains 15 000 well-defined potentially hazardous materials (Christensen, 1971). The poison control centres in some highly industrialized countries in Europe, such as Switzerland and the Federal Republic of Germany, have listed more than 40 000 different toxic agents that may be used in the home (E. G. Krinke, personal communication, 1972).

The magnitude of the problem in industrially advanced countries is well illustrated by the data for the USA provided by the Consumer Protection and Environmental Health Service (1968). The annual total of injuries from toxic products was estimated to be about 1 600 000, with 3000 fatal cases. This estimate includes 25 000 injuries from toxic hazards of recreational equipment, 139 000 from flammable liquids (other than burns), 540 000 from laundering and cleaning products, and 75 000 from pesticides. Ingestions of potentially harmful substances ranged from 500 000 to 1 000 000 incidents, resulting in more than 2000 deaths, 350 of which were in children under five years of age (United States Department of Health, Education and Welfare, 1969). Poisoning is either the second or third most important external cause of fatal domestic accidents in developed countries. It has been found to account for about 9 % of such cases in Canada, 8 % in the USA, 16 % in Japan, over 22 % in England and Wales, and over 30 % in Scotland (Backett, 1965).

It should be realized that the acute toxicity of consumer products and household chemicals and their potential for traumatic injury form only one side of the problem. The other aspect, on which practically no information is available, is the possible deleterious effects of long-term, low-level exposure. Various compounds included in consumer products that can be partially ingested, or substances that may penetrate the skin, may be of particular importance. Examples are rhodamine B used in lipsticks, tri-o-cresyl phosphate used in the manufacture of nail polish, and some organic mercury compounds and female hormones in shampoos and creams. Other potentially dangerous chemicals that have been used in various cosmetic products include p-phenylenediamine, thallium salts, nitrobenzene, and carbon tetrachloride (Truhaut, 1970). There is an urgent need for research in this field, including the development of adequate methodology for epidemiological and other studies (Task Force on Research Planning in Environmental Health Science, 1970).

Generally, the diversity and frequency of accidental intoxications seem to increase with the level of industrial development. There are, however, large variations in this respect from country to country, depending on socioeconomic factors, cultural patterns, geography, and other circumstances. Inter-country comparisons are difficult because of the differences in classification of toxic substances and in reporting schemes. The available statistics reflect the activities of poison centres rather than the actual situation in a community. Although a meaningful comparison of accidental poisoning statistics for different countries is not possible, there is no doubt that drugs used internally or externally, cosmetics, cleaning agents, paints, solvents, and pesticides are high among the leading causes of intoxications. These and other classes of consumer products are complex mixtures of a variety of chemical compounds with widely differing toxicity and modes of action.

Cosmetics

There is a multitude of cosmetics on the market, many of which are potential poisons when ingested in excessive amounts; some of them may affect the skin. They include shampoos, hair curling and straightening solutions, hair dyes, deodorants, and bath additives. The liquid shampoos contain various oils, saponified with an alkali. Dry shampoos usually contain either carbon tetrachloride or alcohols (including methyl and isopropyl alcohol). Surface active agents—salts of sulfonated fats or oils or of sulfonated fatty alcohols—are ingredients of soapless shampoos. Hair curling solutions utilize chemicals (such as morpholine, triethanolamine, ammonium hydroxide, sodium borate, sodium carbonate, and potassium carbonate) that dissolve part or all of the keratin in the hair. "Cold" wave preparations are usually made of the salts of thioglycolic acid, and contain ammonia or sodium hydroxide as well. Hair straighteners contain caustic agents or strong alkaline solutions, and fixatives such as potassium permanganate or formaldehyde are used to hold the hair in a straight position. Hair dyes include the organic vetegable dyes, such as henna, indigo, and wood extracts; metallic preparations containing bismuth, cadmium, cobalt, copper, iron, lead, nickel, silver, and tin; compound dyestuffs utilizing vegetable dyes mixed with any of the metallic preparations; and various synthetic organic dyes, such as p-phenylenediamine used together with an oxidizing agent. Deodorants and bath additives may be dangerous on account of their alkalinity, acidity, and content of alcohol and other additives.

Detergents

Synthetic detergents are household cleaning products based on the non-soap surface active agents. Surface active agents may be anionic, typical examples of which are linear alkylbenzene sulfonates (LAS); they may be non-ionic products of alkylated phenols or fatty alcohols with varying amounts of ethylene oxide; or they may be cationic, as exemplified by the quaternary ammonium compounds. Cationic detergents are more toxic, require special handling, and are therefore restricted mainly to industrial use. In addition to surface active agents, detergent mixtures contain complexing agents, such as polyphosphates, and a variety of other ingredients. Oral LD_{50} values in experimental animals of surface active agents usually present in detergent mixtures are fairly high: for albino rats, 700–4000 mg/kg (Calandra & Fancher, 1969). In general, the alkalinity of household detergents is not so high that they can cause corrosive burns of the mucosa of the oral cavity or of the oesophagus and stomach.

A few household cleaning agents, such as ammonia, are highly alkaline and can cause severe damage to mucosa. Chlorine bleaches are another type of cleaning agent causing fairly frequent intoxications in children.

Out of 84 000 accidental ingestions among all age groups in the USA reported by the poison centres to the National Clearing House for Poison Control Centers in 1967, 11 954 were listed in the broad category of cleaning and polishing agents, and included 10 406 children under 5 years of age. Further breakdown showed that among these there were 3136 cases of accidental ingestion of soaps, detergents, and similar agents (Calandra & Fancher, 1969).

Solvents

Solvents are available in innumerable combinations, and contain alcohols, ethers, aldehydes, ketones and esters, hydrocarbons or nitro-compounds, as well as carbon disulfide, silicones, turpentines, and chlorinated compounds. All of the solvents can act as skin sensitizers. Although they may not cause a rash or "industrial dermatitis" by direct action, they will remove the protective oils from the skin. In severe cases, the skin will crack and fungus and bacterial infections may result. Excessive use of soap and water can have the same effect.

The physiological effects of inhaling or ingesting solvents vary. The chlorinated hydrocarbons can cause anything from mild nose and throat irritation to serious kidney and liver damage. Alcohols generally are eye irritants and in the worst cases may cause irreversible damage to the optic nerve. Methanol is a very cheap solvent, small doses of which may cause severe intoxication.

Many solvents are highly flammable liquids and may cause accidental burns and fires.

Paints

An important cause of acute illness among children in the slum areas of the USA, England, and Australia is the use in the past of lead-based paint and putty (United States Public Health Service, 1972; Committee on Biologic Effects of Atmospheric Pollutants, 1971). Such paints flake readily from wooden buildings, and the flakes are easily ingested by children with pica. In such paints, lead may constitute 5–40 % of the final dried solids. Ninety per cent of the reported cases of lead poisoning were among children who lived in multiple-dwelling, rented housing units. In almost every case of clinical poisoning, old paint could be found on at least one of the surfaces accessible to a young child within the home. Paint with a high lead content was found on the interior surfaces of about 70 % of dwelling units surveyed in selected urban areas of Baltimore, Philadelphia, and London. The number of cases reported depends a good deal on the vigour with which screening is carried out. The fatality rate has tended to decrease in recent years as the frequency of reported cases has gone up. In 1955 the American Standards Association specified that paints for toys, furniture, and the interior of dwellings should not contain more than 1 % lead in the final dried solids of fresh paint, and also limited the content of antimony, arsenic, cadmium, mercury, selenium, and barium in paints. Lead, of course, is only one example of the hazards associated with this type of household chemical.

Pesticides (see also Chapter 12)

The frequency of accidental intoxications by insecticides, fungicides, herbicides, rodenticides, and fumigants varies in different countries from about 2 % to 10 % of the total number of accidental poisonings. An attempt to summarize the available information has been made by Kaloyanova-Simeonova & Fournier (1971). Up-to-date information on pesticide poisoning in the United States has been obtained by the US Environmental Protection Agency (Lisella, F. S. & Courter, R. D., unpublished report, 1972). In 1970, a total of 5729 cases of poisoning were reported, 21 of them fatal. This represented about 5 % of the total number of poisoning cases reported for all categories of chemicals. Of the reported cases of pesticide poisoning, 3887 or 68 % were observed in children up to 4 years of age. About 89 % of poisonings were due to accidental ingestion, and 6 % to inhalation exposure. Agents involved included insecticides (13 deaths), rodenticides (6 deaths), herbicides (1 death) and mothballs (1 death). The situation in some European countries was recently discussed at a conference in Kiev (WHO Regional Office for Europe, 1971). Fatal exposures to organophosphorus compounds in Denmark have been analysed in detail by Juhl (1971). Organomercury compounds used for seed dressing are an important cause of mass poisoning incidents (see pp. 79-80).

Utility gas

The gas piped to houses for heating and cooking, and occasionally for lighting, is a very frequent cause of accidental poisoning in some countries. For example, in England and Wales in 1964, it was responsible for about 60 % of accidental poisonings and 14 % of all accidental deaths at home.

Even in children under 5 years of age it accounted for almost one-third of the poison fatalities, while in people over 60 it caused more than three-quarters (Cargill, 1967). Utility gas may contain up to 10 % of carbon monoxide. In many countries the toxic components, including carbon monoxide, are now removed, or utility gas has been replaced by natural gas, which contains methane (about 85 %), ethane, and hydrogen, or by propane or butane. Aliphatic gaseous hydrocarbons such as propane are physiologically inert at low concentrations. At high concentrations, they may have anaesthetic properties; this is particularly true of unsaturated (olefin) compounds. At very high concentrations, they are simple asphyxiants that may cause death by displacing oxygen in the lungs. Gaseous hydrocarbons are very flammable and can form explosive mixtures with air.

Accidental poisoning by utility gas can occur in a number of ways, particularly through fracture of pipes, faulty apparatus and installation, tampering, temporary interruption of supply, accidental extinguishing of the flame, or the use of cooking or water heating vessels that are too large (incomplete combustion).

Other causes of carbon monoxide poisoning at home include inefficient combustion in heating appliances and emissions from vehicle exhausts in garages. Inefficient heating appliances (stoves, open fires) also produce smoke, which at high concentrations irritates the larynx and bronchi. Continued exposure to smoke may contribute to the development of emphysema (Deichman & Gerade, 1969).

Age patterns

An important fact revealed by the statistics of accidental poisonings by household agents is that children of preschool age (up to 5 years) are at particularly high risk. For example, in 1967 in the USA, approximately 90 % of the accidental poisonings reported to the National Clearing House for Poison Control Centers involved children under 5 years of age. The age at which poisoning among children is most frequent is 18–24 months, when about a quarter of the incidents in children under 5 occur. About three-quarters occur between 12 and 36 months of age. There are differences in the types of products ingested by children in different age groups: 39 % of ingestions of external medications and 46 % of ingestions of internal medications occurred under 5 years of age. However, with increasing age, the emphasis shifts from external to internal medications. Aspirin was involved in about 50 % of the cases where internal medication was ingested. Among older persons, barbiturates are the most frequent type of medication ingested.

Storage facilities

The influence of the surrounding circumstances on the ingestion of poisonous materials by children has been studied recently by a number of authors, but no definite conclusions have been reached. Baltimore & Meyer (1968) found that facilities for storing household poisons did not affect the risk of poisoning in small children. A study carried out on a random sample of 20 % of the 1–2-year-old children in a Swedish town (Berfenstam & Beskow, 1962) showed that either medicines or chemicals were within reach of a child in 99.5 % of the homes. On the other hand, McKendrick (1960) found that in only 12 of 206 incidents was the poison obtained from a room other than that where it was usually kept. A rigorous redesign of the home for definitive and interim storage of poisonous substances and a vigorous campaign of education may help to reduce accidental poisoning in children (R. Neutra & R. McFarland, unpublished observations, 1971).

Prevention programmes

Many countries have initiated home accident prevention programmes. These include epidemiological studies; continuous surveillance of the accident situation; research on etiology, including both the environmental and behavioural aspects; measures to make the home environment safer; education at all levels; and legal and administrative action.

When applied specifically to the prevention and control of hazards arising from chemical consumer products, these programmes may be summarized as follows:

(1) Dissemination of information on the ingredients and toxicity of consumer and household products, within national educational programmes, etc.

(2) Research on the toxicity of consumer and household agents in order to obtain scientific and medical data for enforcement of legislation.

(3) Action to eliminate or minimize the use of hazardous products through regulatory or voluntary action. This includes the labelling of hazardous substances, or, when labelling is not an adequate protection, the prohibition of sale.

(4) Surveillance programmes to detect injuries associated with products.

Many of these activities are conducted by poison control centres that provide information and give first aid and treatment to patients. Such centres have been established in many countries including Algeria, Argentina, Australia, Austria, Belgium, Brazil, Bulgaria, Canada, Colombia, Denmark, Egypt, Federal Republic of Germany, Finland, France, Ireland, Israel, Italy, Japan, Lebanon, Mexico, Morocco, Netherlands, New Zealand, Norway, Panama, Portugal, Romania, Spain, Sweden, the United Kingdom, the USA, the USSR, Venezuela, and Yugoslavia (Sunshine et al., 1966).

REFERENCES

Advisory Committee to the Surgeon General of the US Public Health Service (1964) *Smoking and health*, Washington, D.C., US Government Printing Office (Public Health Service Publication 1103)

Backett, M. E. (1965) *Domestic accidents*, Geneva, World Health Organization (*Publ. Hlth Pap.*, No. 26)

Baltimore, C. L. & Meyer, R. J. (1968) *Pediatrics*, **42**, 312-317

Benjamin, B. (1953) *Brit. J. Tuberc.*, **47**, 4-17

Berfenstam, R. & Beskow, J. (1962) *Brit. J. prev. soc. Med.*, **63**, 123-129

Bernstein, S. H. (1957) *Amer. J. Hyg.*, **65**, 162-171

Blum, B. (1949) *Amer. J. publ. Hlth*, **39**, 1571-1577

Brett, G. Z. & Benjamin, B. (1957) *Brit. J. prev. soc. Med.*, **11**, 7-9

Britten, R. H. (1942) *Amer. J. publ. Hlth*, **32**, 193-199

Britten, R. H. & Altman, I. (1941) *Publ. Hlth Rep.*, **56**, 609-640

Brose, R. (1967) *Accidental fires and explosions in dwelling units (thesis)* University of Pittsburgh (University microfilm No. 64-4389)

Calandra, J. C. & Fancher, O. E. (1969) *Cleaning products and their accidental ingestion*, New York, Soap and Detergent Association (Scientific and Technical Report, No. 5R)

Cargill, D. (1967) *Accidents at home*, London, Hamish Hamilton

Carlestam, G. & Levi, L. (1971) *Urban conglomerates as psychosocial human stressors: general aspects, Swedish trends, and psychological and medical implications*, Stockholm, Royal Ministry for Foreign Affairs and Royal Ministry of Agriculture

Christensen, H. E., ed. (1971) *Toxic substances: Annual List 1971*, Rockville, Md., US Department of Health, Education and Welfare

Committee on Biologic Effects of Atmospheric Pollutants (1971) *Airborne lead in perspective*, Washington, D.C., National Research Council, National Academy of Sciences

Consumer Protection and Environmental Health Service (1968) *Estimates of injuries from consumer products*, Cincinnati, Ohio, US Department of Health, Education and Welfare

Coulter, J. E. (1952) *Milbank mem. Fd Quart.*, **30**, 341-358

de Groot, I., Carroll, R. L. & Whitman, R. M. (1970) *Human health and the spatial environment, an epidemiological assessment.* In: *Proceedings of the First Invitational Conference on Health Research in Housing and Its Environment, Warrenton, Va., 1966*

Deichman, W. B. & Gerade, H. W. (1969) *Toxicology of drugs and chemicals*, New York and London, Academic Press

Ellis, J. M. (1956) *Mortality in Houston, Texas, 1949-1951: a study of socio-economic differentials.* Unpublished Ph. D. dissertation, quoted in Stockwell, E. G. (1962) *Milbank mem. Fd Quart.*, **40**, 101

Ferguson, T. & Pettigrew, M. (1954) *Glasgow med. J.*, **135**, 169-182

Fisher, J. & Pierce, R. C. (1967) *J. Gerontol.*, **22**, 166-173

Foster, D. L. (1970) *J. nat. med. Ass.*, **62**, 95-101

Goromosov, M. S. (1968) *The physiological basis of health standards for dwellings*, Geneva, World Health Organization (*Publ. Hlth Pap.*, No. 33)

Halliday, J. (1928) *Spec. Rep. Ser. med. Res. Coun. (Lond.)*, No. 120

Hart, S. M. (1971) *Food Drug cosmet. Law J.*, **26**, 70-75

Holmes, T. (1956) *Multidiscipline studies of tuberculosis*. In: Sparer, P. J., ed., *Personality stress and tuberculosis*, International Universities Press

Iskrant, A. P. & Joliet, P. V. (1968) *Accidents and homicide*, Cambridge, Mass., Harvard University Press

Juhl, E. (1971) *Dan. med. Bull.*, **18**, Suppl. I, 1-112

Kaloyanova-Simeonova, F. & Fournier, E. (1971) *Les pesticides et l'homme*, Paris, Masson

Kent, A. P. et al. (1958) *Amer. J. publ. Hlth*, **48**, 200-207

Laidlaw, S. (1946) *Edinb. med. J.*, **53**, 49-54

Lemkau, P. V. (1970) *Position paper on mental health and housing*. Abstracted in: *Proceedings of the First Invitational Conference on Health Research in Housing and its Environment, Warrenton, Va., 1966*

Lockhart, R. (1949) *Hlth Bull. (Edinb.)*, **7**, No. 4, p. 76

Loring, W. C. (1964) *J. Hlth hum. Behav.*, **5**, 166-169

Lunn, J. E. (1961) *Scot. med. J.*, **6**, 125-134

Martin, A. E. (1967) *Urban Studies*, **4**, 1-21

Martin, F. M., Brotherson, J. H. F. & Chave, S. P. W. (1957) *Brit. J. prev. soc. Med.*, **11**, 196-202

McKendrick, T. (1960) *Arch. Dis. Childh.*, **35**, 127-133

McKinley, P. L. (1947) *Hlth Bull. (Edinb.)*, **5**, No. 3

McMillan, J. S. (1957) *Brit. J. prev. soc. Med.*, **11**, 142-151

Ryle, J. A. (1946) *J. roy. sanit. Inst.*, **66**, 277-286

Schorr, A. L. (1970) *Housing and its effects*. In: Proshansky, H. M., Ittelson, W. H. & Rivlin, L. G., eds, *Environmental psychology: man and his physical setting*, New York, Holt, Rinehart & Winston, pp. 322-328

Stein, L. (1950) *Brit. J. soc. Med.*, **4**, 143-169

Stein, L. (1954) *Tubercle (Lond.)*, **35**, 195-203

Stockwell, E. G. (1962) *Milbank mem. Fd Quart.*, **40**, 101-119

Sunshine, I., Govaerts, A., Gaultier, M., Roche, L. & Vincent, V. (1966) *Les centres anti-poisons dans le monde*, Paris, Masson

Task Force on Research Planning in Environmental Health Science (1970) *Man's health and the environment—some research needs*, Washington, D.C., US Department of Health, Education and Welfare

Truhaut, R. (1970) In: *The chemical control of the human environment*, London, Butterworth, pp. 419-436

United Nations Conference on the Problems of the Human Environment (1972) *Planning and management of human settlements for environmental quality* (document A/Conf. 48/6)

United States Department of Health, Education and Welfare (1969) *Summary of selected programs related to problems of the human environment* (Document prepared for the purpose of providing background information relevant to planning United States participation in the 1972 United Nations Conference on the Problems of the Human Environment), Washington, D.C.

United States Public Health Service (1972) *Control of lead poisoning in children*, Washington, D.C., Department of Health, Education and Welfare (in preparation)

WHO Expert Committee on the Public Health Aspects of Housing (1961) *First report*, Geneva (*Wld Hlth Org. techn. Rep. Ser.*, No. 225)

WHO Regional Office for Europe (1969) *The prevention of accidents in the home: Report on a Symposium, Salzburg, April 1968,* Copenhagen (document EURO 0345)

WHO Regional Office for Europe (1971) *Modern trends in the prevention of pesticide intoxication: Report on a Conference, Kiev, June 1971,* Copenhagen, (document EURO 7902)

Willie, C. V. (1959) *Social Forces,* **37,** 221-227

Wilner, D. M. (1962) *The housing environment and family life,* Baltimore, Johns Hopkins Press

Worth, R. M. (1963) *Amer. J. Hyg.,* **78,** 338-348

Wright, G. P. & Wright, H. P. (1942) *J. Hyg.,* **42,** 451-473

CHAPTER 7

THE WORK ENVIRONMENT

Occupational hazards are often encountered in industry, agriculture, mining and other working environments. The major categories of environmental stress for the worker are: chemical agents; physical agents and conditions; biological agents and conditions; and psychosocial factors. These may act either singly or in combination. Occupational accidents result from the joint action of both environmental and human factors, and are therefore dealt with separately. The interaction between man and his working environment may lead to betterment of health, when work is fully adapted to human needs and factors, or to ill health, if work stresses are beyond human tolerance. Occupational diseases and injuries result from specific exposures at work. In addition, work exposures may aggravate certain illnesses or be a factor of varying importance in causing diseases of multiple etiology.

The discussion in this Chapter is unavoidably brief and incomplete. A full and up-to-date account of the hazards of the work environment is given by Mayers (1969).

Chemical Agents

In numerous industries, workers must handle potentially toxic chemicals. Many industrial processes involve chemical reactions in which substances toxic or hazardous to man are liberated. However, the degree of risk of handling a given substance depends on the magnitude and duration of exposure. The major hazards arise from dusts, fumes, mists, vapours, gases, and solvents. Detailed information on many of the chemicals involved is given elsewhere in this publication. Major offenders in the working environment are dealt with briefly here.

Dusts

Dusts are solid particles generated by handling, crushing, grinding, and disintegrating organic and inorganic materials, such as rocks, ore, metal, coal, wood, and grains. The exposure of man to dusts can lead to a wide variety of respiratory diseases, including pulmonary fibrosis, obstructive lung disease, allergy and lung cancer. Toxic dusts may produce systemic poisoning after inhalation, or act as skin irritants to produce dermatoses, allergic reactions and cancer.

Silica

Free silica (SiO_2) in the form of quartz, tridymite, or cristobalite, can cause silicosis, whereas silicates do not usually present a significant health hazard. Quartz dust is produced by drilling, crushing, grinding or handling quartz sand. Occupational exposure occurs in mines and quarries, not only where quartz is mined but also in metal mines where the rock between the veins of ore contains free silica. Exposure may also occur in factories where quartz sand is used, e.g., in steel works and iron foundries, and in the ceramics and glass industries.

Entry into the body is by inhalation. Particles larger than 5 microns in size are generally deposited in the upper respiratory tract and bronchi, and are gradually removed by the ciliary epithelium (lung clearance). Smaller particles are deposited in the alveoli of the lungs and then gradually transported to the corresponding lymph nodes. The proportion of the dust that remains in the lungs does so for life, since quartz particles are practically insoluble; connective tissue is then formed around the particles so that nodules are produced. The mechanism whereby this occurs is not fully understood. The nodules may gradually aggregate and massive pulmonary fibroses may develop later and progress over a number of years, leading to emphysema with gradual impairment of lung function. Subjective symptoms, which develop rather late, include cough and shortness of breath (dyspnoea) at effort. Silicosis is often combined with tuberculosis. The disease is gradually progressive and death occurs from right heart failure or from pulmonary tuberculosis (Simonin, 1962).

Asbestos

Asbestos is a mixture of magnesium and iron silicates in fibrous form. It appears as dust in the form of fine fibres in the air.

Occupational exposure occurs in asbestos mines and wherever absestos or asbestos products are used, for instance, in handling asbestos-cement products used in the building industry (roofing sheets, wallboard and pipes). Exposure may also occur in the textile industry in the manufacture of fireproof materials, such as asbestos clothes or brake linings for motor vehicles. Asbestos is also used for insulation and fire protection purposes in ship-building, house-building, and in the undersealing of cars.

Asbestos enters the body by inhalation, and fine dust containing fibres of diameter less than 5 microns and length greater than 5 microns may be deposited in the alveoli. The fibres are insoluble. The dust deposited in the lungs causes fibrosis, pleural plaques, mesothelioma and lung cancer.

Asbestosis results in impaired lung function after five to ten years. The symptoms are shortness of breath, chest pain, and later bronchitis with increased sputum and clubbing of the fingers. Radiography of the lungs shows certain characteristic changes (International Labour Office, 1970).

Other important chemical agents

Lead (see also Chapter 12)

Lead appears as dust or fumes in the air of the work-place. Occupational exposure occurs in mines, but more commonly in lead smelters, where lead is produced from lead ore or scrap, and in occupations where lead or lead compounds are used, such as the production and repair of storage batteries, and the polishing and welding of lead-coated or lead-painted materials. This may occur in shipyards, car factories, glass and ceramic factories, and printing and paint shops.

Solvents

Solvents include aliphatic and aromatic hydrocarbons, alcohols, aldehydes, ketones, chlorinated hydrocarbons and carbon disulfide. The vapours of organic solvents may be toxic.

Occupational exposure can occur in many different processes, such as the degreasing of metals in the machine industry, the extraction of fats or oils in the chemical or food industry, in dry cleaning, painting, the plastics industry, and in the viscose-rayon industry.

Solvent vapours enter the body mainly by inhalation, although some skin absorption may occur. The vapours are absorbed from the lungs into the blood, and are distributed mainly to tissues with a high content of fat and lipids, such as the central nervous system, liver, and bone marrow.

Most solvent vapours have an anaesthetic effect on the central nervous system. Some solvents may, in addition, cause damage to the liver and kidneys (carbon tetrachloride) or to the blood-forming organs (benzene), or contribute to early atherosclerosis. The action on the central nervous system causes nervous symptoms, such as fatigue, headache, and vertigo. Unconsciousness and death may result from short-term exposure to high concentrations. Toxicity to the liver and kidney may cause jaundice and uraemia. Prolonged exposure to benzene may cause leukopenia and anaemia. Carbon disulfide may contribute to a high incidence of atherosclerosis and possibly of ischaemic heart disease, and may also cause severe nervous symptoms, including psychoses (Brieger & Teisinger, 1967).

Carbon monoxide (see also Chapters 1 and 12)

Occupational exposure occurs in mines after explosions, in the iron and steel industry, where carbon monoxide is used to reduce the iron oxide to iron, and in gas plants.

Carbon monoxide enters the body by inhalation, and is quickly absorbed in the blood, where it combines with the haemoglobin. Symptoms of poisoning include headache, dizziness, and unconsciousness. Death may occur within a few minutes on exposure to high concentrations.

Sulfur dioxide (see also Chapter 1)

Occupational exposure may occur in certain mines for sulfur or sulfur-containing ore, in smelters where sulfur-containing ore is roasted, in the paper and pulp industry, in factories manufacturing sulfuric acid, and in some chemical plants where sulfur dioxide is used for organic synthesis.

Sulfur dioxide is a water-soluble gas that acts as a powerful irritant to the mucous membranes of the eyes and the upper respiratory tract. It causes rapid acute irritation of the eyes with tears and redness; its action on the upper respiratory tract causes cough, shortness of breath, and spasm of the larynx.

Skin irritants

Occupational dermatoses may be caused by organic substances, such as formaldehyde, and solvents or inorganic materials, such as acids and alkalis, and chromium and nickel compounds. Skin irritants are usually either liquids or dusts.

Skin irritants may have a primary toxic effect, as with solvents, acids, and alkalis, or produce an allergic reaction after 3–4 weeks of exposure or longer (chromium and nickel compounds, formaldehyde). Dermatosis or eczema develops, mainly on the skin areas exposed at work, such as the hands and forearms, but also on other parts of the body as a result of contact with contaminated clothes. Exposure to fine arsenical powder in the handling of arsenic compounds causes the development of warts on the skin; these may become malignant.

Physical Agents and Conditions

The hazardous physical agents and conditions considered here are the following: vibration; unsatisfactory lighting conditions; ultraviolet radiation; and heat and cold. For information on the effects of ionizing radiation, non-ionizing radiation, noise, and climate and altitude, see Chapters 14, 15, 16 and 8 respectively.

Vibration

Vibration, especially in the frequency range 10–500 Hz, may be encountered in work with pneumatic tools, such as drills, hammers, and chisels, in mines, quarries, foundries or the machine industry, or with other machines, such as those used in the shoe industry, and motor saws in forestry.

Vibration usually affects the hands and arms. After some months or years of exposure, the fine blood vessels of the fingers become increasingly sensitive to spasm, especially after exposure to the cold or to vibration (white fingers). Exposure to vibration may also produce injuries of the joints of the hands, elbows and shoulders. Such symptoms may be very common, e.g., among forestry workers. Vasospastic symptoms occur, however, more often when people are exposed to cold during leisure periods, rather than at work.

Unsatisfactory lighting conditions

The assessment of lighting conditions at work must include not only the light intensity and distribution, but also other characteristics, such as shadows, glare, contrasts, and colour.

The levels of illumination needed for the performance of difficult tasks at work have been defined (Jones, 1959). The desirable quantity of light depends on the fineness of detail and the accuracy required in performance of the task. With regard to the quality of light, many complex factors are involved, such as glare, diffusion of light, direction, uniformity, and distribution.

Dim light associated with high visual demands may lead to eye strain and fatigue. Exposure to the dim light of inadequately illuminated workplaces, or to the partial darkness of a coal mine for eight hours a day over long periods, can cause both acute and chronic effects on health. The former include headache, eye pain, lachrymation, and congestion around the cornea, particularly if the exposure is associated with eye strain from trying to see small objects. The latter include miner's nystagmus.

Natural daylight appears to be best for visual comfort. Artificial lighting may also fulfil the demands of adequate visual performance, if care is taken to secure proper light distribution and to avoid glare. The latter is an important factor in vision. Distraction from visual tasks and loss of concentration may result from "direct glare" This kind of glare is also associated with discomfort, annoyance, and visual fatigue. Intense direct glare may also result in temporary loss of visual ability, as in the case of drivers exposed to direct intense light from on-coming cars at night.

Other kinds of glare include the "indirect glare" from an intense light spot; it may cause blurring of vision. "Reflected glare" from shiny surfaces or dials can obscure details and prevent perception of visual displays. In the occupational environment, intense colours should be avoided as they may result in fatigue of certain retinal cones (Weston, 1962).

Ultraviolet radiation

Occupational exposure to ultraviolet radiation occurs mainly in arc welding. Such radiation mainly affects the eyes, causing intense conjunctivitis and keratitis (welder's flash.) Symptoms are redness of the eyes and pain; these usually disappear in a few days. The welder himself is usually well protected against radiation from his own work. The worker affected by welder's flash will therefore often be found to have been standing next to a welder, and to have been wearing goggles that do not protect the sides of the eyes. No permanent disability appears to result from this occupational disease (Olishifski & McElroy, 1971).

Exposure to heat and cold

Exposure to heat is common in work-places in many branches of industry. Acute disorders may result either from excessive demands on, or failure of, the temperature control mechanism (Leithead & Lind, 1964), or from a combination of the two. The complex interactions between temperature at the work-place, physical work and climatic conditions are such that each of these types of stress reduces the ability to tolerate the other two.

Little is known as to the long-term effects of hot work; no conclusive epidemiological investigations have been carried out to determine the effects of such work on cardiovascular and renal function.

It is known that heat may adversely affect alertness, reaction times, and psychomotor co-ordination; this would account for a higher accident rate among workers exposed to heat (Vernon, 1939). Accidents are particularly frequent among workers who are not acclimatized (Metz, 1967).

Important hazards associated with cold work are chilblains, erythro-cyanosis, immersion foot, and frostbite as a result of cutaneous vaso-constriction. General hypothermia is not unusual. Although it has often been claimed that the frequency of rheumatism and bronchopulmonary disease is greater among those engaged in cold work, this has not been conclusively proved (Goldsmith & Minard, 1971).

Both the reduction in the temperature of the hands and the wearing of protective gloves reduce dexterity and therefore increase the risk of mistakes and accidents.

Biological Agents and Conditions

These may be a part of the total biological environment or may be associated with certain occupations. Biological agents in the work environment include viruses, rickettsiae, bacteria and parasites of various types. In addition, food intake is an important factor in work performance in different occupations.

Diseases transmitted from animal to man in agricultural work are of common occurrence in view of the fact that agriculture is the major economic activity in developing countries. In such work, infectious and parasitic diseases may result from exposure to contaminated water or to insects.

Occupational infectious diseases may also occur in industry and mining. The common infectious and parasitic occupational diseases include anthrax (woolsorting and handling of infected hides), brucellosis (contact with infected animals), tetanus (from infected wounds), ancylostomiasis (hookworm disease) and schistosomiasis (bilharzia). Fungi from organic dusts, such as bagasse and cocoa, may cause myotic respiratory diseases or skin infections.

As an example, the case of schistosomiasis as an occupational disease may be mentioned. In endemic areas in Brazil, workers in plantations are exposed at work to infected water and soil. It was found that the proportion of stool-positive cases was 59 % among exposed workers, as compared with only 10 % among other workers in the same area who did not come into contact at work with infected water or soil (Czapski & Kloetzel, 1971).

Psychosocial Factors

A high degree of mechanization may increase psychosomatic disorders, reduce job satisfaction, and contribute to a higher rate of absenteeism (Gardell, 1971). Factors such as inter-personal relations at work, work stability, shift work, speed, and safety are important. Workers engaged in repetitive tasks, controlled by machines, derive less satisfaction from their work.

Shift work creates a psychosocial working environment that may adversely influence the health of the worker. Night work, and the change of working hours from one shift to another, may subject the workers to certain stresses. Such stresses affect the nervous system, increasing the frequency of peptic ulcer and of nervous symptoms, such as fatigue, nervousness, irritation, and insomnia (Aanonsen, 1959). These nervous symptoms are usually related to lack of sleep, which in turn may be related to housing conditions, and especially to disturbance of sleep by noise during the day, if the worker is on night shift (Andlauer & Metz, 1967).

Gastro-intestinal diseases are of multiple etiology, and the work environment may be a contributing factor, especially where there is emotional or psychological stress at work. Shift workers may have a higher incidence of peptic ulcer than day workers (Aanonsen, 1959). Chronic gastritis and, to some extent, peptic ulcer were found in Egypt among night shift workers, and were attributed to the stress of shift work as well as to dietetic habits (El Batawi & Noweir, 1966).

Effects of Exposure to Combined Stress

Workers are often exposed to stresses of more than one kind; the outcome is then complex. Human tolerance also varies. Workers may be easily affected by minor degrees of stress because of the lowered " vital " status of the exposed individuals. The environmental stress in this case does not cause the illness, but rather brings about, in vulnerable groups a rapid shift from the previously tolerated levels of existing illness, or of subclinical impairment, to a state of disability. Such acute events have often occurred as a consequence of different environmental stress factors acting on individuals with quite different kinds of physiological handicaps. In developing countries, the employment of children, women, the elderly and the partially disabled is common. The degree of tolerance and susceptibility to psychological and physical stresses at work varies in these groups, and may result in health impairment and increased labour turnover.

The stress associated with night work was found, in a study carried out in Egypt, to contribute to a high incidence of high blood pressure; in this study of garage workers, exposure to toxic substances may have contributed to the high incidence of respiratory diseases that was found (El Batawi & Noweir, 1966). In the viscose rayon industry, exposure to carbon disulfide has been associated with an increased incidence of atherosclerosis and cardiovascular diseases, in reports from studies carried out in different countries (Brieger & Teisinger, 1967). The incidence of cardiac deaths among workers exposed to nitroglycol in the dynamite industry is reported to be higher than among the general population (Parmeggiani, 1971). Diet, smoking and mental strain may be a contributing factor in these diseases, although their importance in this connexion remains to be determined.

Occupationally exposed groups are affected by the diseases prevailing in the community and, in some developing countries, by malnutrition. Exposure to dusts or gases, to heat stress, to the stress of physical effort, and to other conditions that are well tolerated by healthy individuals, may cause serious complications among workers suffering from, e.g., pulmonary tuberculosis, cardiovascular disease, damage to organs, such as the liver and the kidneys, as a result of parasitic diseases, or malnutrition. Tuberculous workers suffering from massive pulmonary fibrosis may develop silicosis more quickly than those free of lung disease. Cardiac patients are more liable to heart failure if required to exert considerable physical effort in a hot environment; the diabetic can suffer complications on night-shift work; and the worker whose liver and kidneys are affected by dysentery or other parasitic infestations may suffer from acute degenerative disease if exposed to carbon tetrachloride, mercury, and other toxic substances that may be tolerated by healthy individuals.

Occupational Accidents

Accidents result from both environmental hazards and human factors. The contributing environmental factors include the layout of the workplace, unsatisfactory machine guards, inadequate maintenance of equipment, defective lighting, excessive noise and vibration, unsuitable floors, walls, roofs, etc.   On the human side, we must include poor adaptation to the industrial mechanized environment, a casual attitude towards work, and incorrect methods of work.   In addition, the physical and physiological capacities of the worker may not meet the job requirements; thus his visual acuity may be inadequate, he may suffer from hearing loss or other forms of partial incapacitation, and his psychological state, particularly his alertness, may be unsatisfactory.   Apart from this, failure to observe safe practices and to make proper use of mechanical safeguards and personal protective equipment account for many accidents.   Most authorities consider human factors much more important than environmental hazards in accident causation, the former being possibly responsible for 85 % of all accidents (International Labour Office, 1967).

Maximum Permissible Concentrations

One of the basic principles of the operation of an occupational health programme is that, despite the potential health risk inevitably associated with known poisonous substances, there is for each substance a definable and measurable level of human contact below which there is no significant threat to man's health.   This acceptable level of contact, expressed in appropriate terms of magnitude and duration of exposure to the offending agent, is variously called the threshold limit value (TLV), the maximum allowable concentration (MAC), or the permissible dose.   Since, in most instances, significant contact with toxic substances is by inhalation of airborne dust, fumes, vapours, and gases, these permissible levels are given in terms of atmospheric concentrations, mg/m^3, particles per m^3 (for mineral dusts), or parts per million of air.   Although there are certain differences of detail in the terms given above, all the terms have the same primary purpose: to identify and locate a point on the scale of dose of the offending agent, above which there is increasing probability of injury, overt illness, and even death, but below which the risk is so limited as to impose no serious threat to health, however long the exposure is continued.

Toxicologists seeking stringent criteria on which to base permissible levels, and endeavouring to ensure adequate safety factors in the face of many unknowns, have approached the problem from different directions. One approach has been to start from the higher levels of demonstrable ill effect and work downwards, using increasingly sensitive measures of pre-clinical, physiological, biochemical, and functional disturbance, but always subjecting these to a critical test of usefulness in terms of their significance as predictors of ill health.   Another approach is to start from a known safe level in a healthy animal (or man), and work upwards, including highly sensitive measures of behavioural or other responses; the permissible limit is established just under the lowest level of exposure needed to induce any statistically significant deviation from the normal state of the organism. Two basically different concepts and criteria of health are involved here. In the first case, no serious threat to health is considered to exist so long as the level of exposure does not induce a demonstrable disturbance in the organism of a kind predictive of potential ill health; in the second, a potential for ill health is said to exist as soon as the organism undergoes the first detectable change of whatever kind from its normal state.

In consequence of the differences in approach, it is not at all surprising that the recommended permissible levels in various parts of the world sometimes differ by a facter of 10 or even more.

The Joint ILO/WHO Committee on Occupational Health (1969) proposed a classification of biological effects of occupational exposure to airborne toxic substances, as follows:

Category A (safe exposure zones):
Exposures that do not, as far as is known, induce any detectable change in the health and fitness of exposed persons during their life-time.

Category B:
Exposures that may induce rapidly reversible effects on health or fitness, but that do not cause a definite state of disease.

Category C:
Exposures that may induce a reversible disease.

Category D:
Exposures that may induce irreversible disease or death.

MAXIMUM ALLOWABLE CONCENTRATION OF SOME HARMFUL SUBSTANCES IN VARIOUS COUNTRIES, IN mg/m^3 *

Substance	USSR (1970-71)	USA (1971-72)	Czecho-slovakia (1970-71)	Poland (1970)	Federal Republic of Germany (1971-72)	United Kingdom (1972)	Switzer-land (1971)
Acetone	200	2400	800	200	2400	2400	2400
Xylene	50	435	200	100	870	435	435
Xylidine	3	25	5	—	25	25	25
Methanol	5	260	100	50	260	260	260
Lead	0.01	0.15	0.05	0.05	0.2	0.15	—
Styrene	5	420	200	50	420	420	420
Toluene	50	375	200	100	750	375	380
Trichloroethylene	10	535	250	50	260	535	260
Carbon dioxide	—	9000	9000	—	9000	9000	9000
Carbon monoxide	20	55	30	30	55	55	55
Vinyl chloride	30	770	—	300	260	770	260

* Data from various sources.

Difficulties may be expected in deciding how to classify certain substances encountered in industry in terms of the suggested categories. This is certainly the case with carcinogenic and mutagenic substances where dose/response relationships are not clear. The TLVs set by the American Conference of Governmental Industrial Hygienists (ACGIH) and the MACs prescribed by the health legislation of the USSR are the permissible limits

most widely accepted in other countries.   In the USA, the most recent
list of threshold limit values for airborne contaminants and physical agents
contains permissible limits for almost 600 chemical agents, and thresholds
in exposure to particulate matter and to physical agents including noise,
non-ionizing radiation, and heat stress (American Conference of Governmental Industrial Hygienists, 1971).

The list of MACs of toxic gases in the air of the working environment
adopted in the Soviet Union (USSR Ministry of Health, 1970) contains
almost as many substances, but in many cases there are wide variations in
the permissible limits prescribed in the two countries.   Other countries
have adopted different levels again (see accompanying table), and it does
not seem that international agreement will be possible for many years to
come.   The Joint ILO/WHO Committee noted that a comparison of the
limits established by the USSR and the ACGIH showed close agreement
(difference of less than a factor of two) for 24 industrial and/or agricultural
chemicals.   The Committee recommended safe concentration zones for
international adoption for these 24 substances, as follows:

Substance	Safe concentration zone[1] (mg/m^3)
Hydrogen chloride (hydrochloric acid)	5 – 7
Phosgene	0.4 – 0.5
Hydrogen sulfide	10 – 15
Sulfur dioxide	10 – 13
Sulfuric acid and sulfuric anhydride	1
Ozone	0.1 – 0.2
Ammonia	20 – 35
Arsine	0.2 – 0.3
Ethanol	1000 – 2000
Methyl acrylate	20 – 35
Nitrobenzene	3 – 5
Dinitrobenzene	1
Dinitrotoluene	1 – 1.5
Trinitrotoluene	1 – 1.5
Parathion	0.05 – 0.1
Iodine	1
Beryllium and compounds (as Be)	0.001 – 0.002
Molybdenum, soluble compounds, dust (as Mo)	4 – 5
Vanadium (as V_2O_5)	
dust	0.5
fume	0.1
Ferrovanadium	1
Zinc oxides (fumes)	5
Zirconium and compounds (as Zr)	5
Chlorinated derivatives of diphenyl	1
Chlorinated derivates of diphenyloxide	0.5

[1] The figures given are used by some authorities as maximum values, and by others as time-weighted
average values.

This recommendation, however, is still being debated, particularly with regard to its application in developing countries where these is a wide variation in human susceptibility and tolerance, depending on the general level of health and on other human and environmental factors. Decisions based on epidemiological observations of human exposure to different levels of toxic agents in particular situations are preferable, of course, to those based on extrapolations from animal studies.

Regional and international technical bodies are taking a special interest in maximum permissible concentrations in different parts of the world. These bodies include a technical committee in the Economic Commission for Europe, a subcommittee of the Permanent Commission and International Association on Occupational Health, and the International Union of Pure and Applied Chemistry.

Experience in occupational toxicology and the extensive information derived from laboratory and field studies of industrial toxic agents provide useful background data for criteria and guides, not only for industry and agriculture but also for the community at large.

REFERENCES

Aanonsen, A. (1959) *Industr. Med. Surg.*, **28**, 422-427

American Conference of Governmental Industrial Hygienists (1971) *Documentation on the threshold limit values for substances in workroom air*, 3rd ed., Cincinnati

Andlauer, P. & Metz, B. (1967) *Le travail en équipes alternantes.* In: Scherrer, J., ed., *Physiologie du travail (ergonomie)*, Paris, Masson, Vol. II, pp. 272-281

Brieger, H. & Teisinger, J. (1967) *Toxicology of carbon disulfide*, Amsterdam, Excerpta Medica Foundation

Czapski, J. & Kloetzel, K. (1971) *Schistosomiasis mansoni in workers and as an occupational disease.* In: *XVI. International Congress on Occupational Health, September 22-27, 1969, Tokyo, Japan*, Tokyo, Japan Industrial Safety Association, pp. 273-275

El Batawi, M. A. & Noweir, M. H. (1966) *Industr. Hlth (Kawasaki)*, **4**, 1-10

Gardell, B. (1971) *Production engineering and work satisfaction*, Stockholm, Swedish Council for Personnel Administration

Goldsmith, R. & Minard, D. (1971) *Cold, cold work.* In: *Encyclopaedia of occupational health and safety*, Geneva, International Labour Office, pp. 319-320.

International Labour Office (1967) *Accident prevention. A workers' education manual*, Geneva

International Labour Office (1970) *International classification of radiographs of pneumoconioses*, Geneva (*Occupational Safety and Health Series*, No. 22)

Joint ILO/WHO Committee on Occupational Health (1969) *Sixth report: permissible levels of occupational exposure to airborne toxic substances*, Geneva (*Wld Hlth Org. techn. Rep. Ser.*, No. 415)

Jones, L. V. (1959) *Ann. occup. Hyg.*, **3**, 358

Leithead, C. S. & Lind, A. R. (1964) *Heat stress and heat disorders*, London, Cassel

Mayers, M. R. (1969) *Occupational health, hazards of the work environment*, Baltimore, Williams & Wilkins

Metz, B. (1967) *Ambiances thermiques.* In: Scherrer, J., ed., *Physiologie du travail (ergonomie),* Paris, Masson, Vol. II, pp. 184-200

Olishifski, P. E. & McElroy, F. E., eds (1971) *Fundamentals of industrial hygiene,* Chicago, Ill., National Safety Council

Parmeggiani, L. (1971) *Ethylene glycol dinitrate.* In: *Encyclopaedia of occupational health and safety,* Geneva, International Labour Office, Vol. I, pp. 483-484

Simonin, C. (1961) *Médecine du travail,* 3rd ed., Paris, Maloine

USSR Ministry of Health (1970) [*Maximum allowable concentration of toxic gases, vapours and dusts in the air of workrooms*], Moscow

Vernon, H. M. (1939) *Health in relation to occupation,* London, Oxford University Press

Weston, H. C. (1962) *Sight, light at work,* London, H. K. Lewis

CHAPTER 8

CLIMATE AND ALTITUDE

General Considerations

Climate is a geographical concept representing a summation of the whole range of meteorological phenomena specific to any given region. The many factors making up a climate are subject to individual fluctuations; this accounts for the complexity of their interrelations with living organisms. Biometeorology is the branch of ecology that studies these interrelations (Sergent & Tromp, 1964).

Many classifications of climate have been suggested, depending on whether the subject is being considered from the point of view of meteorology or of flora or fauna. In the case of man, the dominant factors of temperature, air pressure, rain and wind, which all have a direct influence on his physiology, provide a basis for selecting a few main types of climate and a whole range of intermediate categories. The main types comprise:

(1) the hot, dry climates of desert regions, characterized by scanty precipitation and intense solar radiation; and the hot, humid climates, which have a high level of rainfall and no cold season;

(2) the temperate climates (mediterranean, maritime or continental) in all their wide variety;

(3) the polar climates, in which cold is the dominant factor; and the mountain climates, particularly those associated with high altitudes, in which low atmospheric pressure is added to the other climatic factors.

Climate and Adaptability

There is an undoubted relationship between climate and the characteristics of any population. Whether the phenomenon is genetic in nature or not, the human species is characterized by a remarkable adaptability to its environment; this faculty has enabled it to populate nearly all parts of the planet despite the severity of some climates. This adaptability takes the form of an adjustment of physiology and behaviour to environmental conditions. As a result, special morphological features may develop, such as the high ratio of body weight to surface area of the Eskimo (39.14) in comparison with that of the nomad of the hot deserts (32.8), as discussed in the theory of ecological gradients (UNESCO, 1963).

Particularly severe climatic conditions may result in extensive adaptation, as in the case of populations living at the very high altitudes of the Andean plateau. Such populations show a tolerance to hypoxia and a capacity for physical exertion never attained by individuals transferred from elsewhere, even when well acclimatized (Bouloux & Ruffié, 1971; Folk, 1966).

Cyclic climatic changes undoubtedly influence biological rhythms. It is beginning to be realized just how important such biological rhythms are, for they enter into all human functions and activities. Whether daily, monthly or annual, such rhythms are a basic property of all living matter, and are produced by the action of environmental synchronizing mechanisms (Reinberg, 1971), including climate, on the genetic milieu.

Man, however, shows very wide individual variations in adaptability (Sergent & Tromp, 1964; Dill et al., 1964). In addition to differences due to age, sex and the ageing process, the variability of any given characteristic appears to be as great among individuals of the same group as among different ethnic groups. Ethnic differences do appear, however, when the average characteristics of each group are compared (WHO Scientific Group on Optimum Physical Capacity in Adults, 1969).

Types of Climate

Studies of those climatic factors that affect health, the assessment of their relative importance and the analysis of the way in which they operate, are extremely complicated because of the large number of factors involved, each with its own mode of action and each interacting with the others, and the very great difficulty of reproducing them under experimental conditions.

Some climatic factors, such as temperature, pressure, humidity, wind speed and solar radiation, are easy to measure and are, moreover, of fundamental importance. The action of others, such as atmospheric electricity, ionization and solar activity, although possibly producing some effect, are more difficult to interpret (Sergent & Tromp, 1964; Krueger, 1969).

Furthermore, the climatic processes themselves (variations or general trends) are as important as the changes in their constituent elements, particularly where the degree of individual sensitivity is concerned (Sergent & Tromp, 1964; Tromp, 1963).

Finally, while some physical factors, such as temperature or perssure, may affect the body directly, they may also, either separately or in combination, exert an indirect effect, either by acting on an existing pathological state or by creating favourable conditions for the development of parasites or microbes, thus maintaining certain diseases in an endemic state. The presence of such endemic diseases may lead to adaptive selection, as has happened with malaria; the occurrence of an abnormal type of haemoglobin (haemoglobin S), frequently seen in Africa, southern India and other parts of the tropics, is considered to promote "resistance" to the most dangerous form of malaria *(Plasmodium falciparum)* in those areas (Bernard & Ruffié, 1966). However, when the adverse environmental factor is no longer operative this characteristic loses its value and may even become a disadvantage in different surroundings. Haemoglobin S carriers have been unable to settle in the high Andean areas because possession of this characteristic leads to blood disorders, such as splenic infarct, that do not occur at sea level (Pan American Health Organization, 1966). Conversely, when some Andean populations, such as the Aymara Indians, who have lived for a very long time at extremely high altitudes where there are few biological disease agents, try to adapt to a lowland environment, they appear to develop a lower immune response to the disease agents common in the lowlands than do the Quechua, who have become adapted to high altitude more recently. The Aymaras, although perfectly adapted to very high altitudes, seem "trapped" in that environment (Ruffié et al., 1966.)

Climatic factors may also interact with various atmospheric pollutants and increase the hazards associated with them. In particular, geographical macroclimates may be modified by the creation of man-made microclimates, such as those resulting from urbanization and industrialization (Sergent & Tromp, 1964; Rivolier & Rivolier, 1972).

General Effects of Climate on Disease

Although such effects undoubtedly exist, they are not well understood. The epidemiological surveys that have been made are rarely comparable and, in particular, the mechanisms involved are far from being elucidated. Comprehensive reviews made of the subject (Sergent & Tromp, 1964; Tromp, 1963) indicate the harmful effects certain climatic factors may possibly have, mainly on respiratory conditions, rheumatic diseases, skin cancer and malignant melanoma (Blum, 1955a, b; Lee & Merrill, 1970), as well as on cardiovascular disorders. Workers have long described the possible role of certain winds, such as the south wind in France (Piery, 1934) and the Föhn in the Alps (Pasie, 1969; Licht, 1964) as a cause of irritability, depression, headache, malaise, dizziness, haemorrhage, venous insufficiency, embolism, and hypertension.

Further epidemiological research and surveys are needed before the exact contribution of each factor involved can be defined.

Effects of Specific Climates

While it is difficult to determine the general effects of climate on health, it is possible to detect the action of certain basic physical factors, even though the mechanisms involved are not properly understood.

Hot climates

Dry or humid heat is the climatic stress most widely encountered throughout the world since it affects not only many kinds of industrial and agricultural work but also, and more particularly, many developing countries. Acclimatization of the body and its measures to combat heat serve to maintain thermoregulation. The physiological mechanisms involved are very similar to those called upon in physical exertion and compete with them within the physiological limits compatible with safeguarding health (WHO Scientific Group on Health Factors Involved in Working Under Conditions of Heat Stress, 1969).

The human thermoregulatory system is complex and is called upon to maintain thermal equilibrium of the internal tissues within a relatively narrow temperature range. If the core temperature is to be kept steady in this way, then the amounts of heat gained and lost by the organism must be equal.

Three mechanisms are involved:

(1) depending on whether the air temperature is above or below that of the skin, the body will gain or lose heat by convection; any increase in wind speed will increase the rate of such exchanges;

(2) depending on whether the temperature of surrounding surfaces is above or below skin temperature, the body will gain or lose heat by radiation;

(3) the evaporation of sweat causes a loss of body heat; the amount of sweat that can evaporate and the resultant effectiveness of sweating as a cooling mechanism depends on the difference between the ambient vapour pressure and that at the surface of the skin; this difference increases with increasing air movement.

Operating these physiological exchange mechanisms calls for an effort by the whole body and is accompanied by many physiological responses (such as those involving the fluid balance and the humoral functions), which the thermoregulatory system must cope with in a hot climate (WHO Scientific Group on Health Factors Involved in Working Under Conditions of Heat Stress, 1969).

In practice, sweating is the main thermoregulatory mechanism operating in hot climates. It serves to dissipate not only heat received from the environment but also that produced by physical exertion.

The immediate responses to heat are an increase in core temperature, in heart rate, and to a lesser degree, in sweating. Feelings of discomfort or even distress are common.

Acclimatization sets in very rapidly during the first days of exposure to heat and is almost complete by the end of two weeks (UNESCO, 1963; WHO Scientific Group on Health Factors Involved in Working Under Conditions of Heat Stress, 1969). It provides a spectacular illustration of rapid and effective physiological adjustment to an environmental stress. Distress and discomfort disappear, while core temperature and heart rate go down. At the same time, sweating increases and chloride and sodium concentrations fall. Diuria, which is much reduced during the first two days, rises, although remaining at a lower level than is usual in a temperate climate, and is accompanied by an increase in specific gravity of the urine (700 ml/day and s.g. $\geqslant$ 1030). Physical exercise assists acclimatization (Dill et al., 1964; WHO Scientific Group on Health Factors Involved in Working Under Conditions of Heat Stress, 1969). Long and continued exposure to heat apparently provokes more pronounced changes, such as a drop in core temperature during sleep, modification of the electro-cardiogram (flattening of the T wave) and morphological changes (reduction in total fat while body weight is maintained) (Lambert, 1968). Such phenomena are not fully understood and require clarification.

The degree of acclimatization to heat may differ, depending on whether the hot environment is humid or dry, and may be better in the latter case since evaporation is then more effective. In addition, acclimatization disorders seem to be more common in hot, humid environments (Metz, 1967).

Laboratory and field studies have shown that when temperature rises alertness deteriorates and reaction, decision and sensorimotor co-ordination times decrease (Lambert, 1968; Metz, 1967; UNESCO, 1963).

All these processes taken together account in part for the restrictive effect climate may exercise on human activities in hot countries (Hohwü Christensen, 1964; UNESCO, 1963).

When the ambient thermal environment exposes man to too great or too prolonged physiological stress, *acute* or *chronic heat disorders* may result. A comprehensive and practical review of these disorders has been made (Leithead & Lind, 1964), and they can be classified as follows:

1. **Disorders that may result from excessive demands on the thermoregulatory system:**
   (*a*) circulatory instability: heat syncope;
   (*b*) water and electrolyte imbalance: heat oedema, dehydration, salt-depletion, heat cramp.

2. **Disorders that result from failure of thermoregulation:**
   (*a*) heat stroke;
   (*b*) heat hyperpyrexia.

These various disorders may occur in any hot environment, whether climatic or industrial. They are commoner in summer and in the middle of the day. The risk of their occurrence is increased by a heavy physical workload but reduced by acclimatization. Humid heat favours the development of skin diseases.

The long-term effects of hot climates on health are imperfectly understood. The continued demand on the cardiovascular system together with the high urine specific gravity would explain the heart conditions and renal lithiases observed (UNESCO, 1963; Lambert, 1968; Leithead & Lind, 1964), but there are insufficient epidemiological data to give a clear picture of these disorders.

Generally speaking, mortality tends to fall with the annual seasonal rise in temperature (see figure). However, very high temperatures and sudden climatic changes during the hot season result in increased mortality (Licht, 1964; National Center for Air Pollution Control, 1967).

ANNUAL MORTALITY CURVES FOR THREE CITIES IN THE USA *

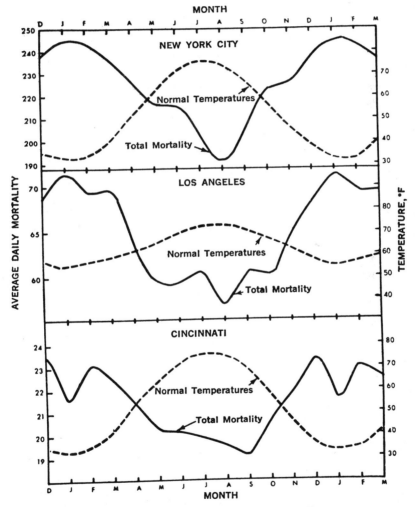

* Reproduced from National Center for Air Pollution Control (1967), p. 83.

Shifts between cold and warm climates can be hazardous for the elderly and for patients with heart disease.

Cold climates and cold environments

These are not as important from the demographic standpoint as hot climates. Like the latter, however, they stimulate thermoregulatory mechanisms, in this case to combat heat loss.

The immediate response to cold is the initiation of the following set of mechanisms to reduce heat loss and increase metabolic heat: peripheral vasoconstriction; increase in breathing and heart rates; piloerection; release by the antehypophysis of hormones stimulating the thyroid and cortico-suprarenal glands; and, lastly, shivering, which is a particularly effective means of increasing heat production. In addition, sleep becomes difficult.

Acclimatization is measured by tests such as immersion of the hand in cold water, temperature at the onset of shivering, and metabolic heat production. By the end of about 10 days, the newcomer to a cold climate shows reduced shivering and metabolic heat production, maintained skin temperature and increased chemical thermogenesis, and he has regained his ability to sleep.

Wide differences in acclimatization, as between African negros and Americans or Europeans, do not seem to exist (Folk, 1966). Nevertheless, some ethnic groups do show special features.

Eskimos, apart from their characteristic morphology (high ratio of body weight to surface area and considerable subcutaneous insulation), have high levels of chemical thermoregulation and skin temperature. The Australian aborigines are unique in their adaptation to cold. They can sleep without protection, their metabolic rate does not increase, they tolerate moderate hypothermia (35 °C) and their insulation from cold is increased by marked vasoconstriction (Folk, 1966).

Adequate protection from cold is generally provided by clothing and shelter. The pathological conditions generally observed are usually the result of accidents (e.g., immersion in cold water).

The acute and chronic disorders due to cold may be divided into two categories:

Disorders resulting from excessive demands on the thermoregulatory system:
(a) superficial: chilblains; erythrocyanosis;
(b) severe: trench or immersion foot; frostbite;

Disorders resulting from breakdown of the thermoregulatory system, e.g., hypothermia (elderly people are particularly susceptible to this condition, which may lead to death when the core temperature falls below 30 °C) (Metz, 1967).

Apart from the above disorders, cold has been shown to increase mortality and morbidity (Licht, 1964), in particular from diseases of the respiratory tract (World Health Organization, 1963). It is also considered that cold may, when associated with humidity, have an effect on rheumatic diseases (Sergent & Tromp, 1964). The influence of the cold of polar climates on tuberculosis requires further clarification (World Health Organization, 1963).

High altitude

This is probably the natural environment of greatest stress for man. In contrast to others, it is permanent, invariable and irremediable. Despite this, millions of men live and work at over 3500 m, or even 4500 m, under conditions of severe hypoxia and very low barometric pressure that create many physiopathological problems.

Sudden exposure to high altitude provokes a wide variety of symptoms such as headache, insomnia, volume changes in the compartments of the lung accompanied by Cheyne-Stokes breathing at night, moderate hyperventilation followed by alkalosis, progressive polycythaemia, and increase in heart rate (Bouloux & Ruffié, 1971; Folk, 1966; Dill et al., 1964).

Acclimatization proceeds fairly rapidly, and, at least as far as concerns the respiratory tract, is attained in three weeks. Heart rate returns to normal, sleep is again possible and without Cheyne-Stokes breathing, the acid-base balance returns to normal and polycythaemia increases (as does the total haemoglobin content and the haematocrit) resulting in better oxygenation of the tissues. However, a person transferred to high altitudes, even when acclimatized, will always show relative hyperventilation, continuing susceptibility to hypoxia, polycythaemia, hyperventilation during muscular exertion, which is limited, moreover, by hypoxia, reduction of skin circulation (which also helps in acclimatization to cold), respiratory and blood redistribution accompanied by enlargement of the pulmonary capillary bed and an increase in the functional residual capacity (Bouloux & Ruffié, 1971; Folk, 1966).

Populations native to high altitudes show a different and at the same time a more varied clinical picture. This can be considered as a true *adaptation* and consists of the following: increase in pulmonary vascular resistance accompanied by pulmonary hypertension; very marked, right ventricular electrocardiographic hypertrophy in childhood (traces similar to those seen in cases of congenital heart disease with pulmonary stenosis), polycythaemia, redistribution of blood, reduction of cerebral and coronary outputs, low arterial pressure, high respiratory function parameters, expanded thoracic cavity, relative hypoventilation, lack of sensitivity to hypoxia and carbon dioxide, and remarkable tolerance to physical exertion so that a given oxygen consumption can be maintained in oxygen-deficient air. Persons indigenous to high altitudes can make use of more oxygen in the air inspired than can acclimatized individuals, and their working capacity is comparable to that of men at sea level (Bouloux & Ruffié, 1971; Folk, 1966; Dill et al., 1964; Pan American Health Organization, 1966).

The pathological symptoms resulting from a high altitude climate are various, and both natives and acclimatized settlers may, although to different extents, be subject to them.

Pulmonary oedema is found in both the indigenous and non-indigenous populations. With the greater accessibility of high mountains as a result of developments in mechanical transport, this serious and sometimes fatal disease has become increasingly prevalent, though still uncommon, among climbers and travellers (*Brit. med. J.*, 1972). Pulmonary hypertension is usual among the indigenous population but its physiological significance is very complex. Monge's disease (chronic mountain sickness) occurs only at high altitudes; it is characterized by congestive symptoms, reduction of the arterial haemoglobin concentration and excessive polycythaemia. The disease is difficult to differentiate from the respiratory insufficiencies caused by the sudden pneumoconioses that are common among the miners of these areas.

There is also an acute form of mountain sickness that attacks acclimatized travellers on their ascent or return to high altitudes.

A high incidence of certain congenital heart diseases such as patent ductus arteriosus has been reported to be directly related to altitude (Pan American Health Organization, 1966; World Health Organization, 1969). On the other hand, arterial hypertension, and very probably cardiac ischaemia also, appears to be very rare among those native to high altitudes (World Health Organization, 1969). Research is at present being carried out with the aim of finding out whether the mechanisms responsible for the curious absence of this type of disease are genetic or biological in nature.

REFERENCES

Bernard, J. & Ruffié, J. (1966) *Hématologie géographique*, Paris, Masson

Blum, H. F. (1955a) *Sunburn.* In: Hollaender, A., ed., *Radiation biology*, Vol. 2, New York, McGraw-Hill, pp. 487-528

Blum, H. F. (1955b) *Ultraviolet radiation and cancer.* In: *ibid.*, pp. 529-559

Bouloux, C. & Ruffié, J. eds (1971) *Pré-adaptation et adaptation génétique*, Paris, Institut national de la Santé et de la Recherche médicale

Brit. med. J., 1972, **3**, 65-66

Dill, D. B., Adolph, E. F. & Wilber, C. G. (1964) *Adaptation to the environment.* In: *Handbook of physiology*, Washington, D.C., American Physiological Society

Folk, G. E. (1966) *Introduction to environmental physiology*, London, Kimpton

Hohwü Christensen, E. (1964) *Man at work: Studies on the application of physiology to working conditions in a subtropical country*, Geneva, International Labour Office (*Occupational Safety and Health Series*, No. 4)

Krueger, A. P. (1969) *Scientia, Paris*, **104**, 1-16

Lambert, G. (1968) *L'adaptation. Physiologie et psychologie de l'homme aux conditions de vie désertique*, Paris, Hermann

Lee, D. H. K. & Merrill, B. A. (1970) *Med. J. Austr.*, **2**, 846

Leithead, C. S. & Lind, A. R. (1964) *Heat stress and heat disorders*, London, Cassel

Licht, S., ed. (1964) *Medical climatology*, New Haven, Conn., Elizabeth Licht

Metz, B. (1967) *Ambiances thermiques.* In: Scherrer, J., ed., *Physiologie du travail (ergonomie)*, Paris, Masson, pp. 184-248

National Center for Air Pollution Control (1967) *Seminar on human biometeorology*, Washington, D.C., US Public Health Service (Public Health Service Publication No. 999-AP-25)

Pan American Health Organization (1966) *Life at high altitudes. Proceedings of the Special Session held during the Fifth Meeting of the PAHO Advisory Committee on Medical Research 15 June 1966*, Washington, D.C.

Pasie, H. (1969) *Int. J. Bioclim. Biomet.*, **13**, suppl. 4

Piery, M. (1934) *Traité de climatologie biologique et médicale*. Paris, Masson

Reinberg, A. (1971) *Recherche*, **2**, 242-250

Rivolier, C. & Rivolier, J. (1972) *Météorologie humaine*, Paris (*Cahiers Sandoz*, No. 22)

Ruffié, J., Larrouy, G. & Vergnes, H. (1966) *Nouv. Rev. franc. Hémat.*, **6**, 544-552

Sergent, II, F. & Tromp, S. W. (1964) *A survey of human biometeorology*, Geneva, World Meteorological Organization (*Technical Note* No. 65; WMO-No. 160. TP. 78)

Tromp, S. W. (1963) *Medical biometeorology*, Amsterdam, Elsevier

UNESCO (1963) *Environmental physiology and psychology in arid conditions. Reviews of research*, Paris (Arid zone research - XXII)

WHO Scientific Group on Health Factors Involved in Working Under Conditions of Heat Stress (1969) *Report*, Geneva (*Wld Hlth Org. techn. Rep. Ser.*, No. 412)

WHO Scientific Group on Optimum Physical Capacity in Adults (1969) *Report*, Geneva (*Wld Hlth Org. techn. Rep. Ser.*, No. 436)

World Health Organization (1963) *Medecine and public health in the Arctic and Antarctic: selected papers from a conference*, Geneva (*Publ. Hlth Pap.*, No. 18)

World Health Organization (1969) *International work in cardiovascular diseases, 1959-1969*, Geneva

CHAPTER 9

TRANSPORT HAZARDS

New advances in the field of transport have exposed users to a whole series of hazards that, although not new, are becoming more and more striking because of the constantly increasing number of persons affected by them.

The rapidity of air transport, for example, results in disturbances of the circadian rhythm in aircrews and passengers who have to travel long distances. In addition there are the difficulties of adapting to sudden changes of climate, way of life, and food, which affect tourists especially.

Variations in pressure during the flight may result in injuries to the ear, the sinuses, and sometimes the teeth (McFarland, 1953). Airsickness, and fainting following hyperventilation provoked by anxiety, are not uncommon (Lavernhe, 1971), but the most frequent hazard is constituted by the accidents, usually slight but sometimes serious, caused by turbulence.

On a more general health level, the contact between distant populations resulting from the growth of air travel facilitates the spread of communicable diseases and raises numerous health problems both in flight and at airports. These problems are dealt with in the *International health regulations (1969)* and the *Guide to hygiene and sanitation in aviation* (World Health Organization, 1960).

Nevertheless, these various risks fade into relative insignificance beside the dramatic toll of road accidents. Indeed, among the accidents resulting from the development of air, land, sea, and river transport, road traffic accidents predominate both in respect of their frequency and seriousness and in terms of human and economic cost: more than 150 000 dead and 6 000 000 injured each year. In 1969 in the USA the total cost of accidents was estimated at $ 25 000 000 000, of which half was accounted for by motor vehicles and slightly more than a third by accidents at work (United States, National Safety Council, 1970).

Consequently road traffic accidents constitute a rapidly spreading "epidemic" from which no country is immune (Norman, 1962). Even though in most countries there seems to have been a relative drop in the number of road deaths in proportion to the number of vehicles on the roads, the absolute number of people killed or injured in these accidents is constantly increasing (United Nations, Economic Commission for Europe, 1970) (see accompanying table).

NUMBER OF PERSONS KILLED (A) OR INJURED (B) IN ROAD ACCIDENTS
PER 100 000 POPULATION AND PER 1 000 000 REGISTERED VEHICLES

Country		Number of persons killed or injured					
		per 100 000 population			per 1 000 000 registered vehicles		
		1950-1952 average	1964-1966 average	Difference (%)	1950-1952 average	1964-1966 average	Difference (%)
Australia . .(1952-1954, 1964-1966)	A	22.0	27.5	+ 25.0	1 012.0	816.0	— 19.4
	B	476.9	675.2	+ 41.6	21 966.3	20 011.5	— 8.9
Canada	A	17.5	25.2	+ 44.0	858.1	736.5	— 14.2
	B	384.4	766.6	+ 99.4	18 835.2	22 428.9	+ 19.1
Federal Republic of Germany .(1953-1955, 1964-1966)	A	23.3	27.7	+ 18.9	2 301.3	1 219.5	— 47.0
	B	656.3	755.0	+ 15.0	64 724.7	33 181.8	— 48.7
France . . .(1950-1952, 1963-1965)	A	8.8	22.9	+ 160.2	1 223.4	711.1	— 41.9
	B	174.2	547.8	+ 214.5	24 242.6	16 991.8	— 29.9
Hungary . .(1951-1953, 1964-1966)	A	5.6	8.8	+ 57.1	—	—	—
	B	39.0	182.4	+ 367.7	—	—	—
Japan	A	5.3	13.5	+ 154.7	8 478.0	866.7	— 89.8
	B	39.4	457.8	+ 1061.9	63 643.8	29 348.2	— 53.9
Norway . .(1950-1952, 1963-1965)	A	4.7	10.6	+ 125.5	954.2	479.2	— 49.8
	B	88.6	215.3	+ 143.0	17 902.6	9 697.5	— 45.8
Poland . . .(1953-1955, 1964-1966)	A	5.4	8.0	+ 48.1	1 215.1	1 215.1	— 75.8
	B	22.3	68.7	+ 208.1	20 669.4	10 454.5	— 49.4
United Kingdom	A	10.2	15.0	+ 47.1	1 146.1	642.1	— 44.0
	B	415.8	725.3	+ 74.4	46 773.5	31 141.3	— 33.4
Yugoslavia .(1954-1956, 1964-1966)	A	2.8	9.1	+ 225.0	—	4 613.1	—
	B	19.7	138.4	+ 602.5	—	69 955.9	—

Source : Wld Hlth Stat. Rep. (1968), pp. 352-353.

A prerequisite for the control of such an "epidemic" is an adequate knowledge of its causes. Unfortunately, the cause of a road accident is often difficult to demonstrate. An accident is very rarely due to a single factor, but generally results from the interaction of a group of factors, including environmental conditions, which affect the driver's behaviour. Neither the mortality statistics, numerous as they are, nor the very fragmentary morbidity statistics permit at present a clear epidemiological analysis of these interactions, since the variation in the definitions and methods applied in different countries is too great.

There is no doubt that the human factor plays a major role. The mortality statistics show the particular proneness of the 15–25-year age group (WHO Regional Office for Europe, 1968); in some countries road accidents account for more than 30 % of all deaths in this age group, where health status is a relatively unimportant factor.

In general, the proportion of accidents attributable to medical causes is very low (less than 2 %), and among these causes defective vision is the most common. On the other hand, sociocultural and psychological factors may make a contribution (dangerous driving, asocial behaviour traits), as may states of physical or mental fatigue or stress.

Certain drugs (hypnotics, tranquillizers, psychotomimetics, stimulants, antihistamines, antiepileptics, antihypertensives) may affect the driver's behaviour. This is a risk element about which little is known as yet, but it needs to be taken into consideration since it is estimated that these drugs are taken by 4–20 % of drivers. Combinations of drugs are particularly dangerous, especially the association of drugs and alcohol (Organisation for Economic Co-operation and Development, 1968).

The United Nations Commission on Narcotic Drugs (1966), which reviewed the problem of the effect of psychoactive drugs on the accident rate in the light of the fourteenth report of the WHO Expert Committee on Dependence-Producing Drugs (1965), concluded that stricter control of the sale and use of such drugs would have a salutary effect.

Many material factors, external to man but on which he is closely dependent, come into play in the complex situations represented by driving a vehicle or by crossing a busy road. By applying ergonomics and bio-engineering (a) to vehicle design in order to improve passive safety (seat belts, collapsible steering columns, head rests, etc.) and active safety (self-inflating bags in the event of a collision, for example) or (b) to the analysis of the driver's "optimum perceptual load", of road signs, and of urban traffic, it should be possible to reduce substantially the risks associated with the man–vehicle–road interface (Adriasola et al., 1972; Michon & Fairbank, 1971), an interface that also includes the physical environment.

The part played in accidents by cold, heat, and inadequate ventilation is well established. These factors may reduce vigilance, and since driving is in any case often a monotonous task, the consequences can be particularly serious.

The incidence of accidents varies according to the time of day and the type of road user. For example, a study in the United Kingdom shows that more adult pedestrians are killed at night than in daytime, whereas the reverse is the case for all other road users.

There are also variations according to the day of the week and the month of the year which do not seem to be attributable solely to fluctuations in traffic density. Apart from meteorological conditions that obviously make driving dangerous (rain, snow, fog, ice), recent studies have shown an apparent link between the incidence of road accidents and the changes in atmospheric pressure associated with cold and warm fronts.

Despite the inadequacy of the data at present available, therefore, it seems that road accidents are rarely due to chance. Human factors are undoubtedly the principal cause, but environmental factors are by no means negligible. In the development of technical and epidemiological studies and of prevention programmes, the interaction of these two types of factor should be taken into account.

REFERENCES

Adriasola, G., Olivares, C. & Diaz-Coller, C. (1972) *Bol. Ofic. sanit. panamer.*, **72,** No. 1

International Health Regulations (1969), Geneva, World Health Organization, 1971

Lavernhe, J. (1971) *Presse méd.*, **79,** 2338

McFarland, R. A. (1953) *The human factor in air transportation*, New York, McGraw-Hill

Michon, J. A. & Fairbank, B. A., jr (1971) *Measuring driving skill.* In: Singleton, W. T., Fox, J. G. & Whitfield, D., eds, *Measurement of man at work*, London, Taylor & Francis

Norman, L. G. (1962) *Road traffic accidents: epidemiology, control, and prevention*, Geneva, World Health Organization (*Publ. Hlth Pap.*, No. 12)

Organisation for Economic Co-operation and Development (1968) *Research on the effects of alcohol and drugs on driver behaviour: a report by an OECD research group*, Paris

United Nations, Commission on Narcotic Drugs (1966) *Report of the Twentieth Session, Geneva, 1965*, New York (document E.4140; E/CN.7/488), pp. 45-46

United Nations, Economic Commission for Europe (1970) *Statistics of road traffic accidents in Europe, 1969*, New York

United States, National Safety Council (1970) *Accident facts—ten-year accident toll*, Chicago

WHO Expert Committee on Dependence-Producing Drugs (1965) *Fourteenth report*, Geneva (*Wld Hlth Org. techn. Rep. Ser.*, No. 312)

WHO Regional Office for Europe (1968) *Human factors in road accidents, Report on a Symposium, Rome, 1967*, Copenhagen (document E-0147)

Wld Hlth Stat. Rep., 1968, **21,** 297-360

World Health Organization (1960) *Guide to hygiene and sanitation in aviation*, Geneva

CHAPTER 10

ENVIRONMENTAL INFLUENCES ON MENTAL HEALTH

Man's physical and mental health depends on the genetic and environmental factors that influence it. How the genes will manifest themselves will depend to a considerable extent on the human genetic constitution as a whole and on a variety of changing environmental factors. It is understandable, therefore, that human behaviour must be considered as a complex product of the interaction between these factors.

From the time of conception, individuals are exposed not only to a physical and chemical environment, and variations in climate, nutrition, and somatic health, but also to a series of social, psychological, and cultural phenomena that influence and enrich the process of learning and determine individual experience, character, and responses.

Living organisms are adjusted or adjust themselves to handling and maintaining a reasonable input of stimuli. If this input is either greater or smaller than that to which the individual organism is adjusted, and the organism's homoeostasis (equilibrium) is disturbed, the excess or lack of stimuli can be considered as stress; this may be, and usually is, multifactorial, i.e., it consists of many similar or dissimilar stimuli. The organism's equilibrium is modified by stress and, if it cannot adjust to the excessive or insufficient load, the result is breakdown or disequilibrium. This may be temporary and reversible (if the organism has the ability to recover from such disturbances or receives treatment from outside), or it may proceed to functional or structural pathology. The mechanisms whereby psychosocial stimuli that cause imbalance can lead to illness are not completely understood. An up-to-date review, together with speculations supported by recent work, is given by Levi (1972).

Stress produced by social or cultural events affects people differently, even in the same group and in a similar environment. Individuals vary greatly in their genetic and constitutional ability to handle stress of all kinds.

The many factors that might modify the amount of mental disorder in a population have been noted in a guide prepared by a committee of the

American Public Health Association (1962). How these factors may actually do this is not in all cases well understood, and continued and more intensive research is essential.

Psychosocial Factors

The term "psychosocial" will be used here to denote all psychological relations between the individual and society.

Demographic factors

Population density

There are some indications from animal experiments that population density in itself may affect mental health. Thus, under conditions of extreme overcrowding, an increase in male aggressiveness and an accompanying decline in the adequacy of maternal behaviour have been observed among rats. When the young were methodically removed from colonies of rats kept at high densities, it was noted in addition that bands of young males assaulted females and that there was an increase in homosexual behaviour (Calhoun, 1963). However, mice brought up under overcrowded conditions showed less stress behaviour than those transferred only later to such conditions (Kessler, cited by Taylor, 1971).

Some epidemiological studies (e.g., Faris & Dunham, 1939; Häfner & Reimann, 1970) have shown higher rates of schizophrenia, crime, suicide, alcoholism, and drug abuse in the central, more crowded areas of old-established cities than in other areas of such cities, but correlations of this kind are by no means clear-cut (see Chapter 27).

There is little evidence that low population density has a detrimental effect on mental health. Small groups in sparsely populated areas are likely to have a well established social structure, which often appears to exert a protective influence on mental health. However, isolated populations may show high rates of certain mental disorders—e.g., mental retardation—as a result of inbreeding (Lopašić & Mikić, 1957), selective emigration, and immigration (Lemkau et al., 1971). Mental deficiency and some mental disturbances may be less apparent and better tolerated in small groups than under crowded conditions.

Age structure

Rapid population expansion has led to an unbalanced age structure in some developing countries, where about half the population is now under 15 years old. This increases the responsibilities of the leaders, educators, and "caretakers" in the countries concerned, and may contribute to social disorganization. In many other parts of the world, the numbers and proportion of old people continue to rise. Certain forms of mental illness become more common from the age of 60 years, and psychogeriatric problems already place a heavy burden on many communities (WHO Expert Committee on Mental Health, 1959; *WHO Chronicle*, 1971).

Population movements

In some highly industrialized countries large proportions of the population change their residence frequently (in the 10 years between 1950 and 1960, for example, 52 million persons in the USA—one in four of the population—moved from one State to another, and about as many moved from one part of a State to another). Moving is likely to cause stress in families, particularly among young children and the aged, who may have considerable difficulty in adapting to new environments and in making new friends. It has been suggested that such stress may result in higher rates of neurosis in housewives who have moved to new towns, but this was not confirmed in two studies (Hare, 1965; Taylor & Chave, 1964).

Uprooting and resettlement is more likely to be traumatic where migration has been involuntary (Malzberg & Lee, 1956), and large populations have been moved in this way during the present century (Murphy et al., 1955; Weinberg, 1961). Migration into new communities poses problems of adaptation to new settings and new people and also breaks up the network of old ties and relationships involving mutual help in times of need (Young & Willmott, 1957). Committees of settlement may help to reduce the consequent mental health problems (Murphy et al., 1955). Movement from close-knit rural villages to industrial communities may lead to increased demands on helping professions, including physicians and mental health personnel, and may actually increase the prevalence of some mental disorders and psychosomatic conditions.

Changing social structures

All cultures in the world are changing, some slowly and others very rapidly, largely as a result of the increasing speed of travel and communications. There is little doubt that this cultural change modifies the previous stereotypes of both individuals and social groups, and fosters different expectations and demands in populations. Whether it also modifies the patterns and incidence of mental illness is highly controversial and requires much further research. As part of this culture modification process, political and economic change—e.g., from a free-enterprise to a centrally controlled economy—may completely alter the perspectives of both individuals and total populations. Whether mental well-being is improved and whether mental illness increases or diminishes as a result is not in fact known. Many studies have been made, but their results are not comparable.

Increased pace

It has many times been claimed that the increased pace and stress of modern times may lead to a higher incidence of mental illness. This has not been proved by quantitative research. From the information currently available, it would appear that psychoses do not increase but that psycho-neuroses may. Under very difficult conditions, such as disasters, riots, and wars, unusual mental syndromes are observed. Some of these may be temporary and quite normal as part of the organism's readjustment phase after disturbed homoeostasis; others may be pathological states precipitated, but probably not actually caused, by severe stress.

Technological change and industrialization

Technology—particularly improvements in communications and trans-port, as also in industry—is continuously changing the patterns of all societies, and modifies psychological attitudes and adjustments in many ways. These changes are reflected to some extent in statistics of absentee-ism, strikes and slow-downs, accidents, etc. (World Federation for Mental Health, 1965a; WHO Study Group on Mental Health Problems of Auto-mation, 1959).

These conditions arise within a complex of social changes involving an increase in the number of highly specialized roles in production and a rapid shift in values. Personal services also become highly specialized and the family and individual lose much of their former self-sufficiency. Investigators have differed in their views as to which of these changes interferes most with healthy mental function. As many millions of people are heading towards such a transformation of their style of living, it is important that we should learn more about what are truly disruptive forces and what can be done to reduce their damaging effects.

Living conditions

Human beings have always lived in groups and, apart from a few nomad tribes, have ordinarily settled in permanent or semi-permanent locations, such as camps, villages, towns, and cities. With rapidly increasing popula-tions, resettlement, and urbanization, administrations are becoming heavily burdened with additional problems of agriculture, housing, traffic move-ment and risks, and of water supplies, sewage disposal, and other matters of hygiene (WHO Expert Committee on Public Health Administration, 1963). These contribute to a variety of mental health problems (World Federation for Mental Health, 1965b).

The ways in which populations use the physical space available for home life, work, and recreation differ widely around the world. Architects and community planners try to find ever more satisfying ways of arranging the physical aspects of our lives. Each culture and civilization expresses its sense of values in these matters. Urban crowding increases the risk of epidemics, but public health measures to counteract this hazard have proved so effective that longevity has greatly increased as the world has become more and more urbanized. Living conditions that may promote an increase in mental disorders have not been identified. But those elements of slum life that are associated with high infant and maternal mortality are also associated with a higher incidence of mental retardation, delinquency, alcoholism, and drug abuse. At the present time there is no reason to think that better architecture alone will be able to prevent these consequences of poverty.

As a practical example of the importance of traffic risks, Selzer et al. (1968) demonstrated that psychopathology and social stress were significantly greater in automobile drivers who had been responsible for fatal accidents than in control drivers.

Economic and sociopolitical conditions

Wealth, its distribution, and the security that it provides may be of importance in relation to mental health problems. Whether poverty itself affects mental morbidity is controversial. There is much interest and concern, but little in the way of clinical or epidemiological facts (Finney, 1969). However, it has been shown that there may be an association between the prevalence of psychosomatic disorders and economic crises (Halliday, 1948).

The availability of structured health services, including mental health services, depends largely on the social, economic, and educational development of an area. The numbers of cases of mental disorder reported tend to rise as treatment facilities improve and then to level off and even decline. Careful surveys in developing areas may reveal a high prevalence of mental disorders for which indigenous treatment is available (Field, 1960; Leighton et al., 1963).

No carefully controlled studies appear to have been made on the effect of political systems on the incidence or prevalence of mental disorders, although notable changes in suicide rates have been reported in relation to specific political events.

The effects of war on mental health are likewise difficult to measure. It has been stated that rates for neuroses decline during times of war and rise abruptly shortly thereafter. However, such changes in reported rates may depend on many factors, such as an increase in death rates and a decrease in the availability of psychiatric services. Yet during both world wars attention was drawn to the high prevalence of "war neuroses" among the armed forces (e.g., among pilots: Reid, 1960). Particularly high rates of mental disorder have been found among war victims who have survived mass ill-treatment (Eitinger, 1964).

Specific cultural settings

A number of "culture-bound" syndromes have been observed. These are symptom complexes seen only in specific culture settings (Yap, 1969; Lehmann, 1967; Ellenberger, 1965; De Reuck & Porter, 1965). Many of these have been described in terms of European or American criteria, and the symptomatology involved reflects the culture in which they are found. Much research is yet needed on this matter.

A number of psychiatric illnesses and behavioural disorders have a particularly profound significance for society as a whole, but the role of social factors in their causation is a matter of controversy. Social factors will permit the *emergence* of many of them but, in the pathogenic sense, would not appear to *cause* them. They include alcoholism, drug addiction, suicidal behaviour, criminality, delinquency, sexual deviation, fanatical behaviour, communicated insanity—e.g., *folie à deux*—and "culture shock"—e.g., displacement syndrome or alien paranoid reactions (Arieti, 1966; Freedman & Kaplan, 1967; Lemert, 1951; Lindzey & Aronson, 1968/69). The controversial issue is whether they are primarily biologically or socially determined.

Physicochemical and Biological Factors

The following are some of the many environmental factors, other than psychosocial ones, capable of producing abnormal human behaviour.

Toxic substances

Technological and social developments have multiplied the hazards to which the population, especially in urban areas, is exposed, such as the harmful effects of chemicals on the central nervous system (CNS). For example, more than one-third of the industrial chemicals listed in the American table of threshold limit values (see pp. 134-135) affect the CNS at the threshold concentration, or at concentrations twice as great or ten times greater than the recommended level (Smyth, 1956).

Many industrial chemicals, such as carbon disulfide, mercury, manganese, tin, lead compounds, trichloroethylene, decaborane, and carbon monoxide have been shown to be selective neurotoxic agents producing neurological and behavioural disturbances (Porter & Birch, 1970). The critical period of vulnerability is during fetal and postnatal life, and infancy; in these stages of cerebral maturation such compounds can produce serious and irreversible damage. The dosage and duration of exposure to chemical agents is also very important. For example, lead poisoning in children can produce irreparable brain damage with permanent mental retardation. Severe exposure often occurs in children from slum areas of industrialized cities and leads to chronic CNS impairment (Caccuri & Pecora, 1965).

Psychotropic substances and other drugs

A large number of psychotropic drugs are now being used therapeutically, some of which have predictable as well as unpredictable and undesirable side effects (Excerpta Medica Foundation, 1968). Since many of these drugs interfere with important enzyme systems if administered for long periods, special attention should be paid to their possible interactions with a large variety of other drugs (Hansten, 1971), or with exposure to chemicals or indirect environmental influences, such as malnutrition. Barbiturates, alcohol, and griseofulvin (an antifungal agent) are among the drugs capable of precipitating attacks of acute and intermittent porphyria, a genetically determined neurometabolic disorder. The clinical picture of the mental disturbances observed in such patients resembles that of some forms of schizophrenia and hysteria. An explosive outbreak of porphyria involving several thousand individuals was reported in 1956 in Turkey as a result of poisoning by hexachlorobenzene, which was being used as a fungicide (Ockner & Schmid, 1961; De Matteis et al., 1961).

Nutritional factors

Physical and mental development, particularly during the early stages of infancy, is handicapped both quantitatively and qualitatively by nutritional deficiencies in proteins, carbohydrates, or vitamins. However, public health workers, psychologists, and educators have only recently become concerned with the problem of potential delay in mental development among malnourished children. Malnutrition modifies the growth and biochemical maturation of the brain in both human beings and animals, and seriously affects the morphological and biochemical processes of the brain's development, with consequent effects on the integration of behaviour (Cravioto, 1968; Scrimshaw & Gordon, 1968). Poor nutrition during early childhood also affects the growth rate and, consequently, adult stature.

The crucial role of vitamins in body metabolism, and particularly their catalytic action on the biochemical processes in the nervous system, is demonstrated by vitamin deficiency, which can be responsible for the production of mental disturbances in man. An example is pellagra psychosis due to nicotinic acid deficiency. Vitamin B_{12} and folic acid deficiency have also been implicated in neuropsychiatric disorders (Davison & Dobbing, 1968).

Pyridoxine is essential for transamination reactions and plays a vital role in amino-acid metabolism in the brain, particularly for the biosynthesis of gamma-aminobutyric acid; when there is a deficiency of pyridoxine, the formation of this acid is affected, resulting in convulsions (Coursin, 1968). Disturbed electroencephalogram (EEG) patterns are a common finding in this deficiency.

The role of thiamine in brain metabolism is also fundamental, and thiamine deficiency causes neurological and mental disturbances. Adult subjects suffering from this type of deficiency show symptoms of anxiety, depression, irritability, and increased sensitivity to noise and pain (McIlwain, 1966). It has been suggested that chronic malnutrition, in both children and adults, produces weakness, apathetic behaviour, and lack of initiative.

Minerals

About 10 % of the world's population live in goitre areas and are thus exposed to the risk of iodine deficiency, which disturbs the relationship between thyroid function and the growth and development of the brain. Neonatal thyroid deficiency can give rise to structural changes in cerebral development, producing mental retardation in children (cretinism) (Cameron & O'Connor, 1964). Myxoedema, due to hypothyroidism in adults, has been associated with some mental disorders. It is probable that a relationship exists between hypothyroid function and schizophrenia (Richter, 1969).

Infective agents

Of the external factors responsible for causing brain damage in infants, one of the most important is infectious disease. Such disease, during the prenatal, perinatal, and postnatal periods of life, may have adverse effects on the brain's development and the integration of mental functions, as shown by the embryopathies caused by viruses, such as those of measles and rubella, The sequelae of meningoencephalitis caused by micro-organisms, e.g., *Listeria*, produce brain damage in children (Crome & Stern, 1967). Herpes simplex and other neurotropic virus infections in the adult can produce encephalopathies leading to the development of psychoses (Bedson et al., 1967). Congenital ocular and brain lesions are produced by toxoplasmosis infection passed from the mother to the fetus during pregnancy. Some parasitic diseases, such as cysticercosis and cerebral trypanosomiasis, and some mycoses, are responsible for producing neurological and mental disturbances in the tropical areas of the world (WHO Scientific Group on Neurology, 1969).

Traumatic factors

Technological development and urbanization have resulted in a great increase in traumatic brain lesions, mainly due to road and occupational accidents. These lesions are often responsible for mood and personality disorders, memory and intellectual impairment, post-traumatic psychoses, and dementia.

Radiation

Radiation exposure has a strong impact on the formation of the nervous system. This system is most sensitive to radiation during the period of neural development, and a large number of congenital anomalies in the CNS produced by ionizing radiation have been observed in both man and animals (Van Cleave, 1963; Haley & Snider, 1964). Experimental investigations in animals have recently demonstrated adverse effects of irradiation on the motivation, emotion, learning, and perception processes (Kinneldorf & Hunt, 1965). Radiation to the whole brain can produce EEG changes (Sams et al., 1964), alteration in the behaviour of experimental animals, and direct stimulation of the autonomic nervous system (Kinneldorf & Hunt, 1964). The normal blood brain barrier is also damaged, thus affecting its permeability to various substances (Clements & Holst, 1954).

Other factors

Seasonal variation seems to play a role in the occurrence and course of some mental disturbances, particularly in the affective disorders and other periodic psychiatric syndromes. These clinical observations have been neglected and merit further research with the aim of elucidating some of the precipitating biological or other external factors in mental illness (Reimann, 1963).

Conclusions

It is clear from this brief review that the environmental influences on mental health are many and profound. The environmental components are often inextricably bound up with the varying biological make-up of individuals, and segregation of the individual factors involved is frequently not possible. Research must be intensified and expanded to improve our present unsatisfactory state of knowledge on this subject.

REFERENCES

American Public Health Association (1962) *Mental disorders: a guide to control methods*, New York, American Public Health Association

Arieti, S., ed. (1966) *American handbook of psychiatry*, New York, Basic Books

Bedson, S., Downie, A. W., MacCallum, F. O. & Stuart-Hams, C. H., ed. (1967) *Virus and rickettsial diseases of man*, 4th ed., London, Arnold

Caccuri, S. & Pecora, L. (1965) *Porphyrins and professional diseases*. In: *International Symposium on Normal and Pathologic Metabolism of Porphyrins*, Torino, Minerva Medica, p. 23

Calhoun, J. B. (1963) *Population density and pathology*. In: Duhl, C. J., ed., *The urban condition*, New York, Basic Books

Cameron, M. P. & O'Connor, M., ed. (1964) *Brain—thyroid relationships* (CIBA Foundation Study Group No. 18), London, Churchill

Clements, C. D. & Holst, E. A. (1954) *Arch. Neurol. Psychiat. (Chic.)*, **71**, 66

Coursin, D. B. (1968) *Vitamin deficiencies and developing mental capacity.* In: Scrimshaw, N. S. & Gordon, J. E., ed., *Malnutrition, learning and behavior*, Cambridge, Mass., M.I.T. Press

Cravioto, J. (1968) *Nutritional deficiencies and mental performance in childhood.* In: Glass, D. C., ed., *Environmental influences*, New York, Rockefeller University Press, pp. 3-51

Crome, L. & Stern, J. (1967) *The pathology of mental retardation*, London, Churchill.

Davison, A. N. & Dobbing, J. (1968) *Applied neurochemistry*, Oxford, Blackwell Scientific Publications

De Matteis, F., Prior, B. E. & Rimington, C. (1961) *Nature (Lond.)*, **191**, 363

De Reuck, A. V. S. & Porter, R., ed. (1965) *Transcultural psychiatry*, London, Churchill

Eitinger, L. (1964) *Concentration camp survivors in Norway and Israel*, London, Allen

Ellenberger, H. F. (1965) *Ethno-psychiatrie.* In: *Encyclopédie médico-chirurgicale*, Paris, Encyclopédie médicochirurgicale (37725 A^{10} & 37725 B^{10})

Excerpta Medica Foundation (1968) *Toxicity and side-effects of psychotropic drugs*, Amsterdam

Faris, N. E. C. & Dunham, H. W. (1939) *Mental disorders in urban areas: an ecological study of schizophrenia and other psychoses*, Chicago, University of Chicago Press

Field, M. J. (1960) *Ethno-psychiatric study of rural Ghana*, London, Faber & Faber

Finney, J. C., ed. (1969) *Culture change, mental health and poverty*, Lexington, University of Kentucky Press

Freedman, A. M., Kaplan, H. I. & Kaplan, H. S., ed. (1967) *Comprehensive textbook of of psychiatry*, Baltimore, Williams & Wilkins

Häfner, H. & Reimann, H. (1970) *Spatial distribution of mental disorders in Mannheim, 1965.* In: Hare, E. H. & Wing, J. K., ed., *Psychiatric epidemiology: Proceedings of the International Symposium, Aberdeen, July 1969*, London, Oxford University Press, pp. 341-354

Haley, T. J. & Snider, R. S. (1964) *Response of the nervous system to ionizing radiation*, Boston, Little, Brown

Halliday, J. L. (1948) *Psychosocial medicine: a study of the sick society.* New York, W. W. Norton

Hansten, P. D. (1971) *Drug interactions*, Philadelphia, Lea & Febiger

Hare, E. H. (1965) *New Soc.*, **125**, 13

Kinneldorf, D. J. & Hunt, E. L. (1965) *Ionizing radiation: neural function and behavior*, New York, Academic Press

Kinneldorf, D. J. & Hunt, E. L. (1964) In: Haley, T. J. & Snider, R. S., ed., *Responses of the nervous system to ionizing radiation*, Boston, Little, Brown, p. 652

Lehmann, H. E. (1967) *Unusual psychiatric disorders and atypical psychoses.* In: Freedman, A. M. & Kaplan, H. I. & Kaplan, H. S., ed., *Comprehensive textbook of psychiatry*, Baltimore, Williams & Wilkins

Leighton, A. M. et al. (1963) *Psychiatric disorder among the Yoruba*, New York, Cornell University Press

Lemert, E. M. (1951) *Social pathology: a systematic approach to the theory of sociopathic behavior*, New York, McGraw-Hill

Lemkau, P. V. et al. (1971) *Epidemiološko ispitivanje psihoza u Hrvatskoj.* In: Peršić, N., ed., *Socijalna psihijatrija*, Zagreb, Pliva

Levi, L., ed. (1972) Stress and distress in response to psychosocial stimuli. *Acta med. scand.*, **191**, Suppl. 528

Lindzey, G. & Aronson, E., ed. (1968/69) *The handbook of social psychology*, Reading, Mass., Addison-Wesley

Lopašić, R. & Mikić, F. (1957) *Duševne poremetnje: Otok Susak*, Zagreb Jugoslovenska Akademija Znanosti i Umjetnosti

Malzberg, B. & Lee, E. S. (1956) *Migration and mental disease*, New York, Social Science Research Council

McIlwain, H. (1966) *Biochemistry and the central nervous system*, 3rd ed., London, Churchill

Murphy, H. B. M. et al. (1955) *Flight and resettlement*, Paris, UNESCO

Ockner, R. K. & Schmid, R. (1961) *Nature (Lond.)*, **189**, 449

Porter, R. & Birch, J. (1970) *Chemical influences on behaviour*, London, Churchill

Reid, D.D. (1960) *Epidemiological methods in the study of mental disorder*, Geneva, World Health Organization (*Publ. Hlth Pap.*, No. 2)

Reimann, H. A. (1963) *Periodic diseases*, Philadelphia, Davis

Richter, D. (1969) *The biochemistry of mental illness.* In: *The biological basis of medicine*, New York, Academic Press, pp. 11-139

Sams, C. F., Aird, R. B., Adams, G. D. & Ellimans, G. L. (1964) In: Haley, T. J. & Snider, R. S., ed., *Response of the nervous system to ionizing radiation*, Boston, Little, Brown, p. 554

Scrimshaw, N. S. & Gordon, J. E. (1968) *Malnutrition, learning and behavior*, Cambridge, Mass., M.I.T. Press

Selzer, M. L., Rogers, J. E. & Kern, S. (1968) *Amer. J. Psychiat.*, **124**, 1028-1036

Smyth, J. F., Jr (1956) *Amer. industr. Hyg. Ass. Quart.*, **17**, 129-185

Taylor, G. R. (1971) *The doomsday book*, Greenwich, Conn., Fawcett, p. 229

Taylor, S. J. C. & Chave, S. (1964) *Mental health and environment*, London, Longmans

Van Cleave, C. D. (1963) *Irradiation and the nervous system*, New York, Rowman & Littlefield

Weinberg, A. A. (1961) *Migration and belonging*, The Hague, Nijhoff

WHO Chronicle, 1971, **25**, 558-566

WHO Expert Committee on Mental Health (1959) *Mental problems of aging and the aged*, Geneva (*Wld Hlth Org. techn. Rep. Ser.*, No. 171)

WHO Expert Committee on Public Health Administration (1963) *Urban health services*, Geneva (*Wld Hlth Org. techn. Rep. Ser.*, No. 250)

WHO Scientific Group on Neurology (1969) *Report* (unpublished WHO document MH/70.6)

WHO Study Group on Mental Health Problems of Automation (1959) *Report*, Geneva (*Wld Hlth Org. techn. Rep. Ser.*, No. 183)

World Federation for Mental Health (1965a) *Industrialization and mental health: Proceedings of the 17th Annual Meeting, Berne, August 1964*, Geneva

World Federation for Mental Health (1965b) *Technical assistance, urbanization and social change*, Geneva

Yap, P. M. (1969) *The culture-bound reactive syndromes.* In: Caudill, W. & Lin, T., ed., *Mental health research in Asia and the Pacific,* Honolulu, East-West Center Press

Young, M. & Willmott, P. (1957) *Family and kinship in East London,* London, Routledge & Kegan Paul

PART II

CHEMICAL CONTAMINANTS
AND PHYSICAL HAZARDS

CHAPTER 11

LABORATORY TOXICITY TESTS

General Considerations

Toxic effects are undesirable disturbances of physiological function caused by poisons, though they may also be the side-effects of some medicines, vaccines, and agricultural, industrial, and other chemicals. As far as medicines are concerned, their acceptability is usually determined by balancing the adverse effects against the therapeutic results achieved.

A distinction must be made between toxicity and hazard. Toxicologists generally consider toxicity as the ability of a chemical to produce an unwanted effect when the chemical has reached a sufficient concentration at a certain site in the body; hazard is regarded as the probability that such an effect will occur. Many factors intervene in both situations: route of entry, dosage, physiological state, environmental variables, and many others. *Complete* non-toxicity and safety for man are fallacious concepts unless applied in a relative sense (Pfitzer, 1972), e.g., the ingestion of too much table salt can be toxic. Risk/benefit judgements for toxicity and hazard apply universally to chemicals, and only experience coupled with increased scientific research can supply the solid base on which such judgements need to be made (see also Chapter 32).

In screening a substance, it is necessary to carry out specific tests for every type of toxicity expected or feared, since all but the most overt effects will demand skilled and specialized investigation (Schubert, 1972). The decisions taken concerning possible environmental pollutants will therefore depend on the kinds of altered physiological response that are unacceptable to a particular community, and on the magnitude of the risk incurred. Thus a country might not be able to satisfy its public opinion unless it banned the use of any chemical that produced an unacceptable toxic effect at the highest dose at which it could be administered to an animal; another country urgently needing to rid itself of a pest or a disease vector, however, might consider that the prevention of death from starvation or disease would still far outweigh the disadvantages of the toxicity of the chemical concerned if it was applied in a way that put, say, only one in ten thousand of the population at risk. Screening programmes are arranged to quantify, if possible, obvious risks.

Because of the very large number of new chemical compounds being introduced into the environment, thorough tests on all of them are impracticable. For mutagenicity tests the use of submammalian test systems and *in vitro* cell cultures (even tests with human cells) should be regarded as ancillary procedures; and although results obtained with viruses and micro-organisms are often not directly relevant to mammals, they may shed light on basic molecular mechanisms (WHO Scientific Group on the Evaluation and Testing of Drugs for Mutagenicity: Principles and Problems, 1971; Hollaender, 1971). Particular attention should be paid to compounds chemically related to known toxic substances. For important chemicals widely used in pharmacy or in industry, tests on animals are essential.

There are obvious difficulties in extrapolating bioassay data from animals to human beings because of differences in species susceptibility, metabolism, and other factors. Neither the adequate bioassay of chemicals nor the surveillance of populations engaged in their manufacture can safeguard against unpredictable, rare, and sometimes serious adverse effects. Prospective surveillance studies on human populations may detect dangerous properties that remained undetected in laboratory testing (see Part III).

Laboratory Tests and their Significance

General aspects

In view of biological variations that influence the reaction to a foreign chemical in different species, it is difficult to duplicate in animal experiments the precise situation to which man may be exposed. Rigidly formulated regulations specifying in detail the test procedures to be performed in toxicological screening may be inadequate and misleading. However, agreement on the basic principles governing the testing of chemicals for their possible adverse effects is desirable, although much disagreement remains on this subject. Such principles should be periodically reviewed in the light of scientific and technological advances, in order not only to abolish unnecessary test procedures, but also to ensure that testing does not give an illusory or erroneous assurance of safety.

Toxicological screening should include both acute single-dose toxicity studies and studies of repeated administration at short intervals. Long-term studies performed during the life span of the animal, and in some instances—if indicated—over several generations, should be part of the complete test programme. The choice of animal is influenced by this programme. Mice, rats, and dogs are frequently used for such studies, but individual animals and species may differ widely in their response to chemicals and in the way in which they are absorbed, distributed, metabolized, and excreted. Early in the development of a specific test programme, preliminary studies are necessary to select species that absorb and metabolize the chemical in ways similar to man.

Acute toxicity studies

The aim of these studies is to define the range of lethal dose, and the effects on important physiological functions. The use of several routes of administration provides some important though preliminary data on the absorption and distribution of the chemical concerned. A route of administration different from that usually used in man, e.g., parenteral administration instead of inhalation or ingestion, may give very misleading results (see below).

Repeated administration

Repeated administration of test substances is practised in toxicity studies where a chemical is to be used over a period of time. Chronic toxicity can also be expected from a single exposure to a substance that remains in the organism for long periods, or indefinitely. Experience has shown that much information can be obtained from studies lasting 3–6 months, but decisions as to the exact duration of such studies must be left to the judgement of experienced investigators and/or national control authorities. Repeated administration is useful in the investigation of such problems as cumulative toxicity, tolerance, and enzyme induction phenomena.

Long-term toxicity studies

Tests of longer duration are necessary for the investigation of all chemicals, but particularly those that persist in the human environment. In addition, they are mandatory for the assessment of the carcinogenic properties of chemicals.

Maximum tolerable doses versus dose-response curves

A number of aspects of the performance and interpretation of screening tests call for some consideration.

The aim of the screening procedure may be to determine whether the compound under test can cause irreversible disease, such as cancer, or congenital abnormalities due either to defects occurring during development or to germ plasm mutations. Preliminary screening procedures may consist in tests on micro-organisms, or on cultured tissue cells or organs.

The screening procedure may then take one of two forms. In one procedure, the maximum tolerated dose for the experimental species would be determined in preliminary trials, and this dose would then be administered to a sufficient number of animals to discover whether undesirable effects occur; proponents of this scheme believe that the use of the compound should be prohibited if the incidence of undesirable effects is significantly greater than in control groups.

The alternative procedure is to dose groups of animals with gradually increasing amounts of the compound and to determine a dose-response curve that can be used to estimate the frequency of the undesirable effect at any dosage level experienced by man, e.g., from medicines; the data can then be extrapolated to dose levels resulting from environmental contamination.

As mentioned previously, whatever the procedure adopted, it should be applied to more than one species of animal, and the animals' metabolic profiles should resemble that of man as closely as possible.

The maximum tolerated dose method is the one most frequently used. Its use has been justified on the grounds that the dose-response curve cannot adequately be extrapolated to man to predict safe dosages, so that little is gained by carrying out the more extensive test procedure (US Department of Health, Education, and Welfare, 1969).

To examine the validity of this point, something must be said about the extrapolation of the dose-response curve. This curve describes the relation between the frequency of occurrence of an undesirable effect in a group of animals and the size of the dose given to each of these animals; its shape can be described in terms of any one of three theoretical models. If these different models are fitted to a set of data for frequencies at different doses, it is possible to estimate at what dose the frequency would be expected to have some acceptable low value, such as one in a million, or less. It has been suggested that the three theoretical models give such widely differing estimates of doses corresponding to these low frequencies that it is not possible to choose the right model for predicting a "safe" dose level (US Department of Health, Education, and Welfare, 1969).

There are a number of important points to be considered here. Firstly, the predictions of dosage level corresponding to a specified low frequency are always in the same ranking order for the three models, whatever the frequency specified. The probit model gives the highest frequency, and the so-called one-hit curve gives a lower estimate of safe dose. The safe strategy would be therefore always to use the "safe" dosage predicted by the one-hit curve.

Secondly, the divergence between the estimated "safe" doses depends very much on the steepness of the curves. The unfavourable conclusion previously mentioned was based on a curve in which the dose had to be increased about one hundred times to increase the frequency of the undesirable effect from 5 per hundred to 95 per hundred (US Department of Health, Education, and Welfare, 1969).[1] For the majority of power-fully toxic substances, the dose would have to be increased only about five-fold to produce this increase in frequency. The change from the low slope to the high one reduces the ratio of the probit estimate to the one-hit estimate of "safe" dose by a factor of 1000. (For further information on the probit model, see: World Health Organization, 1970.)

Dose-response curves have the great merit of showing clearly that the effects of poisons rarely decrease gradually as the dose level falls; they are more likely to decrease quite abruptly, so that at some point in the decreasing scale of dosage, often surprisingly close to that at which half the animals will be affected, it becomes unlikely that any effects of poisoning will be observed, except where synergism takes place.

It is, furthermore, a commonplace in medicine that some substances that are intensely toxic in high doses can be beneficial in lower doses, although this is not observed in the case of man-made chemicals in the environment. However, it is useful to cite an instance where a substance that is of positive benefit can be made to look as though it were unacceptably toxic. The amino-acid leucine is an essential constituent of the diet of all vertebrates in which it has been tested, and an adult rat requires 150–200 mg/kg per day. If 15 mg/kg per day are injected intraperitoneally into pregnant rats, however, a high proportion of abnormal fetuses is produced (Persaud, 1969). It is not possible to ban leucine on the basis of this evidence; we cannot live without it, and neither can the pregnant rat.

This example indicates that observations of a toxic effect consequent on an abnormal route of administration of a substance may not constitute an acceptable basis for a judgement regarding the safety of that substance; it also helps to support the view that it may not always be sound to extra-polate from the effects of a maximally tolerated dose of any toxic agent in order to estimate the magnitude or even the nature of the hazard at lower doses. It is most desirable, therefore, that dose-response curves should be established as part of the testing of compounds for undesirable effects, and that careful extrapolations should be made from such curves in order to establish whether the effects could constitute an environmental hazard.

The cost of determining a dose-response curve with sufficient accuracy is much greater than that of performing a maximum tolerable dose screening operation, but such curves provide much more information, and form a better basis for comparisons between species. Full dose-response relation-ships should be required as part of the assessment of the safety of important agricultural, industrial, or other chemicals.

Final tests on suspected carcinogens, as mentioned previously, require long-term observations. It must be realized that the evaluation of car-

---

[1] This report is mainly concerned with tests of pesticides for carcinogenic action. Both this subject and the safety evaluation of food additives are dealt with in: US Food and Drug Administration (1971).

cinogenic hazards is different from other toxicological exercises, and that the determination of zero hazard is impossible.   The problem is complicated because of lack of information on the factors involved in co-carcinogenesis and anti-carcinogenesis (Falk, 1971).

Even assuming it were possible to extrapolate from a specific strain of mouse to all species including man, taking into consideration such factors as weight, surface area, metabolic profiles, genetic susceptibilities, and lack of idiosyncrasies, and accounting for differences in age, inter-current disease, and drug-induced changes in metabolism, it might still not be possible to reach justifiable conclusions because of the existence of synergism.   One of the best examples is the effect of cigarette smoking on the lung: the synergistic action of unknown components increases many times over the carcinogenic activity of trace amounts of polycyclic hydro-carbon and other carcinogens.

In the laboratory the augmentation of effects of common carcinogens by common promoters has been studied in some detail, and can be as great as 1000-fold.   It may therefore be inappropriate to use the best fitting curve to extrapolate to the limit of the hazard for man, if the ubiquitous existence of co-carcinogenesis is ignored.

Summary

In summary, toxic effects must be viewed from many angles: the nature and interpretation of laboratory tests in animals, about which much controversy remains; the validity of extrapolation of results of such tests to man; observations on man himself of the total body burden of substances derived from many sources and correlation with toxic effects, although such data are often hard to obtain (see Part III); and, finally, the risk/benefit ratio selected by the authorities concerned, which may vary widely from country to country.   Balanced judgements with regard to all these factors are often very difficult to make, and will remain so until much more knowledge accrues.   The inadequacy of our information on many of these points is reflected in the chapters that follow.

REFERENCES

Falk, H. L. (1971) *Progr. exp. Tumor Res. (Basel)*, **14**, 105-137

Hollaender, A., ed. (1971) *Chemical mutagens*, New York, Plenum Press

Persaud, T. V. (1969) *Naturwissenschaften*, **56**, 37-38

Pfitzer, E. A. (1972).   In: Lee, D. H. K., ed., *Metallic contaminants in human health*, New York and London, Academic Press, pp. 1-14

Schubert, J. (1972) *Ambio*, **1**, 79-89

US Department of Health, Education, and Welfare (1969) *Secretary's Commission on Pesticides and their Relationship to Environmental Health.   Report*, Washington, D.C., US Government Printing Office

US Food and Drug Administration, Advisory Committee on Protocols for Safety Evaluation, Panel on Carcinogenesis (1971) *Toxicol. appl. Pharmacol.*, **20**, 419-438

WHO Scientific Group on the Evaluation and Testing of Drugs for Mutagenicity: Principles and Problems (1971) *Report*, Geneva (*Wld Hlth Org. techn. Rep. Ser.*, No. 482)

World Health Organization (1970) *Health aspects of chemical and biological weapons*, Geneva, pp. 85-86

CHAPTER 12

SELECTED ENVIRONMENTAL POLLUTANTS

A number of environmental pollutants have already been discussed in the context of air, water, and food (Chapters 1, 2, and 3). A few of them have been selected for further study in this chapter in order to illustrate better the circumstances under which certain substances become environmental pollutants; how different pollutants behave in the environment; and how their physicochemical properties and toxicity characteristics determine their pollution potential. The emphasis in this chapter is on the principal sources of intake, on the observed body burdens, and on known and suspected effects on the community at large of low-level, long-term exposure. The mechanism of biological action is indicated, together with the early physiological and biochemical signs of excessive exposure. Data on acute toxicity obtained from animal experiments are omitted, because they are usually of little relevance in predicting the possible effects of long-term, low level exposure to environmental pollutants.

Because of space constraints, only the highlights of this extensive subject can be dealt with here. Sources of further information are indicated in the lists of selected references at the end of each section.

Arsenic

Arsenic occurs in almost all soils in small amounts. It is also found in variable quantities in natural waters, depending on geographical location. Air also contains arsenic, but usually in very small concentrations (see Chapter 1).

Environmental pollution by arsenic may arise from agricultural practices (weed-killers, fungicides, sheep dips, rodenticides, insecticides), and from industry. Arsenic in topsoils is exposed to atmospheric oxygen and is usually present in pentavalent form. Industrially produced arsenic is in the more toxic trivalent form (Schroeder & Balassa, 1966).

Arsenic may be present in small amounts in drinking-water, and a tentative limit of 0.05 mg/l is recommended by WHO (*International Standards for Drinking-Water*, 1971). Organic arsenic was detected in shrimps as long ago as 1935 in amounts of 42–174 mg/kg. There is some controversy as to whether organic or inorganic arsenic compounds are the more toxic (US Consumers Union, 1972; *Chem. Engng News*, 1971).

Arsenic is not an essential element for human physiology, but it is regularly found in human tissues in very small quantities.

Arsenic is a cumulative, potent, protoplasmic poison that inhibits SH-groups in enzymes. The salts are readily absorbed from the gastrointestinal tract, but elemental arsenic is not. Arsenic is also absorbed through the lungs and skin.

In short-term and long-term studies in experimental animals, a variety of arsenic compounds have been administered orally or by inhalation. The results have generally paralleled the toxic reactions seen in man (Bencko & Symon, 1969a, 1969b, 1970; Bencko et al., 1968; Bencko, 1972).

Chronic poisoning leads to loss of appetite and weight, diarrhoea alternating with constipation, gastrointestinal disturbance, peripheral neuritis, conjunctivitis, hyperkeratosis and melanosis of the skin, and sometimes skin cancer (Browning, 1969).

In 1900 in Manchester and Liverpool, some 7000 clinical cases of subacute poisoning and 70 deaths were attributed to the consumption of beer containing more than 15 mg/litre of arsenic (Kelynack et al., 1900).

Arsenic poisoning has been observed in wine-growers (Roth, 1957). Autopsies on wine-growers have shown that chronic poisoning progresses, even if no more arsenic can be found in the body. Late stages are characterized by skin changes, especially severe hyperkeratosis, necrotic cirrhosis of the liver, and an unusually high incidence of malignant tumours of the skin and internal organs (e.g., liver, lung, bile ducts, and oesophagus). Chronic exposure to arsenic from water in certain geographical areas has been referred to in Chapter 2.

Arsenic is usually considered carcinogenic for man, although various factory studies have produced conflicting data. It produces lung and skin cancer, depending on the type of contact (Lee & Fraumeni, 1969; Snegireff & Lombard, 1951; Tseng et al., 1968). It is of interest that similar results have not been obtained in experimental bioassays in animals.

At present, arsenic is not considered as an environmental pollutant of more than local significance (Smith, 1972).

REFERENCES

Bencko, V. (1972) *J. Hyg. Epidem. (Praha)*, **16** (1)

Bencko, V., Nejedlý, K. & Somora, J. (1968) *Čs. Hyg.* **13**, 344-347

Bencko, V. & Symon, K. (1969a) *J. Hyg. Epidem. (Praha)*, **13**, 248-253

Bencko, V. & Symon, K. (1969b) *J. Hyg. Epidem. (Praha)*, **13**, 1-6

Bencko, V. & Symon, K. (1970) *Atmosph. Environm.*, **4**, 157-161

Browning, E. (1969) *Toxicity of industrial metals*, London, Butterworth

Chem. Engng News, 1971, July 5, pp. 22-34

International Standards for Drinking-Water, 1971, 3rd ed., Geneva, World Health Organization

Kelynack, T. N., Kirkby, W. & Delépine, S. (1900) *Lancet*, **2**, 1600-1602

Lee, A. M. & Fraumeni, J. F., Jr. (1969) *J. nat. Cancer Inst.*, **42**, 1045-1052

Roth, F. (1957) *Germ. med. Mth.*, **2**, 172-175

Schroeder, H. A. & Balassa, J. J. (1966) *J. chron. Dis.*, **19**, 85-106

Smith, R. G. (1972) In: Lee, D. H. K., ed., *Metallic contaminants and human health*, New York & London, Academic Press

Snegireff, L. S. & Lombard, L. M. (1951) *A.M.A. Arch. industr. Hyg.*, **4**, 199-205

Tseng, W. P., Chu, H. M., How, S. W., Fong, J. M., Lin, C. S. & Shu Yeh (1968) *J. nat. Cancer Inst.*, **40**, 453-463

US Consumers Union (1972) *Consumer reports*, January

Cadmium

Cadmium is not essential for the human body. It is present in the soil, in vegetation, and in man's food. It enters the human environment as a contaminant from mining and metallurgy, chemical industries, scrap metal treatment, electroplating, superphosphate fertilizers, and cadmium-containing pesticides. Cadmium is accumulated in certain marine animals, but very little is known about environmental transformations. Human intake of cadmium is chiefly through the food chain—about 40 μg/day. Analysis of necropsy material shows that smokers accumulate much more cadmium than non-smokers (Lewis et al., 1972). Cadmium metal is soluble in acid solutions encountered in many food products containing organic acids. (For environmental levels of cadmium, see Chapters 1, 2, and 3.)

The total body burden of the average man is about 30 mg, about a third in the kidney and a sixth in the liver. The quantity in liver increases shortly after exposure. The kidney burden increases with age (Friberg et al., 1971).

Chronic cadmium poisoning produces proteinuria and affects the proximal tubules of the kidney, causing the formation of kidney stones (Kazantzis et al., 1963). Administration of cadmium to laboratory animals has demonstrated that the element accumulates in the kidney (Axelsson & Piscator, 1966). The toxic effect on the mammalian testis has been well established since it was first observed by Parízek & Záhor (1956). The toxic effects of cadmium have been attributed to its action on the sulfhydryl groups of essential enzymes (Granata et al., 1970).

Zinc appears to give some protection against the toxic effects of cadmium. The reported hypertensive effect of cadmium in man has been associated with a high cadmium/zinc ratio in kidneys (Schroeder et al., 1967). Two studies (Caroll, 1966; Hickey et al., 1967) on air pollution have shown that the cadmium concentration in air is positively correlated with heart disease, hypertension, and arteriosclerosis. There is, however, some doubt regarding these correlation studies (Friberg et al., 1971).

A specific disease, observed in Toyama City in Japan, has been attributed to cadmium. The epidemic was related to exposure to cadmium released from a nearby mining complex, resulting in contamination of water and rice paddies. It is known as "itai-itai" (ouch-ouch) disease because of the painful symptoms from multiple fractures arising from osteomalacia. It appears to be largely confined to post-menopausal women who have experienced several deliveries, and this suggests that other factors besides cadmium are involved. Initial symptoms are lumbar pains and myalgia in the legs. Later, skeletal deformation takes place, with marked decrease in body height, proteinuria, and glaucoma. There is an increase in serum-alkaline phosphatase, and a decrease in inorganic phosphorus. In the terminal stage, multiple fractures occur after very mild exertion, such as coughing (Murata et al., 1970). Histological findings at autopsy are similar to those associated with osteomalacia (Kono et al., 1961). Hereditary (Dent & Harris, 1956) and dietary factors, such as vitamin D deficiency (Toyama Prefectural Health Authorities, 1956), may help to induce this disease. The disease follows a prolonged course, perhaps lasting more than 12 years. It is estimated that 100 deaths due to the disease have occurred over the past 35 years (Friberg et al., 1971). There was no means of establishing the total amount of cadmium in the victims' diet, but it seems that the chronic dose capable of causing the disease was much higher than the estimated daily intake (0.6 mg per day) of the inhabitants in the affected areas in Fuchu-cho in 1969 (Yamagata & Shigematsu, 1970).

There is some evidence that cadmium may be carcinogenic to experimental animals. It has been implicated in human prostate carcinoma (Kipling & Waterhouse, 1967).

REFERENCES

Axelsson, B. & Piscator, M. (1966) *Arch. environm. Hlth*, **12**, 360

Caroll, R. E. (1966) *J. Amer. med. Ass.*, **198**, 267

Dent, C. E. & Harris, H. (1956) *J. Bone Jt Surg.*, **38**, 204

Friberg, L., Piscator, M. & Nordberg, G. (1971) *Cadmium in the environment*, Stockholm, Karolinska Institute

Granata, A., Barbaro, M. & Maturo, L. (1970) *Arch. Mal. prof.*, **31**, 357-364

Hickey, R. G., Schoff, E. P. & Clelland, R. C. (1967) *Arch. environm. Hlth*, **15**, 728

Kazantzis, G., Flynn, F. V., Spowage, J. S. & Trott, D. G. (1963) *Quart. J. Med.*, **32**, 165

Kipling, M. D. & Waterhouse, J. A. H. (1967) *Lancet*, **1**, 730

Kono, M. et al. (1961) *Seikei Geka (Tokyo)*, **12**, 405

Lewis, G. P., Jusko, W. S., Coughlin, L. L. & Hartz, S. (1972) *Lancet*, **1**, 291

Murata, I., Hirano, T., Saeki, Y. & Nakagawa, S. (1970) *Bull. Soc. int. Chir.*, **1**, 34

Pařízek, J. & Záhoř, Z. (1956) *Nature*, **177**, 1036

Schroeder, H. A., Mason, A. P., Tyston, I. H. & Balassa, J. J. (1967) *J. chron. Dis.*, **20**, 179

Toyama Prefectural Health Authorities (1956) *Survey 1955-56.* Cited in: Friberg et al. (1971), pp. 8-14

Yamagata, N. & Shigematsu, J. (1970) *Koshu-Eisei-In-Kenkyu-Hokoku, Bull. Inst. publ. Hlth*, **19**, 1-27

Lead

Hazards of industrial exposure to lead are well documented, but the significance of general community exposure to lead in the environment has been a controversial subject for a number of years. The concentration of lead in soil, food, water, and air is highly variable, but the total body burden of lead found in man appears to vary within the comparatively narrow limits of 100–400 mg (Smith, 1966).

Lead occurs naturally in plants and in soils throughout the world (8–20 mg/kg in virgin soils, up to 300 mg/kg in cultivated areas), and has always been present in man's environment. Man-made sources include lead smelting and refining, brass manufacture, the combustion of leaded fuels, the production of storage batteries, the manufacture of alkyl lead and lead paints, and the agricultural application of lead arsenate, the burning of lead-painted surfaces and the incineration of leaded plastics and other material. Lead-glazed earthenware (particularly when used for cooking) and flaking lead paints in old houses are possible sources of lead exposure in the domestic environment.

High lead contents (up to 1000 mg/kg or more) have been found in soils near industrial sources such as lead smelters and storage battery works and in roadside dust in the vicinity of heavy traffic.

Lead is added to automobile fuel in organic form (tetraethyl or tetramethyl lead) as an "antiknock" agent. It is released into the air, principally as inorganic lead salts and oxides, in aerosol form. Measurements in England on main roads in urban areas have shown monthly or quarterly averages of 2.5–4.5 $\mu g/m^3$ (Bullock & Lewis, 1968); in nearby areas with comparatively little traffic, the concentrations were not more than 0.25–1.2 $\mu g/m^3$. Daily averages were sometimes as high as 24 $\mu g/m^3$ on busy highways, which is comparable to values observed near lead smelting plants. In most cities covered by the US National Air Surveillance Networks, the annual averages in the 1957-1966 period ranged from 1–3 $\mu g/m^3$, in non-urban stations from 0.1–0.5 $\mu g/m^3$ (Committee on Biologic Effects of Atmospheric Pollutants, 1971). Short-term averages recorded in the United States during rush hours on roads with dense traffic were occasionally as high as 50 $\mu g/m^3$ (Working Group on Lead Contamination, 1965). In addition to being a source of immediate inhalation exposure, airborne lead is important for the environmental transport of the pollutant to other areas and media.

The lead content in most waters is well below the tentative limit for lead in drinking-water of 0.1 mg/litre (*International Standards for Drinking-Water*, 1971), and ranges from 1 to 10 µg/litre. Problems exist, however, in areas with soft, slightly acid water, which may dissolve lead from the lead pipes that are still used in many community water supplies. In areas where plumbosolvency exists, the lead intake from water supplies may contribute an appreciable amount of the total intake.

The average content of lead in food is about 0.2 mg/kg (Schroeder et al., 1961; Warren & Delavault, 1962). This has been confirmed by an extensive survey of the lead contents of British foods involving over 3000 separate analyses. Average levels of 0.17 mg/kg were found in cereals, 0.17 mg/kg in meat and fish, 0.08 mg/kg in fish alone, 0.08 mg/kg in fats, 0.12 mg/kg in fruits and preserves, 0.20 mg/kg in root vegetables, 0.24 mg/kg in green vegetables, and 0.03 mg/kg in milk (Working Party on the Monitoring of Foodstuffs for Mercury and other Heavy Metals, 1972). According to some authors, the levels of lead in milk have risen slightly over the past 20–30 years (Lewis, 1966), but there is no convincing evidence of any real increase in dietary lead during recent decades.

The major source of intake of lead in adults who are not occupationally exposed is food. It has been estimated that the dietary intake averages about 300 µg per day, with a range of 100–500 µg per day (Committee on Biologic Effects of Atmospheric Pollutants, 1971; Joint FAO/WHO Expert Committee on Food Additives, 1967). The average daily intake in drinking-water is about 20 µg (Committee on Biologic Effects of Atmospheric Pollutants, 1971), with a range of 10–100 µg (Working Group on Lead Contamination, 1965). The dietary intake of children aged 1–3 years is about 140–200 µg per day (King, 1971). Only a fraction of the lead ingested in the diet is absorbed. For adults, the absorption from the gastrointestinal tract over long periods of time averages about 5–10 %, if intakes are not excessive (Kehoe, 1961). Faecal output of lead provides a good estimate of the dietary intake, since about 90 % of lead is excreted in this way (Kehoe, 1961).

The contribution of airborne lead to the total daily absorption is more difficult to estimate. The concentration is not the only significant parameter to be considered; the particle size distribution and the solubility of lead in airborne particles must also be taken into account. For a typical airborne lead concentration of 2 µg/m³, and assuming 30 % respiratory deposition, the absorption would be about 14 µg per day. However, this may be an overestimate. Recent work by Lawther et al. (1972) indicates that the particles of lead emitted in motor vehicle fumes are much smaller than was previously thought, and they are aggregated, probably on carbon filaments. Even these aggregates are so small (mostly of the order of 0.1 µm) that the amount retained in the alveoli will probably be less than 10 %. Solubility tests showed that the lead was in a very insoluble form.

Although all organs contain some lead, about 90 % is found in the skeleton (Engel et al., 1971). Blood contains slightly less than 1 %. The lead level in blood is influenced by recent intake (e.g., during the first 24 h) and by release of lead from the skeletal system. Individuals with a low level of exposure have 10–30 µg of lead per 100 g of blood. Highly exposed individuals often have more than 100 µg per 100 g of blood. Blood levels of 40 µg per 100 g or more are considered excessive and indicative of undue absorption of lead, even if no symptoms are detected. A survey in the United States of the lead content in the blood and urine in three urban areas showed that only 4 of 2342 individuals had blood levels equal to or in excess of 60 µg per 100 g. There was a definite gradation in lead levels between urban and rural areas. Women tended to show lower levels than men, and smokers slightly higher levels than non-smokers (Working Group on Lead Contamination, 1965). Statistically significant differences of lead in blood between rural and urban populations have been observed in other countries as well (Vouk et al., 1955). These findings are in general agreement with those of a study carried out in co-operation with WHO (Goldwater & Hoover, 1967), which examined the results of blood and urinary lead determinations in 15 countries throughout the world. Another conclusion of the WHO study was that these levels did not change significantly in three decades. All were below levels bordering on lead intoxication.

Although symptoms of clinical lead poisoning in adult individuals do not appear at levels in the whole blood below about 80 µg per 100 g,[1] the inhibition of certain enzymes involved in the synthesis of haem can be shown to occur at lower levels, starting with δ-aminolaevulinic acid dehydratase (cf. Waldron, 1966). Epidemiological evidence suggests that such inhibition is demonstrable at lead blood levels considered to be within "normal" limits, i.e., < 30–40 µg per 100 g (Hernberg & Nikkanen, 1970). Various other tests are also used as indicators of lead absorption (De Bruin & Hoolboom, 1967; Nakao et al., 1968; Lane, 1968).

Lead accumulates in hair, providing a convenient indicator for estimating lead exposure or body burden (Kopito et al., 1967). Radiography in young children may reveal excessive storage of lead in the form of bands of increased density at the metaphysis of the long bones (cf. Goyer & Chisholm, 1972). Russian workers have reported changes in conditioned reflexes at low levels of exposure to lead (Gusev, 1960).

Young children in some urban and industrial areas represent high-risk groups with respect to environmental, non-occupational exposure to lead. Mass screening programmes in New York and Chicago showed that 1–2 % of the children in low-income areas had blood levels indicative of lead poisoning; a further 25 % had levels above 40 µg per 100 g (Blanksma

---

[1] In children the levels may be lower (Bradley et al., 1956).

et al., 1969; Hunt et al., 1971). Direct ingestion of lead pigment paints is no doubt the main source of exposure. Industrial emissions and the ingestion of roadside dust are other possible sources. A recent study in London showed that 40.9 % of children living within 100–400 m of a lead factory had blood lead levels over 40 µg per 100 g; at a range of 400–500 m the figure was 13.7 %. Raised blood levels are also found in children of lead workers—"take home" lead on hair and underclothing in spite of complete changing and showering facilities (E. Martin, personal communication, 1972).

The possibility of a causal relationship between lead absorption and mental retardation has been suggested, but some investigations of blood levels in mentally handicapped children have not confirmed this (Gordon et al., 1967). However, acute encephalopathy in young children is followed by permanent neurological consequences in at least 25 % of cases (Byers, 1959; Chisholm & Harrison, 1956).

Organic lead compounds are primarily neurotoxic and cause no anaemia. Most of the tetraethyl lead in petrol is converted to inorganic lead in the process of combustion. Some tetraethyl lead may escape into the atmosphere as a result of evaporation from the carburettor or from spillage, but the amounts in the atmosphere will probably be small (G.J. Stopps, unpublished data, 1968); there is little information on the actual concentrations in air. No evidence exists that lead alkyl compounds are synthesized in nature, as are the corresponding mercury compounds (Goyer & Chisholm, 1972).

The significance of the present average lead body burden to human health is not known but watch must be kept for possible long-term effects. Lead bound in bone seems not to be toxic but in certain cases it may be released by infection or biochemical stress and produce overt signs.

Lead salts are not carcinogenic to man. In the rat, they produce kidney tumours (Van Esch & Kroes, 1969), and tetraethyl lead may cause hepatomas in young mice (Epstein & Mantel, 1968).

REFERENCES

Blanksma, L. A., Sachs, H. K., Murray, E. F. & O'Connell, M. J. (1969) *Pediatrics*, **44**, 661-667

Bradley, J. E., Powell, A. E., Nierman, W., McGrady, K. R. & Kaplan, E. (1956) *J. Pediat.*, **49**, 1-6

Bullock, J. & Lewis, W. M. (1968) *Atmosph. Environm.*, **2**, 517

Byers, R. K. (1959) *Pediatrics*, **23**, 585-603

Chisholm, J. J., Jr & Harrison, H. E. (1956) *Pediatrics*, **18**, 948-957

Committee on Biologic Effects of Atmospheric Pollutants (1971) *Airborne lead in perspective*, Washington, D. C., National Academy of Science, National Research Council

De Bruin, A. & Hoolboom, H. (1967) *Brit. J. industr. Med.*, **24**, 203

Engel, R. E., Hammer, D. I., Horton, R. J. M., Lane, N. M. & Plumlee, L. A. (1971) *Environmental lead and public health*, Research Triangle Park, N. C., US Environmental Protection Agency

Epstein, S. & Mantel, N. (1968) *Experientia*, **1**, 580-581

Goldwater, L. J. & Hoover, A. W. (1967) *Arch. environm. Hlth*, **15**, 60-63

Gordon, N., King, E. & Mackay, R. I. (1967) *Brit. med. J.*, **2**, 480

Goyer, R. A. & Chisholm, J. J. (1972). In: Lee, D. H. K., ed., *Metallic contaminants and human health*, New York & London, Academic Press

Gusev, M. I. (1960) [*Maximum permissible concentration of lead in the air of inhabited areas*]. In: Rjazanov, V. A., ed. [*Maximum permissible concentrations of atmospheric pollutants*], vol. 4, Moscow, Medgiz

Hernberg, S. & Nikkanen, J. (1970) *Lancet*, **1**, 63

Hunt, W. F., Jr, Pinkerton, C., McNulty, O. & Creason, J. P. (1971) *A study in trace element pollution of air in seventy-seven mid-western cities*. In: Hemphill, D. D., ed., *Trace substances in environmental health, IV*, New York, Columbia University

International Standards for Drinking-Water, 1971, 3rd ed., Geneva, World Health Organization

Joint FAO/WHO Expert Committee on Food Additives (1967) *Tenth report*, Geneva (*Wld Hlth Org. techn. Rep. Ser.*, No. 373)

Kehoe, R. A. (1961) *Pure appl. Chem.*, **3**, 129-144

King, B. G. (1971) *Amer. J. Dis. Childh.*, **122**, 337

Kopito, L., Byers, R. K. & Schwachman, H. (1967) *New Engl. J. Med.*, **276**, 949

Lane, R. E. (1968) *Brit. med. J.*, **4**, 501

Lawther, P. J., Cummins, B. T., McK. Ellison, J. & Biler, B. (1972) *Airborne lead and its uptake by inhalation*. In: *Proceedings of a Conference on Lead in the Environment, London, January 1972* (in preparation)

Lewis, K. H. (1966) *The diet as a source of lead*. In: *Symposium on Environmental Lead Contamination*, Washington, D.C., US Department of Health, Education, and Welfare (USPHS Publication No. 1440)

Nakao, K., Wade, O. & Yano, Y. (1968) *Clin. chim. Acta*, **19**, 319-325

Schroeder, H. A., Balassa, J. J., Gibson, F. S., Valanju, S. N., Brattleboro, V. & Hanover, N. H. (1961) *J. chron. Dis.*, **14**, 408-425

Smith, H. A. (1966) *How sensitive and how appropriate are our current standards of normal and safe body content of lead*. In: *Symposium on Environmental Lead Contamination*, Washington, D.C., US Department of Health, Education, and Welfare (USPHS Publication No. 1440)

Van Esch, G. J. & Kroes, R. (1969) *Brit. J. Cancer*, **23**, 765

Vouk, V. B., Voloder, K., Weber, O. A. & Purec, L. (1955) *Arch. hig. rada.*, **6**, 277-287

Waldron, H. A. (1966) *Brit. J. industr. Med.*, **23**, 83-100

Warren, H. V. & Delavault, R. E. (1962) *J. Sci. Food Agric.*, **13**, 96-98

Working Group on Lead Contamination (1965) *Survey of lead in the atmosphere of three urban communities*, Cincinnati, Ohio, US Public Health Service, Division of Air Pollution

Working Party on the Monitoring of Foodstuffs for Mercury and other Heavy Metals (1972) *Survey of lead in food*, London, HM Stationery Office

Mercury

The health effects of mercury in certain population groups (through occupational exposure or therapeutic application) have been recognized for many years, but the concern with mercury as a general environmental contaminant is new (cf. Study Group on Mercury Hazards, 1971; Friberg & Vestal, 1971; Wood, 1971).

Mercury occurs naturally in the human environment; annual erosion and weathering are estimated to contribute some 5000 tons to the sea. Another 4000–5000 tons of mined mercury (about half the annual world production of 9000 tons) are lost to sea, soil and the atmosphere (Goldberg, 1970). Man-made sources of mercury include mining and refining processes, chlorine-alkali plants, pulp and paper, plastics and electronics industries, hospitals, agricultural practice, and drugs. Burning of fossil fuels appears to add large quantities of mercury to the environment (Grant, 1971).

Mercury is discharged into the environment as metallic mercury, as inorganic mercury compounds, or as alkyl, alkoxy, aryl or other organic mercury compounds. Once in the environment, mercury compounds are capable of a variety of transformations. It has recently been recognized that inorganic mercury can be transformed under certain conditions into methylmercury and dimethylmercury by the action of micro-organisms, particularly in sediments. Some recent laboratory studies have confirmed the non-enzymatic and enzymatic methylation of mercury (Wood, 1971). Methylmercury can enter food chains through uptake by aquatic plants, algae, low forms of animal life, and fish (Jensen & Jernelöv, 1969; Larsson, 1970). The concentration factor in fish may exceed 3000. Methylmercury compounds are much more toxic compared with all other forms of mercury and it is therefore important to know the fraction of the total mercury in the diet that exists in the methylmercury form.

Concentrations of mercury in air are low; in large industrial cities 24-hour averages may approach 1 $\mu g/m^3$ (United States Environmental Protection Agency, 1971), but are usually much lower. Mercury concentrations in surface sea-water are about 0.1 $\mu g/litre$ (Food and Agriculture Organization, 1971), in rain-water about 0.5 $\mu g/litre$ (Study Group on Mercury Hazards, 1971), and in surface waters generally below 1 $\mu g/litre$ (*International Standards for Drinking-Water*, 1971). Insufficient information is available to ascertain what proportion of mercury in water or other environmental media is in the form of methylmercury.

The estimation of the total amount of mercury that the human organism is likely to take up through air, water, and food poses many problems. Food seems to be the major source of intake. Levels of mercury in different food items are very variable (Study Group on Mercury Hazards, 1971). Samples of Japanese rice have been found to contain as much as 200–1000 $\mu g/kg$

(Smart, 1968); Swedish chicken eggs examined in 1966 contained about 0.02 μg of mercury per g of egg white (Westöö, 1969). The total mercury content of total diet samples examined in the United Kingdom was generally below 5 μg/kg; in fish, however, values up to 200 μg/kg were found (Working Party on the Monitoring of Foodstuffs for Mercury and other Heavy Metals, 1971). The expected mercury intake from average diets, over a considerable period of time, is about 10 μg per day (United States Environmental Protection Agency, 1971); but diets containing contaminated fish may lead to the intake of 30 μg per day or higher, much more than the intake from water and air. Increased levels are consistently found in fish where the water is contaminated with mercury from industrial and mining processes. The methylmercury to total mercury ratio is often high, particularly when the total mercury level itself is high. In fish from unpolluted waters, which comprise most of world's main fishing areas, mercury levels are generally low.

The level in the blood is considered to be a good indicator of the quantity of mercury in the body. The concentrations in the blood reported to be associated with identifiable symptoms are 20–60 μg/100 ml (Berglund & Berlin, 1969; Berglund et al., 1971; Hammond, 1971). It is estimated that a steady daily intake of about 0.3–1.0 mg of mercury for a 70-kg man would result in this level.

The Joint FAO/WHO Expert Committee on Food Additives (1972) assessed the lowest Hg levels at the onset of poisoning in adults with neurological involvement as 50 mg per g hair and 0.4 mg per g blood cells. The Committee set the provisional tolerable weekly intake at 0.3 mg total Hg, of which no more than 0.2 mg should be in the form of methylmercury.

Absorption in the organism depends on the chemical form of the mercury. For inorganic compounds, such as mercuric chloride and mercuric acetate, the absorption of dietary mercury is about 2 % and 50 % respectively (Fitzhugh et al., 1950). For phenylmercury, the absorption may range from 50–80%, and for methylmercury it may exceed 90 % (Fitzhugh et al., 1950; Berglund & Berlin, 1969). The metabolism of organic mercury compounds also depends on the chemical form. There are marked differences in the metabolism and excretion of alkyl and aryl mercury compounds. The rate of conversion of organic compounds to inorganic mercury is an important factor in their tissue distribution and excretion. Because of their non-polar nature, alkylmercury compounds easily pass biological membranes and are distributed throughout the body (Wood, 1971). According to Suzuki and his collaborators (1967), the concentration of mercury in brain tissue required to produce clinical effects is of the order of 20 μg/g. The passage of organomercury compounds across the placenta and their concentration in the fetus presents a special problem.

Mercury combines with sulfhydryl groups; for this reason, soluble mercuric salts are toxic to all cells. The high concentrations attained during renal excretion lead to specific damage to renal glomeruli and tubules.

There is some evidence that in certain plants and *Drosophila* organic mercury can produce genetic mutations and chromosomal aberrations, but the significance of this for man is difficult to assess (cf. Study Group on Mercury Hazards, 1971). The same applies to chromosomal aberrations observed in a limited group of individuals with high blood levels of mercury (Skerfving et al., 1970).

The first reported major incident of mercury poisoning arising from the discharge of industrial wastes occurred in the Minamata Bay area in Japan. The first case of an unidentified disease of the central nervous system was noticed in April 1956. By February 1971 the total number of cases was 121, including 22 cases of congenital Minamata disease (M. Hashimoto, personal communication, 1972). It was ascertained that the disease was caused by methylmercury—a waste product of the acetaldehyde manufacturing process in which an inorganic mercury catalyst is used—contained in plant effluent and polluted water. The methylmercury was present in the water at an undetectably low level, but was taken up by fish and shellfish and biologically concentrated (Study Group on Minamata Disease, 1968). In some instances the concentration of mercury (as total mercury) in fish and shellfish exceeded 10 mg/kg. Minamata disease occurred among heavy fish eaters, mostly in fishermen's families. Twenty-two infants with cerebral involvement (palsy and retardation) were born to mothers who had ingested methylmercury fish protein, which indicates that there was transplacental fetal damage. Since the mothers were mostly symptom-free, this may point to preferential concentration in the fetus. Minamata disease was again reported in 1964-65 in the area of the Agano river, Niigata Prefecture, Japan; this time 49 persons were affected, of whom 6 died (Tsuchiya, 1969; M. Hashimoto, personal communication, 1972).

The use of mercury compounds in agriculture is the second major aspect of environmental pollution by mercury. As reported by Smart (1968) the use of mercury pesticides in the world amounts to about 2000 metric tons a year. A variety of inorganic and organic (alkyl-, alkoxy-, and aryl-) mercury compounds have been used to treat seed potatoes, flower bulbs, and especially grain seed (wheat, rice, barley, oats, etc.). Several outbreaks of poisoning have been described as a consequence of such use of mercury compounds. Several hundred persons have become poisoned and many have died in Guatemala, Iraq, and Pakistan, following the consumption of treated seed (Ordóñez et al., 1966; Jalili & Abbasi, 1961; Haq, 1963). More recently (1971-1972) a new poisoning outbreak occurred in Iraq involving several thousand persons and causing more than 200 deaths (*New York Times*, 1972). The major food pathway to man was apparently the preparation of home-made bread from wheat.

In addition to concern as to the direct health effects of environmental pollution by mercury, there has also been much concern with ecological effects (Larsson, 1970). Since the early 1950s comprehensive documentation has been collected showing the relationship between the use of alkylmercury-treated seed and the increased content of mercury in the feathers and livers of birds, particularly birds of prey. Populations of a number of species seemed to decline. As a result of these observations the use of phenyl-mercury for seed treatment was prohibited in Sweden in 1966. Extended investigation showed increased mercury content in sediments and fish in areas subject to mercury pollution from industrial discharges. Nevertheless, the effects on aquatic invertebrates and fish are poorly understood. A recent report indicated that very low mercury concentrations (of the order of 0.1 µg/litre, often found in coastal waters) could inhibit photosynthesis in phytoplankton (Harris et al., 1970).

REFERENCES

Berglund, F. & Berlin, M. (1969) *Risk of mercury cumulation in men and mammals and the relation between body burden of methylmercury and toxic effects.* In: Miller, M. W. & Berg, C. G., eds, *Chemical fallout*, Springfield, Ill., Thomas

Berglund, F., Berlin, M., Birke, G., von Erler, V., Friberg, L., Holmstedt, B., Jonsson, E., Ramel, C., Skerfving, S. et al. (1971) *Nord hyg. T.*, Suppl. 4, 1-364

Fitzhugh, O. G., Nelson, A. A., Laug, E. P. & Kunze, F. M. (1950) *Arch. industr. Hyg.*, **2**, 433-442

Food and Agriculture Organization (1971) *Report of the Seminar on Methods of Detection, Measurement and Monitoring of Pollutants in the Marine Environment, Rome, 4-10 December 1970*, Rome (*FAO Fisheries Reports*, No. 99), Suppl. 1

Friberg, L. & Vestal, J., eds (1971) *Mercury in the environment: a toxicological and epidemiological appraisal*, Research Triangle Park, N.C., US Environmental Protection Agency, Office of Air Programs

Goldberg, E. D. (1970) In: Singer, S. F., ed., *Global effects of environmental pollution*, Dordrecht, Reidel

Grant, N. (1971) *Environment*, **13**, No. 11, 2-15

Hammond, A. L. (1971) *Science*, **171**, 788-789

Haq, I. V. (1963) *Brit. med. J.*, **1**, 1579-1582

Harris, R. C., White, D. B. & Macfarlane, R. B. (1970) *Science*, **170**, 736-737

International Standards for Drinking-Water, 1971, 3rd ed., Geneva, World Health Organization

Jalili, M. A. & Abbasi, A. H. (1961) *Brit. J. ind. Med.*, **18**, 303-308

Jensen, S. & Jernelöv, A. (1969) *Nature (Lond.)*, **223**, 753-754

Joint FAO/WHO Expert Committee on Food Additives (1972) *Sixteenth report*, Geneva (*Wld Hlth Org. techn. Rep. Ser.*, No. 505)

Larsson, J. E. (1970) *Environmental mercury research in Sweden*, Stockholm, Swedish Environmental Protection Board

New York Times, 1972, 9 March

Ordóñez, J. V., Carrillo, J. A., Miranda, C. M. & Gale, J. L. (1966) *Bol. Ofic. sanit. panamer.*, **60**, 510-517

Skerfving, S., Hansson, K. & Lindsten, J. (1970) *Arch. environm. Hlth*, **21**, 133-139

Smart, N. A. (1968) *Residue Rev.*, **23**, 1-36

Study Group on Mercury Hazards (1971) *Environm. Res.*, **4**, 1-69

Study Group on Minamata Disease (1968) *Minamata disease*, Kumamato University

Suzuki, T., Matsumoto, N., Miyama, T. & Katsunuma, H. (1967) *Industr. Hlth (Kawasaki)*, **5**, 149-155

Tsuchiya, K. (1969) *Keio J. Med.*, **18**, 213-227

United States Environmental Protection Agency (1971) *Proposed national emission standards for hazardous air pollutants: asbestos, beryllium, mercury—background information*, Research Triangle Park, N.C., Office of Air Programs

Westöö, G. (1969) *Vår Föda*, **7**, 137-154

Wood, J. M. (1971) *Advanc. environm. Sci. Technol.*, **2**, 39-56

Working Party on the Monitoring of Foodstuffs for Mercury and other Heavy Metals (1971) *Survey of mercury in food*, London, HM Stationery Office

Other Metallic Contaminants

In addition to the metallic contaminants discussed in the preceding sections, a number of other metals and their compounds are of potential importance as environmental hazards to the general community. The principal toxic effects on man of some of these substances are summarized below.

Substance	Sources	Toxic effects in man
Antimony (Sb)	Industrial metals; safety matches	Very rarely, antimony can produce toxic effects in man through contamination of food containers. Chronic poisoning is very similar to chronic arsenic poisoning but vomiting is more violent and continuous, accompanied by watery diarrhoea, much weakness, and collapse with slow or irregular respiration and a lowered temperature (Browning, 1969).
Barium (Ba)	Rodenticides (accidental intake)	Acid-soluble barium salts (in rodenticides) are very toxic, whereas insoluble compounds (medium for roentgenography) are benign. The oral lethal dose of barium chloride is about 1 g. Symptoms of poisoning: hyperstimulation of smooth, striated, and cardiac muscles, violent peristalsis, arterial hypertension, muscular twitching, convulsions, and cardiac disturbances. The CNS may first be stimulated and then depressed; kidney damage (Takagi & Takayanagi, 1962; Arena, 1970).

Substance	Sources	Toxic effects in man
Beryllium (Be)	Production of beryllium and its alloys	Occupational exposure may produce two kinds of disease: (a) acute pneumonitis; and (b) berylliosis, a chronic progressive disease located primarily in the alveolar walls. Berylliosis has been observed in individuals not occupationally exposed, i.e., "neighbourhood" cases (Hardy et al., 1967). Beryllium may be a local air pollution problem.
Cobalt (Co)	Water and food chain	Fatal poisoning has been caused by drinking beer containing 1.2–1.5 mg/litre of cobalt (J. Amer. med. Ass., 1966). Ingestion of 0.25 mg per day had no observable adverse effects. Ingestion of higher doses of Co over a period of some days affects haemoglobin content, and produces polycythaemia and hyperlipaemia (Arena, 1970; Davis & Fields, 1955). Cobalt is considered to be a goitrogenic agent (Arena, 1970). The principal symptoms of poisoning are cardiac insufficiency and myocardial failure (National Institute of Environmental Health Sciences, 1970).
Manganese (Mn)	Soils, fertilizers, fuel oil	Mn in the air may have adverse effects on health (Lee, 1972). Chronic poisoning (through ingestion) takes the form of progressive deterioration in the CNS (Dreisbach, 1971), lethargy, and symptoms simulating Parkinson's syndrome (cf. Lee, 1972).
Nickel (Ni)	Airborne industrial effluent; direct contact	Nickel dust or the nickel of asbestos dust inhaled in occupational exposure may produce bronchial cancer in man (Loken, 1950; Mastromatteo, 1967). Dermatitis due to direct contact with nickel is described by Fisher (1967).
Selenium (Se)	Marine sediments; drinking-water	Se is found in abnormally high concentrations in the urine of residents of seleniferous regions; it can cause poisoning in grazing cattle. A causal relationship between the high incidence of certain disorders (intestinal disturbances, enlargement of liver, dermatitis, and arthritic symptoms) and elevated selenium intake has not been established (National Institute of Environmental Health Sciences, 1970).
Tin (Sn)	Food chain (canned food and beverages)	Acute accidental intoxications are very rarely reported. The toxic dose in food is 2–3 g: this causes severe headache, vomiting, vertigo, photophobia, abdominal pain, dehydration, and retention of urine (Alajouanine et al., 1958).

Substance	Sources	Toxic effects in man
Vanadium (V)	Fuel oils (exhaust from combustion); air of most cities	Ash and exhausts arising from the combustion of fuel oils containing relatively high concentrations of vanadium oxides present public health hazards (National Institute of Environmental Health Sciences, 1970). The effects on man following exposure to V_2O_5 dusts include: conjunctivitis, nasopharyngitis, and persistent cough (Mountain et al., 1955). Carcinogenicity has not been proved (Lee, 1972).

REFERENCES

Alajouanine, T., Dérobert, L. & Thiéffry, S. (1958) *Rev. neurol.*, **98**, 85-96

Arena, J. M. (1970) *Poisoning*, 2nd ed., Springfield, Ill., Thomas

Browning, E. (1969) *Toxicity of industrial metals*, London, Butterworths

Davis, J. E. & Fields, J. P. (1955) *Fed. Proc.*, **14**, 331-332

Dreisbach, R. H. (1971) *Handbook of poisoning*, Los Altos, Calif., Lange Medical

Fisher, A. A. (1967) *Contact dermatitis*, Philadelphia, Lea & Febiger

Hardy, H. L., Rabe, E. W. & Lorch, S. (1967) *J. occup. Med.*, **9**, 271-276

J. Amer. med. Ass. (1966) **197**, 25 July, p. 27

Lee, D. H. (1972) *Metallic contaminants and human health*, New York & London, Academic Press

Loken, A. C. (1950) *T. norske Lægeforen.*, **70**, 376-378

Mastromatteo, E. (1967) *J. occup. Med.*, **9**, 127-136

Mountain, J. T., Stockell, F. R. Jr & Stokinger, H. E. (1955) *A. M. A. Arch. industr. Hlth*, **12**, 494-502

Takagi, K. & Takayanagi, T. (1962) *Arch. int. Pharmacodyn.*, **135**, 223-234

US National Institute of Environmental Health Sciences (1970) *Man's health and the environment—some research needs: report of the Task Force on Research Planning in Environmental Health Science*, Washington, D.C., Department of Health, Education, and Welfare

Asbestos

Nearly all the evidence indicating an association between asbestos and disease has been derived from occupational exposure. Recently, however, it has been recognized that the general public can be exposed to asbestos, and several reviews have examined the possible hazards arising from such exposure (Committee on Biologic Effects of Atmospheric Pollutants, 1971; Cooper, 1967; Gilson, 1966; Hardy, 1965; Martin, 1970; Selikoff & Hammond, 1968; Selikoff et al., 1970; Sullivan & Athanassiadis, 1969; Tabershaw, 1968; Wright, 1969).

Asbestos is a generic name for a class of natural fibrous hydrated silicates of different chemical composition and with different physical properties, such as range of fibre diameter, flexibility, tensile strength, and surface properties.   They consist of 40–60 % of silica (SiO_2) in combination with oxides of iron, magnesium, and other metals.   The most important forms are chrysotile (white asbestos, which accounts for 95 % of world production) and the amphiboles, which occur in different varieties, e.g., crocidolite (blue), amosite (brown), and anthophyllite (white).

There has been a very rapid expansion in the use of asbestos.   In 1924 the world production was 300 000 tons of chrysotile, 5000 tons of crocidolite, and 3000 tons of amosite; the corresponding figures in 1964 were 3 000 000, 120 000, and 80 000 tons respectively (Wagner et al., 1971). As there are over a thousand uses of asbestos (Hendry, 1965), the number of occupations in which exposure may occur and the number of possible sources of exposure of the general population are also very large.   Asbestos fibres can become airborne during road building, soil tilling, and by erosion and weathering.   Air pollution may also result from mining and milling, transportation of asbestos ore and asbestos-containing products, and ventilation of asbestos manufacturing plants.   Asbestos cement, floor tiles, heat and electric wire insulation, brake linings, asbestos cloth and paper, pipe and furnace fittings, sprayed fireproofing materials, and paint filters represent sources of environmental pollution of varying importance. Other sources are the demolition of industrial and commercial buildings and practices for the disposal of solid wastes.   As pointed out in Chapter 1, there is very little information on the levels of airborne asbestos.   Asbestos may be found also in water (asbestos pipes) and in beverages such as beer (asbestos filters).   A study of river water showed that asbestos fibres were almost universally present, although in small amounts (Wright, 1969).

The evidence for non-occupational exposure to asbestos is derived from three sources (Committee on Biologic Effects of Atmospheric Pollutants, 1971):

(1)   Asbestos fibres have been demonstrated in the lungs of persons not occupationally exposed (Langer et al., 1971; Pooley et al., 1970).

(2)   Asbestos fibres have been demonstrated in ambient air (Selikoff et al., 1970; Alcocer et al., 1970).

(3)   In a few geographical areas, pathological changes regarded as indicating a reaction to asbestos—such as pleural calcification—have been identified in persons with no obvious occupational exposure (Meurman, 1968).

Such evidence was obtained in Finland in the vicinity of asbestos mines (Kiviluoto, 1960; Raunio, 1966); in the German Democratic Republic near an asbestos factory (Anspach, 1962); in Bulgaria in rural populations in relation to asbestos in the soil (Zolov et al., 1967); and in rural districts of Czechoslovakia (Hromek, 1962; Marsová, 1964; Rous & Studeny, 1970).

Different types of asbestos do not seem to be equally hazardous, and in considering the effects of exposure it is essential to know both the type of asbestos and the circumstances of exposure.   It has also been pointed out that the biological effects of asbestos fibres may depend not only on the physical and chemical properties of the fibres themselves, but also on their contamination with other chemical substances (Stokinger, 1969; Committee on Biologic Effects of Atmospheric Pollutants, 1971) and on the smoking habits of the exposed population groups.

Asbestosis is an occupational disease, and in most cases heavy exposure over many years is required to produce this condition. Cases have been reported in which asbestosis resulted after comparatively short exposure (cf. Elmes, 1966), but this seems to be exceptional. The disease is characterized by extensive fibrosis of the lungs, with pronounced shortness of breath, and in severe cases is often fatal. Asbestosis has been produced experimentally in various animal species such as rats, guineapigs, rabbits, and monkeys (cf. Wagner, 1963). Using quantitative inhalation techniques, Wagner & Skidmore (1965) and Morris et al. (1966) have shown that chrysotile produces less fibrosis than an equal dose of amosite or crocidolite; this appears to be due to different rates of elimination. The importance of particle length is not yet quite clear, but some authors (Wagner, 1965; Holt et al., 1964; Davis, 1964) have shown that in several species fibrosis of the lung is produced by fine particles or very short fibres.

The association of lung cancer with asbestos exposure was first suggested by Lynch & Smith (1935) but convincing epidemiological evidence was not provided until Merewether (1949) reported 31 cancers of the lung among 235 persons who died of occupationally acquired asbestosis in the United Kingdom between 1924 and 1946. Further studies in many countries, including the United Kingdom, the USA, South Africa, Canada, Finland, Australia, the USSR, and Italy (cf. Wagner et al., 1971; Committee on Biologic Effects of Atmospheric Pollutants, 1971) have confirmed the association between occupational exposure to asbestos and an excess incidence of bronchogenic cancer. It is difficult to establish whether an increased rate of lung cancer may result from exposures that are insufficient to cause asbestosis, but it is certain that the risk of bronchial cancer is exceptionally high if occupational exposure to asbestos is combined with cigarette smoking (Selikoff et al., 1970; Wagner et al., 1971). There is no evidence so far that non-occupational exposure to asbestos may increase the risk of lung cancer (US Environmental Protection Agency, 1971a). Evidence for an association between asbestos exposure and cancer of the gastrointestinal tract and other sites is inconclusive (Martin, 1970; Wagner et al., 1971).

Mesothelioma, a rare form of cancer of the pleura and peritoneum, has been shown to have a strong association particularly with one form of asbestos, crocidolite. Wagner et al., (1960) found that 32 of 33 patients dying of mesothelioma had been exposed to crocidolite during childhood. Other evidence from, South Africa, Canada, and Australia points in the same direction (Martin, 1970; Wagner et al., 1971). A characteristic feature of the disease is a long latent period of 30–40 years. Approximately 80 % of cases of mesothelioma of the pleura and peritoneum are associated with asbestos, either directly in industrial exposure or indirectly in home contacts or in people living near asbestos factories. A number of mesotheliomas reported by Wagner et al. (1960) could be attributed to household and neighbourhood exposures in a crocidolite producing area. A study of 76 patients with mesothelioma in the London Hospital from 1917 to 1964 (Newhouse & Thompson, 1965) showed that 31 had occupational exposure to asbestos, 9 had a relative who worked with asbestos, 11 lived within 800 metres of an asbestos factory, and 25 had no known exposure. These and other studies (cf. Bohlig et al., 1970; Lieben & Pistawka, 1967) also suggest that mesothelioma might be the most important potential hazard associated with exposure of the general public to asbestos, since it appears that "mesothelioma may be caused by the inhalation of a very small number of fibres" (Martin, 1970).

Most evidence for the adverse effects on health of asbestos exposure is derived from occupational exposure, and great caution must be observed in extrapolating to the general population.

In comparison with the occupational hazards, the risk to the general public from exposure to asbestos is small; however, the evidence is incomplete and this makes it difficult to assess the risk accurately. The occurrence of mesothelioma in neighbourhood cases indicates that a risk exists, and in one country asbestos has been declared a "hazardous air pollutant" for which national emission standards have been proposed (US Environmental Protection Agency, 1971b).

REFERENCES

Alcocer, A. E., Murchio, J. & Mueller, D. K. (1970) *Asbestos content of some urban air samples*, Berkeley, State of California Department of Health (AIHL Report 90, revised)

Anspach, M. (1962) *Int. Arch. Gewerbepath. Gewerbehyg*, **19**, 108-120

Bohlig, H., Dabbert, A. F., Dalqhen, P., Hain, E. & Hinz, I. (1970) *Environm. Res.*, **3**, 365-372

Committee on Biologic Effects of Atmospheric Pollutants (1971) *Asbestos: the need for and feasibility of air pollution controls*, Washington, D.C., National Academy of Sciences

Cooper, W. C. (1967) *Arch. environm. Hlth*, **15**, 285-290

Davis, J. M. G. (1964) *Brit. J. exp. Path.*, **45**, 634-641

Elmes, P. C. (1966) *Postgrad. med. J.*, **42**, 623

Gilson, J. C. (1966) *Trans. Soc. occup. Med.*, **16**, 62-74

Hardy, H. L. (1965) *Amer. J. med. Sci.*, **250**, 381-389

Hendry, N. W. (1965) *Ann. N. Y. Acad. Sci.*, **132**, 12-22

Holt, P. F., Mills, J. & Young, D. K. (1964) *J. Path. Bact.*, **87**, 15-23

Hromek, J. (1962) *Rozhl. Tuberk.*, **22**, 405-418

Kiviluoto, R. (1960) *Acta radiol.*, Suppl. 194, 1-67

Langer, A. M., Selikoff, I. J. & Sastre, A. (1971) *Arch. environm. Hlth*, **22**, 348-361

Lieben, J. & Pistawka, H. (1967) *Arch. environm. Hlth*, **13**, 559-563

Lynch, K. M. & Smith, W. A. (1935) *Amer. J. Cancer*, **14**, 56-64

Marsová, D. (1964) *Z. Tuberk.*, **121**, 329-334

Martin, A. E. (1970) *Hlth Trends*, No. 1, 19-21

Merewether, E. R. A. (1949) *Annual Report of the Chief Inspector of Factories for the Year 1947*, London, H.M.S.O.

Meurman, L. O. (1968) *Environm. Res.*, **2**, 30-46

Morris, T. G., Roberts, W. H., Silverton, R. E., Skidmore, J. W. & Wagner, J. C. (1966) In: *Proceedings of the Second International Symposium on Inhaled Particles and Vapours, Cambridge, 1965*, London, Pergamon

Newhouse, M. L. & Thompson, H. (1965) *Ann. N. Y. Acad. Sci.*, **132**, 579-588

Pooley, F. D., Oldham, P. D., Um, C. H. & Wagner, J. C. (1970) In: Shapiro, H. A., ed., *Pneumoconiosis: Proceedings of the International Conference, Johannesburg, 1969*, Cape Town, Oxford University Press

Raunio, V. (1966) *Ann. Med. intern. Fenn.*, **55** (Suppl. 49), 1-61

Rous, V. & Studeny, J. (1970) *Thorax*, **25**, 270-284

Selikoff, I. J. & Hammond, E. C. (1968) *Amer. J. publ. Hlth*, **59**, 1658-1666

Selikoff, I. J., Nicolson, W. J. & Langer, D. M. (1970) *Asbestos air pollution in urban areas* (Paper presented at the American Medical Association Air Pollution Medical Research Conference, New Orleans)

Stokinger, H. E. (1969) *Amer. industr. Hyg. Ass. J.*, **30**, 195-217

Sullivan, R. J. & Athanassiadis, Y. C. (1969) *Preliminary air pollution survey of asbestos: a literature review*, Raleigh, N. C., National Air Pollution Control Administration (Publication APTD 69-27)

Tabershaw, I. R. (1968) *J. occup. Med.*, **10**, 32-37

US Environmental Protection Agency (1971a) *Background information: proposed national emission standards for hazardous air pollutants: asbestos, beryllium, mercury*, Research Triangle Park, N. C., Office of Air Programs

US Environmental Protection Agency (1971b) *Federal Register*, **36**, 23239-23256

Wagner, J. C. (1963) *Brit. J. industr. Med.*, **20**, 1-12

Wagner, J. C. (1965) *Ann. N. Y. Acad. Sci.*, **132**, 575-578

Wagner, J. C., Gilson, J. C., Berry, G. & Timbrell, V. (1971) *Brit. med. Bull.*, **27**, 71-76

Wagner, J. C. & Skidmore, J. W. (1965) *Ann. N. Y. Acad. Sci.*, **132**, 77-86

Wagner, J. C., Sleggs, C. A. & Marchand, P. (1960) *Brit. J. industr. Med.*, **17**, 260-271

Wright, G. W. (1969) *Amer. Rev. resp. Dis.*, **100**, 467-479

Zolov, C., Bourilkov, T. & Babadjov, L. (1967) *Environm. Res.*, **1**, 287-297

Carbon Monoxide

Carbon monoxide (CO) results from the incomplete combustion of carbonaceous materials. A major source is the petrol engine. Industrial plants, such as power stations or steel mills, can also produce CO. Other important sources that are frequently overlooked are cigarette smoke, which may contain up to 4 % CO, and poorly adjusted home heating devices.

Carbon monoxide is absorbed in the lungs, where it combines reversibly with the haemoglobin in the blood and some extravascular haemo-proteins. This results in a reduction of the oxygen carrying capacity of the blood, and also interferes with the release of the oxygen that is carried to the tissues. Carbon monoxide has an affinity for haemoglobin 240 times greater than that of oxygen, and carboxyhaemoglobin is therefore a more stable compound than oxyhaemoglobin.

Carbon monoxide is not a cumulative poison, but is excreted or absorbed, depending upon its partial pressure in the ambient air and the percentage saturation of the haemoglobin. Some hours are required for equilibrium to be reached. Important factors in the absorption or excretion of CO, therefore, are the level of CO in the ambient air, the amount of carboxyhaemoglobin (COHb) in the blood, the duration of the exposure, and the rate of ventilation of the lungs. These interrelationships have been worked out by a number of authors (Forbes et al., 1945; Bender et al., 1971; Peterson & Stewart, 1970), and are indicated in the accompanying table. Assuming that the individual has a basal carboxyhaemoglobin content and is breathing ambient air at sea level, 50 % of the equilibrium value is reached after about three hours (Bender et al., 1971; Peterson & Stewart, 1970).

Ambient CO		Carboxyhaemoglobin %		
ppm	mg/m³	after 1 hour	after 8 hours	at equilibrium
100	117	3.6	12.9	15
60	70	2.5	8.7	10
30	35	1.3	4.5	5
20	23	0.8	2.8	3.3
10	12	0.4	1.4	1.7

In a non-smoker, the normal background of carboxyhaemoglobin is about 0.5 % and varies from 0.4 to 0.8 %; these levels are attributed mainly to endogenous sources, such as heme catabolism (Sjostrand, 1949; Coburn et al., 1969). Smokers, however, have much higher values, with a median value of 5 % and a maximum over 15 %. Thus a person with a low COHb level, e.g. 0.5 %, who is continuously exposed to 35 mg/m³ of CO will absorb CO until a level of 5 % COHb is reached. Conversely, a heavy smoker with a COHb level of 10 %, who ceases to smoke and is exposed to the same level of CO (35 mg/m³), will excrete CO until he attains the same equilibrium value of 5 % (Lawther & Cummins, 1970; Goldsmith, 1970; WHO Expert Committee on Air Quality Criteria and Guides, 1972).

The symptoms observed in man are directly related to the actual blood levels of carboxyhaemoglobin, both in experimental and in epidemiological studies.

The biological effects of carbon monoxide were intensively reviewed at a meeting sponsored by the New York Academy of Sciences in 1970. There is no doubt that saturations of 20 % in the blood can cause symptoms and impairment of performance. In general, symptoms such as lassitude, headache, and impaired co-ordination are not reported until saturations exceed 10 % (Lindgren, 1961; Stewart et al., 1970). Much attention has been given to the possible relevance of concentrations too low to cause symptoms. Bender et al. (1971) exposed volunteers to 100 ppm CO (117 mg/m^3) or ambient air for 2½ hours (blind trial) and subsequently applied a battery of psychological tests. At 7.2 % saturation, a significant diminution of visual perception, manual dexterity, and ability to learn and perform certain "intellectual" tasks was reported. Guest et al. (1970), using a double blind technique, studied critical flicker fusion and auditory flutter fusion thresholds after administration of 500 ppm CO (585 mg/m^3) for 1 hour (or 8 % saturation) to 20 volunteers and found no effect, whereas thresholds were increased by 60 mg phenobarbitone. Stewart et al. (1970) have studied the effects of various levels of carboxyhaemoglobin on many indicators of performance and perception, and have demonstrated that 15–20 % saturations are associated with headache and impairment of manual co-ordination. Further studies by Hosko (1970) have shown that the visual evoked response changed with carboxyhaemoglobin levels over 20 % but that spontaneous EEG activity remained unaffected until saturation approached 33 %.

When assessing the results of these tests of psychomotor function, it must be remembered that concentrations too low to give measurable results when administered alone may eventually be shown to have effects on subjects who have taken alcohol, sedatives, antihistamines, or hypotensive drugs.

The effect of carbon monoxide on the cardiovascular system and on the oxygenation of tissue other than that of the central nervous system may be important. Chevalier et al. (1966) studied the reactions of non-smokers to carbon monoxide, and demonstrated an increase in oxygen debt with exercise in healthy men at saturations of about 4 %. Ayres et al. (1965, 1969) have reported decreased arterial and mixed venous Po$_2$ in men with about 9 % carboxyhaemoglobin, and they claim that this could explain cardiac changes and the observed increased oxygen debt. Ayres et al. (1970) found that coronary arteriovenous oxygen differences were uniformly increased and that coronary artery blood flow was also increased when carboxyhaemoglobin saturation was raised to 5–10 %, while significant myocardial changes were seen in patients with carboxyhaemoglobin saturation above 6 %. Obviously there will be patients in the general population who already have impaired myocardial function and to whom lesser saturations would be harmful. Extrapolation on a quantitative basis is difficult, but clearly there are patients with many diseases who could not tolerate any further hypoxia.

The possible role of carbon monoxide in the genesis of disease, as distinct from its role in the exacerbation of existing illness or other impairment of function, is a separate problem. The work of Astrup et al. (1967, 1970) on rabbits may be of great assistance in understanding the etiology of some cardiovascular diseases: an increased incidence of atheroma was demonstrated in cholesterol-fed rabbits that were also exposed to carbon monoxide, and the changes produced in the vessel walls led the authors to suggest that the observed relationship between cardiovascular disease and cigarette smoking may well be explained in terms of chronic or repeated exposure to carbon monoxide. Following the experiments on rabbits, 1000 Copenhagen factory workers chosen at random were examined, and a clear relationship demonstrated between high carboxyhaemoglobin concentrations after smoking and the occurrence of arteriosclerotic disease (Kjeldsen, 1969).

REFERENCES

Astrup, P., Kjeldsen, K. & Wanstrup, J. (1967) *J. Atheroscler. Res.*, **7**, 343-354

Astrup, P., Kjeldsen, K. & Wanstrup, J. (1970) *Ann. N. Y. Acad. Sci.*, **174**, 294-300

Ayres, S. M., Giannelli, S. & Armstrong, R. G. (1965) *Science*, **149**, 193-194

Ayres, S. M., Giannelli, S. & Mueller, H. (1970) *Ann. N. Y. Acad. Sci.*, **174**, 268-293

Ayres, S. M., Mueller, H. S., Gregory, J. J., Gianelli, S. & Penny, J. L. (1969) *Arch. environm. Hlth*, **18**, 699-709

Bender, W., Göthert, M., Malorny, G. & Sebbesse, P. (1971) *Arch. Toxikol.*, **27**, 142-158

Chevalier, R. B., Krumholz, R. A. & Ross, J. C. (1966) *J. Amer. med. Ass.*, **198**, 1061-1064

Coburn, R. F., Blakemore, W. S. & Forster, R. E. (1969) *J. clin. Invest.*, **42**, 1172-1178

Forbes, W. H., Sargent, F. & Roughton, F. J. W. (1945) *Amer. J. Physiol.*, **143**, 594-608

Goldsmith, J. R. (1970) *Ann. N. Y. Acad. Sci.*, **174**, 122-134

Guest, A. D. L., Duncan, C. & Lawther, P. J. (1970) *Ergonomics*, **13**, 587-594

Hosko, M. J. (1970) *Arch. environm. Hlth*, **21**, 174-180

Kjeldsen, K. (1969) *Smoking and atherosclerosis* (thesis) Copenhagen, Munksgaard

Lawther, P. J. & Cummins, B. T. (1970) *Ann. N. Y. Acad. Sci.*, **174**, 135-147

Lindgren, S. A. (1961) *Acta med. scand.*, **167** (Suppl. 356), 1-135

Peterson, J. E. & Stewart, R. D. (1970) *Arch. environm. Hlth*, **21**, 165-171

Sjostrand, T. (1949) *Scand. J. clin. Lab. Invest.*, **1**, 201-204

Stewart, R. D., Peterson, J. E., Baretta, E. D., Bachand, R. T., Hosko, M. J. & Herrman, A. (1970) *Arch. environm. Hlth*, **21**, 154-164

WHO Expert Committee on Air Quality Criteria and Guides (1972) *Report*, Geneva (*Wld Hlth Org. techn. Rep. Ser.*, No. 506)

Ozone and Photochemical Oxidants

The oxidizing type of air pollution found in many urban areas results from the chemical combination of reactive hydrocarbons, with nitrogen oxides in the presence of sunlight; this results in the production of ozone, peroxyacyl nitrates, aldehydes, and other chemical compounds. Sunlight is essential, as it supplies the energy necessary for the chemical reactions to take place. The hydrocarbons come primarily from gasoline and motor vehicle exhaust, while the nitrogen oxides are emitted not only from motor vehicles but also from stationary combustion sources. The photochemical oxidants are ozone, peroxyacyl nitrates, and other oxidizing products of the complex atmospheric reaction. These products are measured by various methods, but are expressed in terms of ozone (O_3).

The interpretation of the results of studies is complicated by the complex nature of the pollutants, and it has not always been possible to separate the effects of ozone, oxides of nitrogen, oxidant precursors, and by-products of reactions in the atmosphere. It has therefore become customary to refer to total oxidant level as a gross indicator of these various components. Laboratory studies on human beings have assessed the effects of specific pollutants, such as ozone (Silverman et al., 1970; Young et al., 1964) or peroxyacyl nitrates (Smith, 1965). Some concern has been expressed about the possible mutagenic effects of ozone and also as to whether it can produce effects directly on tissues even at low concentrations. More data on this are needed. In studies in Los Angeles, no association has been shown between increased mortality and the "alert days" when the levels of oxidants are 1000–1700 $\mu g/m^3$ (0.50–0.85 ppm).

Acute effects of the oxidizing type of air pollution include eye, nose, and throat irritations. Reasonably precise dose-response curves have been developed for eye irritation (Richardson & Middleton, 1958), but attempts to develop such curves for other symptoms have not been very successful.

A statistically significant association has been shown between asthmatic attacks and days when oxidant levels were above 500 $\mu g/m^3$ (0.25 ppm), but no such association was shown for days with mean levels of 260 $\mu g/m^3$ (0.13 ppm) (Schoettlin & Landau, 1961). The number of persons who had attacks on days when plant damage occurred at official monitoring stations was significantly greater than on other days. The number of persons affected was not significantly correlated with levels of carbon monoxide and particulates.

Persons with chronic pulmonary disease have experienced a decrease in pulmonary function when exposed to photochemical smog (Motley et al., 1959), with oxidant levels of 390–1370 $\mu g/m^3$ (0.2–0.7 ppm). These changes were reversible, and disappeared when the patients were exposed to "clean" filtered air. Rokaw & Massey (1962) carried out a similar study at much lower levels of oxidant (120 $\mu g/m^3$ or 0.06 ppm) and found no effect on pulmonary function in patients with chronic lung disease.

Schoettlin (1962) studied elderly males in the Los Angeles area. In those with pre-existing pulmonary disease, 30 % of the changes in symptoms were associated with the maximum levels of oxidant precursor. Oxidant levels, which were in the range 60–1350 $\mu g/m^3$ (0.03–0.69 ppm), were associated with 11 % of the symptoms and 13 % of the clinical signs.

In a number of studies it was not possible to demonstrate any effects of oxidants on health (McMillan et al., 1969; Wayne & Wehrle, 1969; Pearlman et al., 1971). These observations may be valid, but on the other hand they may be due to insensitivity of the test, inadequate sample size, or a limited range of relatively low oxidant levels.

The effects of oxidant on athletic performance have been examined by Wayne et al. (1967), who compared the times of long-distance runners at different meetings in the Los Angeles area. They found that, if the oxidant level during the hour before the race was above 200 $\mu g/m^3$ (0.1 ppm), a significant number of the runners had increased (i.e., poorer) times, whereas the values for three or two hours before, or during the race, had no such association. Other air pollutants, such as oxides of nitrogen, carbon monoxide, and suspended particulates, had no effect over the ranges studied.

In laboratory studies, human subjects who inhaled ozone at a concentration of 1200–1600 $\mu g/m^3$ (0.6–0.8 ppm) for two hours showed decreases in diffusing capacity for carbon monoxide, in dynamic compliance, in vital capacity, and in $FEV_{0.75}$ (forced expiratory volume in 0.75 seconds) in comparison with pre-exposure values (Young et al., 1964; Silverman et al., 1970).

Smith (1965) studied the effect of peroxyacyl nitrate on oxygen consumption in male college students at rest and during a 5-minute exercise test on a bicycle ergometer. He used only one level of peroxyacyl nitrate, 1480 $\mu g/m^3$ (0.3 ppm), which was rather high in relation to usual ambient levels, and a work-load of 900 kg/m^2 min. The oxygen consumption was higher than the control value at work, but not at rest.

Animal experiments (Coffin et al., 1968; Coffin, 1970; Gardner et al., 1971) have indicated that exposure to ozone at 160 $\mu g/m^3$ (0.08 ppm) for three hours or more leads to increased mortality when infectious aerosols are subsequently introduced. Bacteria that showed this effect in several animal species were *Streptococcus* (group C), *Klebsiella pneumoniae*, and *Diplococcus pneumoniae*. The phenomenon seems to be attributable to a reduction of specific antibacterial defences of the lung, leading to slowed bacterial inactivation, enhanced growth, and more rapid invasion of the bloodstream. As a result of exposure to ozone, pulmonary macrophages are reduced in number, their phagocytic ability is lessened, and their lysosomal enzyme competence and life span *in vitro* are reduced.

It is not known whether human beings are capable of developing a tolerance to oxidants (ozone), as has been reported for animals (Stokinger &

Scheel, 1962).   The development of such a tolerance could account for the relatively few changes associated with repeated chronic exposure at the levels of oxidant air pollution that occur in Los Angeles, but there is no evidence to support this hypothesis.

REFERENCES

Coffin, D. L. (1970)   In: *Inhalation carcinogenesis: Proceedings of a Conference, Gatlin-burg., Tenn., 1969,* Springfield, Va., US Atomic Energy Commission (*AEC Symposium Series,* 18) pp. 259-264

Coffin, D. L., Gardner, D. E. & Holzman, R. S. (1968) *Arch. environm. Hlth,* **16,** 633-636

Gardner, D, E., Pfitzer, E. A., Christian, R. T. & Coffin, D. L. (1971) *Arch. intern. Med.,* **127,** 1078-1084

McMillan, R. S., Wiseman, D. H., Hanes, B. & Wehr, P. F. (1969) *Arch. environm. Hlth,* **18,** 941-949

Motley, H. L., Smart, R. H. & Leftwich, C. I. (1959) *J. Amer. med. Ass.,* **171,** 1469-1477

Pearlman, M. E., Finklea, J. F., Shy, C. M., Van Bruggen, J. B. & Newill, V. A. (1971) *Environm. Res.,* **4,** 129-140

Richardson, N. A. & Middleton, W. C. (1958) *Heat., Pip. Air Condit.,* **30,** 147-154

Rokaw, S. N. & Massey, F. (1962) *Amer. Rev. resp. Dis.,* **86,** 703-704

Silverman, F., Bell, G. M., Burnham, C. D., Hazucha, M., Mantha, J., Pengelly, L. D. & Bates, D. V. (1970) *Physiologist,* **13,** 309

Schoettlin, C. E. (1962) *Amer. Rev. resp. Dis.,* **86,** 878-897

Schoettlin, C. E. & Landau, E. (1961) *Publ. Hlth Rep.,* **76,** 545-548

Smith, L. (1965) *Amer. J. publ. Hlth,* **55,** 1460-1468

Stokinger, H. E. & Scheel, L. D. (1962) *Arch. industr. Hlth,* **4,** 327-333

Wayne, W. S. & Wehrle, P. F. (1969) *Arch. environm. Hlth,* **19,** 315-322

Wayne, W. S., Wehrle, P. F. & Carroll, R. F. (1967) *J. Amer. med. Ass.,* **199,** 901-904

Young, W. A., Shaw, D. B. & Bates, D. V. (1964) *J. appl. Physiol.,* **19,** 765-768

Oxides of Nitrogen

Oxides of nitrogen are produced during combustion processes at temperatures higher than about 1000 °C, the most important of these oxides being NO and NO_2; they are expressed in terms of NO_2.   Their principal source is the internal combustion engine and their major role in air pollution appears to be as components in the reactions of photochemical pollution, although they may occur separately around plants producing explosives or power stations.   When oxides of nitrogen are associated with photochemical air pollution, their level tends to drop as the ozone level rises, in such a way that the total level of the two pollutants remains approximately constant.

Nitrogen dioxide has distinct biological effects apart from those associated with photochemical pollution.   It can exist as a primary pollutant in areas not experiencing such pollution, and should therefore be considered as a discrete pollutant requiring independent exposure guidelines. There are very few epidemiological data specifically concerned with oxides of nitrogen.

Studies of exercising men exposed to simulated air pollution consisting of irradiated automobile exhaust at levels of 1320–1880 $\mu g/m^3$ (0.7–1.0 ppm) NO_2 and 470–710 $\mu g/m^3$ (0.38–0.58 ppm) NO showed no effect (Holland et al., 1968). This exposure involved a complex mixture of compounds.

In contrast, a study of schoolchildren aged 6–8 years has shown what appears to be an effect of oxides of nitrogen (Pearlman et al., 1971; Shy et al., 1970). In this study, four areas were selected around Chattanooga (Tenn., USA): a "high" NO_2 area close to a TNT plant, two control areas with "low" NO_2 and low suspended particulates, and a fourth area with "high" suspended particulates. In the "high" NO_2 area there was significantly more respiratory illness than in the control areas. An increased occurrence of lower respiratory tract infections, such as bronchitis, was seen in children exposed for the first 2–3 years of life in the "high" NO_2 area (Pearlman et al., 1971), but not in those exposed for a year or less. A similar increase was also reported in primary schoolchildren. Croup and pneumonia did not show an association. A dose-response gradient across the levels of pollution encountered in the investigation could not be demonstrated.

These findings deserve further study and verification. The levels at which changes were reported are lower than the oxidant levels associated with effects on health, although no really comparable study has been made of oxidant exposure. In the area of "high" NO_2, 190 $\mu g/m^3$ (0.10 ppm) NO_2 was exceeded on 40 %, 18 %, and 9 % of days at the three monitoring stations; in one of the control areas, this level was exceeded on 17 % of days, but at only one station. For oxides of nitrogen, peak exposures may be of more importance than average values.

Nitrogen dioxide has been shown to be toxic to a number of animal species; the acute manifestations are generally similar to those of ozone, but at a somewhat higher threshold. A two-hour exposure to 6580 $\mu g/m^3$ (3.5 ppm) and higher levels of NO_2 increased the mortality of animals (mice) infected with *Klebsiella pneumoniae*. Exposure to NO_2, 24–48 hours after exposure to monkey-adapted influenza virus, resulted in increased mortality in squirrel monkeys (Ehrlich & Henry, 1968; Henry et al., 1970). Pathological effects on lung mast cells (Thomas et al., 1967) and other pulmonary cells (Gardner et al., 1969) have also been reported.

Continuous exposure to various levels of NO_2 for 6 months or longer has produced a sequence of lesions in the lungs of rats, beginning at 3760 $\mu g/m^3$ (2 ppm) or possibly below; these lesions consist of subtle changes in the epithelium of the terminal airway, enlargement of the pulmonary air space, and degenerative changes in the lung collagen

(Freeman et al., 1968). Changes resembling those seen in human emphysema have been reported in mice exposed 6–24 hours daily for a period of 3–12 months to 940 $\mu g/m^3$ (0.5 ppm) NO_2 (Blair et al., 1969).

Although care is required in extrapolating these results from animals to man, the findings indicate the high biological activity of NO_2 in producing animal diseases that have human counterparts. This should serve as a warning of its potential toxicity.

REFERENCES

Blair, W. H., Henry, M. C. & Ehrlich, R. (1969) *Arch. environm. Hlth*, **18**, 186

Ehrlich, R. & Henry, M. C. (1968) *Arch. environm. Hlth*, **17**, 860

Freeman, G., Stevens, R. J., Crane, S. C. & Furiosi, H. J. (1968) *Arch. environm. Hlth*, **17**, 181

Gardner, E. E., Holzman, R. S. & Coffin, D. L. (1969) *J. Bact.*, **98**, 1041

Henry, M. C., Findlay, J., Spangler, J. & Ehrlich, R. (1970) *Arch. environm. Hlth*, **20**, 566

Holland, G. J., Benson, D., Bush, A., Rich, G. Q. & Holland, R. P. (1968) *Amer. J. publ. Hlth*, **58**, 1684

Pearlman, M. E., Finklea, J. F., Creason, J. P., Shy, C. M., Young, M. M. & Horton, R. J. M. (1971) *Pediatrics*, **47**, 391

Shy, C. M., Creason, J. P., Pearlman, M. E., McClain, K. E. & Benson, F. B. (1970) *J. Air Pollut. Control Ass.*, **20**, 539, 583

Thomas, H. V., Mueller, P. K. & Wright, G. (1967) *J. Air Pollut. Control Ass.*, **17**, 33

Fluorides

Fluorine compounds are found in nature (in soil, water, and food) and in the human body in the form of fluorides. They are present in sea-water, in some supplies of drinking-water, in mineral deposits of fluorspar (CaF_2), and in surface dusts found close to mineral deposits. The fluoride ion is physiologically very active. The entire question of the effects of fluorides on human health has been extensively reviewed by the World Health Organization (1970).

Fluorine compounds are used in a number of industries, and may lead to pollution of air, water, soil, and plants in the vicinity of aluminium works, fertilizer factories, and brick and ceramics factories (see also pp. 35 and 59). The combustion of coal also introduces fluorides into the atmosphere. In some countries industrial waste liquors and slurries containing sodium and potassium fluorosilicate, hydrofluoric acid, and fluorosilic acid are often disposed of in the sea or in large settling ponds. Fluorides vaporizing from such ponds may cause considerable pollution of the surrounding atmosphere (National Academy of Sciences, 1971).

Fluorine accumulates in the young organism more readily than in the adult (Macúch et al., 1963). The newborn infant's skeletal tissues are relatively free of fluorides and therefore pick them up more readily. As the concentration in the skeleton increases, the rate of accumulation drops. The fluoride content in human bones tends to increase with age and with fluoride intake (Smith et al., 1960). Higher fluoride values were found in the maternal blood and placental tissue of pregnant women living in an area with drinking-water containing 1 mg fluoride per litre than in those living in a fluoride-free area (Gardner et al., 1952; Gedalia et al., 1964; Ericsson & Malmnäs, 1962). Individuals with pulmonary and renal dysfunction may be especially susceptible to fluoride intoxication (National Academy of Sciences, 1971).

It has been reported that in an area with fluoride pollution from industry, children had a decreased haemoglobin and increased erythrocyte level, in some cases with increased fluoride in their teeth, fingernails, hair, and urine (Balazova et al., 1967). However, experience in the United Kingdom shows that where proper pollution control methods are adopted there is no hazard to man, although emissions cannot always be brought down to a level where there is no risk to farm animals.

Small doses of fluoride (1 mg/litre in drinking-water) benefit dental health, resulting in a lower incidence of carious teeth, a smaller number of cavities, and slower decay (World Health Organization, 1970; Blaney & Hill, 1967). Higher doses can be toxic for man when taken over a long period, apparently with depression of collagen formation (Nichols & Flanagan, 1966), bone resorption, and an increase in bone crystal (Neer et al., 1966). Aortic calcification was found to be decreased in residents of communities with high environmental fluoride levels (Bernstein et al., 1966).

The additive and synergistic interaction between fluorides and other airborne pollutants should not be neglected (Adams et al., 1952; van Raay, 1969).

REFERENCES

Adams, D. F., Mayhew, D. J., Gnagy, R. M., Richey, E. P., Koppe, R. K. & Allen, I. W. (1952) *Industr. Engng Chem.*, **44**, 1356

Balazova, G., Lezovic, J., Macúch, P. (1967) In: *Proceedings of the First Meeting of the International Society for Fluoride Research, Frankfurt, 1967*, International Society for Fluoride Research

Bernstein, D. S., Sadowsky, N., Hegsted, D. M., Guri, C. D. & Stare, F. S. (1966) *J. Amer. med. Ass.*, **198**, 499

Blaney, J. R. & Hill, I. D. (1967) *J. Amer. dent. Ass.*, **74**, No. 2

Ericsson, Y. & Malmnäs, C. (1962) *Acta obstet. gynec. scand.*, **41**, 144-158

Gardner, D. E., Smith, F. A., Hodge, H. C., Overton, D. E. & Feltman, R. (1952) *Science*, **155**, 208-209

Gedalia, I., Brzezinski, A., Zukerman, H. & Magersdorf, A. (1964) *J. dent. Res.*, **43**, 669-671

Macúch, P., Balážová, G., Bartošová, L., Hluchán, E., Ambruš, J., Janovicová, J. & Kirilčuková, V. (1963) *J. Hyg. Epidem. (Praha)*, **7**, 389-403

National Academy of Sciences (1971) *Fluorides*, Washington, D. C.

Neer, R. M., Zipkin, I., Carbone, P. P. L. & Rosenberg, L. E. (1966) *J. clin. Endocr.*, **26**, 1059-1068

Nichols, G., Jr & Flanagan, B. (1966) *Fed. Proc.*, **25**, 922

Smith, F. A., Gardner, D. E., Leone, N. C. & Hodge, H. C. (1960) *A. M. A. Arch. industr. Hlth*, **21**, 330-332

Van Raay, A. (1969) In: *Air pollution: Proceedings of the First European Congress on the Influence of Air Pollution on Plants and Animals, Wageningen, 1968*, Wageningen, Centre for Agricultural Publishing and Documentation, pp. 319-328

World Health Organization (1970) *Fluorides and human health*, Geneva (*Monograph Series*, No. 59)

Nitrates, Nitrites, and Nitroso Compounds

Reviews of the health hazards arising from the presence of nitrates, nitrites, and nitrosamines in water and food have recently been published by Lee (1970) and Wolff & Wassermann (1972).

Inorganic nitrates and nitrites are a health hazard because they may contaminate deep-well drinking-water. Infant methaemoglobinaemia resulting from the consumption of food made with water with high nitrate concentrations was recognized many years ago. Clinical cases have been reported, but are very rare in areas with less than 45 mg/litre of NO_3 in the water (Knotek & Schmidt, 1964). Various endogenous forms of methaemoglobinaemia are known. Nitrates do not directly convert haemoglobin to methaemoglobin, but they can be converted to nitrites by intestinal microflora, with subsequent formation of methaemoglobin (cf. Sander & Seif, 1969; Gruener & Shuval, 1969). Nitrate fertilizers and animal wastes are sources of nitrates and nitrites formed by bacterial reduction. These environmental sources are particularly dangerous in farming communities using individual water wells.

Nitrosamines are formed by the reaction of secondary amines with nitrites. The carcinogenicity in laboratory animals of several nitroso compounds has been known for some years (Druckrey et al., 1961; Druckrey & Preussmann, 1962), and the subject has recently been reviewed (Magee, 1971). Many of the nitrosamines and nitroso-ureas are extremely potent carcinogens in many species of animal, and tumours have been found in a variety of organs, including the liver, kidney, trachea, oesophagus, and lungs. The liver appears to be the initial site but, after damage by necrosis, tumours appear elsewhere (Magee & Barnes, 1962). The simplest nitrosamine, dimethylnitrosamine, has been found to be carcinogenic to all species of animal tested. It is highly hepatotoxic to sheep; a single dose of 5 mg per kg body weight or 12 doses of 0.5 mg per kg body weight proved lethal (Sakshaug et al., 1965). The formation of lethal concentrations of dimethylnitrosamine in fishmeal preserved with sodium nitrite and used for feeding sheep in Norway has been reported (National Research Council, Committee on Environmental Physiology, 1970).

The possible formation of nitrosamine carcinogens in the stomach of man is of particular concern, and there is substantial evidence that the low pH of the mammalian stomach favours the formation of nitrosamines from secondary amines and nitrites (Sander, 1967; Lijinsky & Epstein, 1970). In one study, 31 human subjects were given sodium nitrate and diphenyl-amine intragastrically, and the presence of diphenylnitrosamine was demon-strated in the stomach contents (Magee, 1971). No tumours were induced in rats that ingested diethylamine and nitrites (Druckrey et al., 1963), but malignant tumours have been found in rats fed morpholine or N-methyl-benzylamine and sodium nitrite (Sander & Burkle, 1969).

A number of nitroso compounds have been found to be mutagenic in all the usual microbial systems, in several plants, and in *Drosophila* (Magee & Barnes, 1967; Pasternak, 1964). However, dimethylnitrosamine was reported to be active only in *Drosophila*, suggesting that activation is essential and may be dependent on the metabolic system that is present in the insect but absent in the micro-organisms (Pasternak, 1964).

N-nitrosomethylurea and N-nitrosoethylurea are potent teratogens, and both can induce tumours in the progeny of rats treated during pregnancy (Kreybig, 1965; Druckrey et al., 1966). The high incidence of tumours of the central and peripheral nervous systems induced by N-nitrosoethylurea is noteworthy. By contrast, dimethylnitrosamine is reported not to have any teratogenic action in rats but to induce renal and other tumours in the progeny of females treated during the third week of pregnancy (Alexandrov, 1968).

REFERENCES

Alexandrov, V. A. (1968) *Nature (Lond.)*, **218**, 280

Druckrey, H., Ivankovic, S. & Preussmann, R. (1966) *Nature (Lond.)*, **210**, 1378

Druckrey, H., Preussmann, R., Schmähl, D. & Blum, G. (1961) *Naturwissenschaften*, **48**, 722

Druckrey, H., Steinhoff, D., Benthner, H., Schneider, H. & Klärner, P. (1963) *Arzneimittel-Forsch.*, **13**, 320

Druckrey, H. & Preussmann, R. (1962) *Nature (Lond.)*, **195**, 1111

Gruener, N. & Shuval, H. I. (1970) *Health aspects of nitrates in drinking-water*. In: *Developments in water quality research: Proceedings of the Jerusalem International Conference on Water Quality and Pollution Research, 1969*, Ann Arbor and London, Ann Arbor-Humphrey Science Publishers, pp. 89-106

Knotek, Z. & Schmidt, P. (1964) *Pediatrics*, **34**, 78

Kreybig, T. von (1965) *Z. Krebsforsch.*, **67**, 46

Lee, D. H. K. (1970) *Environm. Res.*, **3**, 484-511

Lijinsky, W. & Epstein, S. S. (1970) *Nature (Lond.)*, **225**, 21

Magee, P. N. (1971) *Food Cosmet. Toxicol.*, **9**, 207

Magee, P. N. & Barnes, J. M. (1962) *J. Path. Bact.*, **84**, 19

Magee, P. N. & Barnes, J. M. (1967) *Advanc. Cancer Res.*, **10**, 163

Pasternak, L. (1964) *Arzneimittel-Forsch.*, **14**, 802

National Research Council, Committee on Environmental Physiology (1970) *Physiology, environment and man*, New York, Academic Press

Sakshaug, J., Sognen, E., Hansen, M. A. & Koppang, N. (1965) *Nature (Lond.)*, **206**, 1261

Sander, J. (1967) *Arch. Hyg. (Berl.)*, **157**, 23

Sander, J. & Seif, F. (1969) *Arzneimittel-Forsch.*, **19**, 1091

Sander, J. & Bürkle, G. (1969) *Z. Krebsforsch.*, **73**, 54

Wolff, I. A. & Wassermann, A. E. (1972) *Science*, **177**, 15-19

DDT and Related Compounds

The significance of environmental pollution by pesticides, particularly DDT and its analogues, has been a controversial subject for many years, and a number of excellent reviews are available (US Department of Health, Education and Welfare, 1969; Agricultural Research Council, 1970; Gillet, 1970; Kaloyanova-Simeonova & Fournier, 1971; Ling et al., 1972).

Pesticides are deliberately released into the environment for agricultural and public health purposes; they become environmental pollutants if they are transferred outside the area of intentional application, and if they persist in the environment longer than necessary. Other sources of pollution are accidental releases and the uncontrolled disposal of wastes from manufacturing plants or by agricultural and industrial users.

A large variety of compounds are used as insecticides, fungicides, herbicides, and rodenticides. They include inorganic compounds such as copper sulfate, lead arsenate, and mercuric chloride; organochlorine compounds like DDT, dieldrin, aldrin, heptachlor, and gamma-HCH; organophosphorus compounds such as parathion, dimethoate, and malathion; carbamates; chlorinated phenoxyacetic acids; organic mercury compounds (see pages 183-187); and others.

Local pollution problems of a transient nature may arise from any of these compounds, particularly if released accidentally; however, extensive pollution can be caused only by a few classes of compounds that are sufficiently resistant to chemical and biochemical degradation, i.e., some organochlorine compounds, notably DDT and its analogues, and compounds that contain toxic metals in their molecule. The total amount of the compound used is of course another factor that determines the pollution potential. Since DDT and related compounds are by far the most important pesticides from the standpoint of large-scale environmental pollution, it is with these substances that this section is principally concerned.

The outstanding property of DDT and dieldrin is their chemical stability. Gamma-HCH is more easily transformed into non-toxic substances; the degradation products of aldrin and heptachlor are very stable substances themselves, as are some degradation products of DDT, such as DDE. Generally, chlorination of a hydrocarbon increases the resistance of the compound to both chemical and biochemical degradation. When a molecule such as p,p'-DDT includes chlorinated aromatic groups, its persistence in the environment increases from months to years (cf. Robinson, 1971). Rates of biochemical degradation vary for different compounds, and the time required for a 50 % change may range from about 2 weeks to 2 years; the period may be much longer in abiotic components of the environment, such as water.

Organochlorine compounds are very slightly soluble in water (DDT, for example, has a solubility of about 0.04 ppm); on the other hand, they are very soluble in fatty substances. For this reason they tend to be stored in fatty tissues of birds, fish, and man, at levels that depend on the intake and metabolic peculiarities of the species concerned (cf. Moriarty, 1972). Some aquatic organisms may have levels of organochlorine compounds exceeding 10 000 times that in the water in which they live (Agricultural Research Council, 1970). An additional property associated with low solubility in water is their tendency to adsorb on suspended particulate matter in water, on bottom sediments, and on organic matter in soil.

DDT and other organochlorine compounds generally have a very low vapour pressure, but when an extensive surface is exposed appreciable amounts of vapour find their way into the air.[1] These vapours in turn condense on colloidal particles suspended in air or coalesce into aerosol droplets, and thus can be transported over considerable distances. This may be one of the important mechanisms by which DDT (and also some other pollutants) are transported from the land to the sea (cf. Joint Group of Experts in Scientific Aspects of Marine Pollution, 1971).

An important question in relation to pesticides in the environment is whether or not they are present in concentrations sufficient to produce biological effects. In general the concentration of organochlorine compounds found in the environment can be measured in parts per million at most, and more often in parts per hundred million or parts per thousand million (cf. Edwards, 1970; see also Chapters 1–3). For DDT, concentrations range from 1×10^{-6} ppm (air, sea-water) to 10 ppm (some tissues of predatory birds.) Data on levels in ambient air (remote from areas of application) are scarce; concentrations have been found ranging from 0.1 to about 20 ng/m^3, but these levels do not present a health hazard from inhalation. The levels of DDT and related compounds in natural water bodies extend from less than 0.001 µg/litre to about 1 µg/litre. Pesticide levels in cultivated soils depend on the amounts applied.

---

[1] Aerial application is of course another possible source of airborne material.

Food is the main source of exposure, and according to some estimates accounts for more than 90 % of the total intake of DDT by man (Campbell et al., 1965).   The contributions from drinking-water supplies and air are of minor significance.

Trace amounts of DDT and its analogues are found in human fat. Because of its lipophilic property DDT is found mainly in adipose tissue. Accumulation in the individual organs is proportional to the neutral fat content of the organs.   As more sensitive analytical methods are developed the list of organochlorine insecticides found in human fat is growing, but DDT and its metabolite DDE are the compounds that have been most extensively studied.   Results from human monitoring surveys are now available from more than 20 countries, and a review covering the period 1960-1970 is given by Kaloyanova-Simeonova & Fournier (1971).   The mean levels of DDT and its analogues in human body fat vary from country to country, while age, sex, race, and social class have been described as important demographic variables influencing the frequency distribution of DDT residue in the general population.   The high residue levels in India and Israel, where the mean levels for total DDT are 30.2 ppm and 19.2 ppm respectively, can be attributed to a particularly high rate of DDT application.   In the Federal Republic of Germany an average DDT content of 2.3 ppm was measured in the population in 1958-1959, at a time when DDT was used only for a few agricultural pests.   More recent studies in some countries suggest that the level of DDT and its metabolites in man is tending to fall rather than rise.

While for the majority of the population the body content of DDT is probably derived mainly from the diet, other sources of DDT in the immediate human environment, such as insecticidal vaporizers, may be a major determinant of body content in some groups or individuals.

The residues of DDT in tissues do not continually increase with continued uptake; an upper uptake level is reached in man after about a year (Hoffman et al., 1964; Hayes et al., 1956).   Investigations by Hayes et al. (1958) confirmed that the uptake capacity is limited: in 342 subjects the DDT residues did not increase from 1950 to 1958.

There is no evidence that the presence of DDT in human fat, even at levels very much greater than those found in the general population, affects the metabolic behaviour of the fat itself, nor is there any evidence that the DDT in fat causes any injury to health.

A direct correlation between the quantity of DDT stored in the fat and exposure was found by Hayes et al. (1956) in man and by Durham et al. (1963) in monkeys.   The results of studies in volunteers given known doses of DDT make it possible to calculate the daily intake that will give rise to the levels found in the fat.   The dosage-response to DDT in man is shown in the accompanying table; the data show that dosages hundreds of times greater than those encountered by the general population have been tolerated by volunteers for more than a year (Hayes, 1971) and by factory workers for as long as DDT factories have existed, i.e., about one-fourth of the human life span (Orteler, 1958; Laws et al., 1967). Over 150 persons with heavy and prolonged occupational exposure to DDT have been subjected to exhaustive medical examinations, but the only relevant findings were those that could be predicted, i.e., increased storage and excretion of DDT and its metabolites and a mild stimulation of the microsomal enzymes of the liver (Poland et al., 1970). A level as high as 1131 ppm has been observed in the fat of a man occupationally exposed to DDT, without symptoms of poisoning (Hayes et al., 1956). The negligible hazard to man resulting from the use of DDT against malaria has been discussed by Hayes (1971).

DOSAGE-RESPONSE OF DDT IN MAN *

Dosage (mg/kg/day)	Remarks
Unknown[a]:	Fatal
16-286[a]	Prompt vomiting at higher doses (all poisoned, convulsions in some)
10[a]	Moderate poisoning in some
6[a]	Moderate poisoning in one man
0.5	Tolerated by volunteers for 21 months
0.5	Tolerated by workers for 6½ years
0.25	Tolerated by workers for 19 years
0.004	Dosage of population in Delhi area, India, 1964—combined intake from living in sprayed houses and from food
0.0025	Dosage of general population of United States of America, 1953-1954
0.0004	Current dosage of general population of United States of America

* From *Off. Rec. Wld Hlth Org.* (1971).
[a] One dose only (accidental or suicidal).

Blood concentrations of DDT are significantly correlated with adipose tissue concentrations; recent exposure is reflected by a comparatively high proportion of DDT as such, lifelong exposure by a high proportion of DDE, the major metabolite of DDT.

Those who oppose the use of DDT suggest that it may present a hazard as a carcinogen and a mutagen. The limited experimental data relating to the mutagenicity of DDT are inconclusive. Although there is definite evidence that DDT in large doses increases the incidence of hepatomas in mice (Innes et al., 1969), the significance of this finding for man cannot yet be assessed. The present controversy is not only concerned with DDT as a potential carcinogen but raises the whole question of hepatoma induction in mice. The evaluation of DDT storage levels in mouse and human tissues, which has also been performed by the International Agency for Research on Cancer (IARC), indicates a difference in storage levels and metabolic patterns between man and mouse.

Epidemiological studies on the effects of long-term exposure of man to DDT are being carried out on malaria control spraymen in Brazil, with WHO support, and in India by WHO and the Indian Council for Medical Research. No adverse findings have yet emerged from these studies. Other epidemiological studies have been carried out by the IARC, and no clear relation between cancer patterns in different countries and the level of DDT in human fat has yet been demonstrated. There appears to be no evidence of an increase of primary carcinoma in man in the last 25 years in North America or Western Europe, that is from the time DDT was introduced into the human environment.

Ecological aspects of environmental pollution by DDT have received much attention in recent years. DDT has long been known to affect crustaceans and fish at rather low levels, but direct evidence of the harmful effects of DDT and other organochlorine insecticides on aquatic organisms is not easy to obtain, except when massive accidental pollution occurs, since the death of large quantities of fish may be due to a variety of causes other than poisoning. However, experimental studies and field observations seem to indicate that prolonged exposure to water containing DDT and dieldrin at concentrations exceeding 0.1 µg/litre constitutes a significant hazard to freshwater fish (Agricultural Research Council, 1970).

Another problem that has received much publicity is the effects of DDT on bird populations. There is experimental evidence that sufficiently high but sublethal concentrations of DDT may cause delay in sexual maturity and particularly by changes in land use. A United Kingdom committee observed in certain predatory bird populations, but whether the DDT was the dominant factor causing the reduction in number of a particular species is not certain. Bird populations may be reduced for other reasons as well, and particularly by changes in land use. A United Kingdom committee concludes that DDT must be regarded as a significant hazard to predatory birds that can accumulate residues in high concentrations (Agricultural Research Council, 1970).

REFERENCES

Agricultural Research Council (1970) *Third report of the Research Committee on Toxic Chemicals*, London, HM Stationery Office

Campbell, J. E., Richardson, L. A. & Schafer, M. L. (1965) *Arch. environm. Hlth*, **10**, 831-836

Durham, W. F., Ortega, P. & Hayes, W. J., jr (1963) *Arch. int. Pharmacodyn.*, **141**, 111-129

Edwards, C. A. (1970) *CRC Crit. Rev. environm. Control*, **1**, 7-67

Gillet, J. W., ed. (1970) *The biological impact of pesticides in the environment.* In: *Proceedings of a Symposium, Oregon State University, 1970*, Cornwallis, Oreg. (*Environmental Health Sciences Series*, No. 1)

Hayes, W. J., jr, Durham, W. F. & Cueto, C. (1956) *J. Amer. med. Ass.*, **162**, 890-897

Hayes, W. J., jr, Quinby, G. E., Walker, K. C., Elliott, J. W. & Upholt, W. M. (1958) *A.M.A. Arch. industr. Hlth*, **18**, 398-406

Hayes, W. J., jr (1971) *Bol. Ofic. sanit. panamer.*, **72**, 481-499

Hoffman, W. S., Fishbein, W. J. & Andelman, M. B. (1964) *Arch. environm. Hlth*, **9**, 387-394

IMCO/FAO/UNESCO/WMO/WHO/IAEA/UN Joint Group of Experts on the Scientific Aspects of Marine Pollution (GESAMP) (1971) *Report of the Third Session, Rome, 1970*, Geneva, Word Health Organization (unpublished document WHO/W. POLL/ 71.8; GESAMP 111/19)

Innes, J., Ulland, B. M., Valerio, M., Petrucelli, L., Fishbein, L., Hart, E. R., Pallotta, A. J., Bates, R., Falk, H., Gat, J., Klein, M., Mitchell, J. & Peters, J. (1969) *J. nat. Cancer Inst.*, **42**, 1101-1114

Kaloyanova-Simeonova, F. & Fournier, E. (1971) *Les pesticides et l'homme*, Paris, Masson

Laws, E. R., Curley, A. & Biros, F. J. (1967) *Arch. environm. Hlth*, **15**, 766-775

Ling, L., Whittemore, F. W. & Turtle, E. E. (1972) *Persistent insecticides in relation to the environment and their unintended effects*, Rome, Food and Agriculture Organization (unpublished document AGPP:MISC/4)

Moriarty, F. (1972) *New Scientist*, **53**, March

Off. Rec. Wld Hlth Org., 1971, **190**, 176-182

Ortelee, M. F. (1958) *A.M.A. Arch. industr. Hlth*, **18**, 433-440

Poland, A., Smith, D., Kuntzman, R., Jacobson, M. & Conney, A. H. (1970) *Clin. Pharmacol. Ther.*, **11**, 724-732

Robinson, J. (1971) *Chemistry in Britain*, **7**, 472-475

US Department of Health, Education and Welfare (1969) *Report of the Secretary's Commission on Pesticides and their Relationship to Environmental Health, Parts I and II*, Washington, D.C., US Government Printing Office

Polychlorinated Biphenyls

Polychlorinated biphenyls (PCBs) have recently given rise to great concern with respect to environmental contamination (Jensen, 1966; Holden & Marsden, 1967; Koeman et al., 1969; Lichtenstein et al., 1969; Duke et al., 1970; Sweden, National Environment Protection Board, 1970). They are used commercially in plasticizers, dielectrics, lubricants, hydraulic fluids, heat exchange media, and flame retardants. They are extremely resistant to biological degradation, and although characterized by a very low water solubility, have become widespread in the environment. Like DDT, the PCBs are stored in fatty tissue.

The commercially produced PCBs are mixtures; the highly chlorinated PCBs seem to persist in the environment much longer and are less toxic than the low-chlorine forms, which are more rapidly degraded. Some PCB mixtures may contain traces of dibenzofurans (Vos et al., 1970) or other extremely toxic impurities, including dioxins, which are difficult to detect in small amounts by current analytical procedures (Meselson & Baughman, 1971). The impurities may account for some of the toxic effects ascribed to the PCBs themselves.

The only information about the harmful effects of PCBs on man is derived from an accidental poisoning episode in Japan in 1968, which affected about a thousand people. The illness was named "Yusho" oil disease, and was caused by the ingestion of rice bran oil that had become contaminated with a commercial PCB mixture through a heat exchanger (Kuratsune et al., 1969; Hammond, 1972). The victims developed severe acne, eye discharge, and darkened skins. They consumed an average of 2 g of PCB, but about 0.5 g was sufficient to cause some symptoms. PCBs can pass through the placenta, and infants of apparently unaffected mothers were born with "Yusho" symptoms. Symptoms were still present in some individuals three years later. It is not known whether the PCB mixture contained dibenzofurans or other impurities. In biological systems, it seems that PCBs principally affect the liver tissue and a variety of enzyme systems (Hammond, 1972).

Recent studies in laboratory animals reveal liver damage and some reproduction abnormalities (Nishizumi, 1970; Hammond, 1972; US Food and Drug Administration Laboratories, unpublished report, 1971). PCB residues found in human tissue are presumably derived from food (Hammond, 1972), especially from fish because of their ability to concentrate PCBs in their organs and tissues (F.G. Lee & H.E. Stokinger, unpublished data, 1970). Fish-eating birds have also been found to contain relatively high concentrations of PCBs.

REFERENCES

Duke, T. W., Lowe, J. I. & Wilson, A. J., Jr (1970) *Bull. environm. Contam. Toxicol.*, **5**, 171-180

Hammond, A. L. (1972) *Science*, **175**, 155

Holden, A. V. & Marsden, K. (1967) *Nature (Lond.)*, **216**, 1274-1276

Jensen, S. (1966) *New Scientist*, **32**, 612

Koeman, J. H., ten Noever de Brauw, M. C. & de Vos, R. H. (1969) *Nature (Lond.)*, **221**, 1126-1129

Kuratsune, M. et al. (1969) *Fukuoka Acta med.*, **62**, 513

Lichtenstein, E. P., Schulz, K. R., Fuhremann, T. W. & Liang, T. T. (1969) *J. econ. Entomol.*, **62**, 761-765

Meselson, M. & Baughman, R. (1971) *An improved analysis for 2, 3, 7, 8-tetrachlorodi-benzen-p-dioxin.* In: *Proceedings of the 162nd National Meeting of the American Chemical Society*, Washington, D.C., American Chemical Society

Nishizumi, N. (1970) *Arch. environm. Hlth*, **21**, 620

Sweden, National Environment Protection Board (1970) *PCB Conference, Stockholm, 1970*, Solna

Vos, J. G., Koeman, J. H., van der Maas, H. L., ten Noever de Brauw, M. C. & de Vos, R. H. (1970) *Food Cosmet. Toxicol.*, **8**, 625

CHAPTER 13

SPECIAL PROBLEMS:
MUTAGENS; CARCINOGENS; TERATOGENS

General Considerations

A mutagen acts by changing the genetic material that is transferred to daughter cells when cell division occurs, with the result that the new cells have new heritable characters. The changes in the genetic material may consist in the alteration of one or a few nucleotides, or in chromosomal alterations, resulting in an altered number of chromosomes or an altered chromosomal structure (Kalter, 1971).

If a mutagen acts on the *germ* cells (spermatozoa or ova) of man (or any other sexually reproducing organism) some of the offspring will carry the mutant genes in all their cells. The mutant may be so disadvantageous that death occurs before birth, and if this occurs at a very early stage of fetal growth, the pregnancy may not even be detected. If pregnancy goes to term, however, an abnormal offspring may be born, but the appearance of such an offspring is not in itself evidence that a mutation has occurred, since it may also be due to teratogenesis.

This is the name given to the creation of congenital malformations resulting from interference with normal embryonic development by an environmental agent. Such malformations are not hereditary. In contrast, the congenital malformations resulting from changes in the genetic material are mutations, and are hereditary.

A mutagen may have an effect on *somatic* cells, and not on germ cells. In this case its effects are not passed on to offspring, but depend on the kind of cell affected. For example, the cells of the bone marrow go on multiplying throughout life and shed the products of division into the blood, where they function for a time as red and white blood cells before they are removed and replaced. Gross interference with the genetic material of such cells may make cell division ineffective in one way or another, and the outcome is no different from that of suppressive poisoning of the bone marrow by any other means. Another type of interference with the genetic material of these cells, e.g., theoretically by a virus or chemical, may make them capable of more rapid growth and multiplication, so that they are formed far more rapidly than they can be removed from the blood, where they interfere with normal body functions: if the white cells are affected in this way, the outcome is a leukaemia.

Similar interference with the genetic material could theoretically start up cell division in cells that do not normally divide during adult life. If the products of such division displace or invade normal tissues, the result is a cancer.

In both these instances, the mutagen responsible would have manifested activity as a *carcinogen*. A gross similarity between mutagenesis and carcinogenesis can be said to exist, since both these processes produce heritable changes in the phenotype (Miller & Miller, 1971). The mutation theory of carcinogenesis, first formulated by Boveri (Boveri, 1929), has recently received more support as a consequence of the demonstration that several chemical carcinogens or their metabolites have mutagenic properties. In the present state of our knowledge, we can say only that some chemicals have mutagenic, teratogenic and carcinogenic effects, but that no evidence exists that all chemicals exerting one of these three effects are necessarily also able to exert either or both of the other two.

From the point of view of protecting mankind from health hazards, it is the outcome of the action of these agents rather than the fundamental mode of action that is of importance. If a chemical proves to exhibit any of these three kinds of effect, however, it should be carefully tested for evidence of ability to produce either or both of the others.

A. Mutagens

Mutagens are feared because it is assumed that any altered genetic properties of the germ cells will always be disadvantageous and that they may not be detected until a considerable period of time, perhaps several generations, has elapsed. It is theoretically possible, however, for mutations to be neutral or even advantageous: evolution is assumed to be the outcome of the natural selection of advantageous mutations.

The number of possible mutations is immense, because of the genetic complexity of man, but there is no reliable information regarding recent changes in human mutation rates. Geneticists usually estimate such rates from retrospective studies, and the estimated values vary greatly and are affected by differences in the procedures used for this purpose. Furthermore, no systematic population monitoring has been performed in the past on any appreciable scale, whether in terms of numbers or the period of time covered. It is thus not possible to give an exact figure for the rate of either spontaneous or induced mutations in man (Sutton & Harris, 1972). Research to define the base-lines is the primary requirement.

Though it is not known to what extent, if any, gene mutations in the germ or somatic cells of man are due to chemicals present in the environment, a number of observations (WHO Scientific Group on the Evaluation and Testing of Drugs for Mutagenicity: Principles and Problems, 1971; Hollaender, 1971) speak for the existence of a potentially serious problem:

(1) many substances have been shown to cause gene mutations in micro-organisms and in insects;

(2) the induction of mutations by some drugs has been demonstrated in the laboratory in mammalian systems *in vivo*, and in human somatic cells;

(3) in man, chromosome aberrations have been observed with significant frequency in spontaneous abortions and in newborn infants, although it is not known what part chemicals might have played; and

(4) the use of chemicals that affect nucleic acids, the basic component of chromosomes, is increasing in the human environment.

An ideal strategy to minimize possible mutagenic hazards due to chemical substances in the human environment would require the testing of all such substances for mutagenicity in man. This is not feasible or possible, and a realistic programme must necessarily be more restricted in scope. Such a programme has recently been outlined with special reference to drugs (WHO Scientific Group on the Evaluation and Testing of Drugs for Mutagenicity: Principles and Problems, 1971). The difficulties involved in drawing up an ideal strategy are the result, however, not only of the enormous number of potential mutagens, but also of other factors, all subject to wide variation, including the concentrations of these substances and the period for which they are present in the environment, the size of the population group exposed to any particular substance, and the age-group structure of this group. Finally, risk/benefit ratios will no doubt vary according to value judgements based upon observed need in different countries.

The following should receive special attention (WHO Scientific Group on the Evaluation and Testing of Drugs for Mutagenicity: Principles and Problems, 1971; Schubert, 1972; Sutton & Harris, 1972):

(1) compounds that are chemically, pharmacologically and biochemically related to known or suspected mutagens;

(2) compounds that exhibit certain toxic effects in animals, such as depression of bone marrow; inhibition of spermatogenesis or oogenesis; inhibition of mitosis; teratogenic effects; carcinogenic effects; causation of sterility or semi-sterility in reproduction studies; stimulation or inhibition of growth or synthetic activity of a specific cell or organ; inhibition of immune response; and

(3) compounds that are likely to be continuously absorbed into the body and retained by it for long periods.

Testing for mutagenic activity should be considered as part of the overall toxicological procedure, and since no single test or battery of tests can be expected to detect and characterize all mutagenic agents, the use of several tests is essential. It is most desirable that the mutagenic test species should be mammalian. The use of submammalian test systems and *in vitro* cell cultures (even tests with human cells) should be regarded as ancillary procedures.

Representative examples of mutagenic tests include the dominant lethal test, *in vivo* cytogenetic methods, and host-mediated assays, using micro-organisms or mammalian cells in a mammalian host.

In the dominant lethal test, male rodents are fed with food including the mutagen under test. Each male is caged with virgin females. All females are autopsied 13 days from mid-week of their mating. At autopsy, animals are scored for total implantations, early deaths, and late deaths.

A mutagenic index (M.I.) reflecting the incidence of dominant lethal mutations in the experimental group of animals is conventionally calculated as follows:

$$\text{M.I.} = \frac{\text{deciduomata} + \text{late deaths}}{\text{total implantations}} \times 100$$

In the host-mediated assay, indicator micro-organisms or mammalian cells are incorporated intraperitoneally within a mammalian host. Direct administration of the compound to the host allows the animal to activate or deactivate the potential mutagen before it encounters the cell or micro-organism in the peritoneum. After an incubation period, the micro-organisms or the cells are removed from the peritoneum and plated on minimal and complete media in order to determine the ratio of mutants to wild type. The resulting mutant frequency is compared to that occurring spontaneously, and thus serves as an indicator of relative mutagenicity.

In vivo cytogenetic methods are based on a comparison between the number of chromosome breaks in the cells of treated and control animals.

Each test has advantages and disadvantages that must be weighed when selecting a panel of tests. Almost all experimentally tested alkylating compounds, derivatives of nitrogen mustard, ethyleneimine, certain derivatives of sulfonic acid, several *N*-nitrosamines and hydrazine derivatives, as well as the natural compounds aflatoxin, cycasin and their metabolite methylazoxymethanol, show mutagenic activity in the dominant lethal test (Frohberg, 1971).

The mutagenic indices of certain environmental pollutants, as indicated by the results of the dominant lethal test in an experimental group of mice, have been determined by a few authors (Epstein et al., 1970; Ehling et al., 1968; Vogel, 1971). The information obtained from such an index, however, is of limited value in the assessment of risk, since large sex and strain differences in response to the same compound exist in mice (Generoso

& Russell, 1969). Furthermore, the finding that a substance is mutagenic in one species does not necessarily mean that it is mutagenic in all species, although the basic chemical components of hereditary material are the same in all organisms.

MUTAGENIC INDICES OF ENVIRONMENTAL POLLUTANTS [1]

Compound	Dose (mg/kg)	Mutagenic index (M.I.)[2]
Cumene hydroperoxide	34	3
I, I, I-Trichloro-2, 2-bis (p-chlorophenyl) ethane (DDT)	105	3
Acrolein	1.5	5
Aflatoxin [3]	68	11
Benzo[a]pyrene	750	11
Tris (I-aziridinyl) phosphine sulfide (THIOTEPA)	5	18
Triethylene melamine (TEM)	0.2	26
Tris (2-methyl-I-aziridinyl) phosphine oxide (METEPA)	40	27
Methylmethanesulfonate (MMS)	50	29
Tris (I-aziridinyl) phosphine oxide (TEPA)	7	38

[1] From Epstein & Shafner (1968).

[2] As determined from the results of the dominant lethal test in mice treated with the median lethal dose (LD$_{50}$) of the compound concerned.

$$M.I. = \frac{deciduomata + late\ deaths}{total\ implantations} \times 100$$

The value of the M.I. was I in mice used as controls.

[3] In dimethylsulfoxide suspension.

A positive finding in one species (see table) should thus be considered as an indication of potential mutagenic activity in man, unless relevant differences in metabolism, toxicological behaviour and/or other effects can be demonstrated between the species used and man, although the failure to demonstrate such differences does not mean that they do not exist. If, however, such differences are demonstrated, the relevance to man of the positive mutagenic findings should be further questioned (WHO Scientific Group on the Evaluation and Testing of Drugs for Mutagenicity: Principles and Problems, 1971).

As in other areas of toxicological testing, the dose-response relationship is important (see Chapter 11). It is also important to correlate mutagenic dose-response curves with those of other important biological effects (WHO Scientific Group on the Evaluation and Testing of Drugs for Muta-genicity: Principles and Problems, 1971). Dose-dependent mutagenic effects have been demonstrated in the dominant lethal test for the oral or parenteral administration of trimethylphosphate—a gasoline additive—to male mice (Generoso & Russell, 1969), N-propylmethanesulfonate, iso-propylmethane-sulfonate, ethylmethanesulfonate and methylmethanesulfonate (Epstein et al., 1970).

The assumption that mutagenic activity in animals is relevant to man presents problems similar to those in some other fields of toxicology. The assessment of the risk to man is difficult because the pharmacokinetic behaviour and metabolism of a chemical may vary from one species to another and this increases the difficulty of predicting its effects in man. The confirmation in man of a positive mutagenic finding in tissue culture or in experimental animals is very difficult. It may be more difficult to confirm than a negative finding.

Studies in man can be of two types: (1) the examination of individuals; and (2) epidemiological. The design is often complicated by uncontrollable variables (WHO Scientific Group on the Evaluation and Testing of Drugs for Mutagenicity: Principles and Problems, 1971). Monitoring of human populations for mutagenic effects on the genome is subject to difficult and, as yet, mostly unsolved problems (Vogel, 1971; Sutton & Harris, 1972).

Whatever the system of testing potential mutagens adopted, it can never be perfect. It will still be necessary to decide whether and when to use chemicals of known or unknown mutagenic potency. Where there is a choice of several equally effective compounds of different mutagenic potential, the compound with the smallest mutagenic risk for the individual and the population, as determined by whatever tests are available, should naturally be chosen. With this approach in mind, protection against genetic hazard need not (and cannot) await a complete bioassay on all chemicals. Substantial progress has already been made in this field, and research must be continued and expanded, for it will undoubtedly contribute significantly to the development of testing methods, and thus to better assessments of the risk connected with the use of chemicals in the human environment (Sutton & Harris, 1972).

REFERENCES

Boveri, T. (1929) *The origin of malignant tumors*, Baltimore, Williams & Wilkins Co.

Ehling, U. H., Doherty, D. G. & Malling, H. V. (1968) *Differential mutagenic action of N- and iso-propyl methanesulfonate in mice.* In: *Proceedings of the XII International Congress of Genetics*, Vol. 1, Tokyo, The Science Council of Japan, p. 103

Epstein, S. S., Bass, W., Arnold, E. & Bishop, Y. (1970) *Science*, **168**, 584

Epstein, S. S. & Shafner, H. (1968) *Nature (Lond.)*, **219**, 385-387

Frohberg, H. (1971) *Arch. Toxikol.*, **28**, 135-148

Generoso, W. M. & Russell, W. L. (1969) *Mutation Res.*, **8**, 589-598

Hollaender, A., ed. (1971) *Chemical mutagens*, New York/London, Plenum Press

Kalter, H. (1971) *Correlation between teratogenic and mutagenic effects of chemicals in mammals.* In: Hollaender, A., ed., *Chemical mutagens*, New York/London, Plenum Press, pp. 57-82

Miller, E. C. & Miller, J. A. (1971) *The mutagenicity of chemical carcinogens: correlations, problems and interpretations.* In: Hollaender, A., ed., *Chemical mutagens*, New York/London, Plenum Press, pp. 83-119

Schubert, J. (1972) *Ambio*, **1**, 79-89

Sutton, H. E. & Harris, M. I. (1972) *Mutagenic effects of environmental contaminants*, New York/London, Academic Press

Vogel, F. (1971) *Monitoring of human populations.* In: Vogel, F. & Röhrborn, G., eds, *Chemical mutagenesis in mammals and man*, Berlin/Heidelberg/New York, Springer

WHO Scientific Group on the Evaluation and Testing of Drugs for Mutagenicity: Principles and Problems (1971) *Report*, Geneva (*Wld Hlth Org. techn. Rep. Ser.*, No. 482)

B. Carcinogens

Introduction

It has been estimated that a large proportion of human cancers are directly associated with environmental agents (US Congress, Senate, Government Operations Committee, 1971; Higginson, 1969; Clayson, 1962), and it is necessary to determine if these agents can be identified and quantified. While no association has as yet been found between biological environmental agents and cancer in man, such an association has been proved for certain chemical and physical agents.

A situation where an identified population group is exposed to an identified carcinogen is obviously the most easily controlled and offers the best possibility for prevention. An increased incidence of tumours occurring at a particular site or at an unusual rate has generally given the alarm in such a situation, and has been followed by investigations to determine the chemical responsible (WHO Expert Committee on the Prevention of Cancer, 1964). However, for the investigations to be successful, the chemical must be present at such a high level that its action obscures the effect(s) of other environmental factors to which the same population group may be exposed.

A much more difficult situation exists in respect of the general population, where exposure to a multitude of recognized, suspected or unknown carcinogenic hazards must be assumed. The quantitative assessment of the total environmental carcinogenic load to which man is exposed in his environment remains the ultimate goal. This is the total of all the identified carcinogens that are ingested, inhaled, percutaneously absorbed or occasionally introduced by medical or accidental injection, implantation or mucosal absorption. In our present state of knowledge of many of these factors, the practical implication is that the assessment of the carcinogenic load must be restricted to the evaluation of known carcinogenic agents, including both those for which human data exist and those for which experimental data alone are available.

Up to the present, it has been assumed that a "no-effect" level cannot be determined for carcinogenic substances. This concept is based on experimental animal studies showing that, unlike other forms of intoxication, carcinogenesis is the result of an accumulation of irreversible cellular damage rather than an accumulation of a toxic substance (Foulds, 1969).

Quantitative information on identified carcinogens in the human environment is incomplete. This is partly due to the lack of adequate analytical methods and/or the great variations in the levels of accuracy of the analytical methods available (US Food and Drug Administration, 1971).

Two programmes currently being carried out by the International Agency for Research on Cancer (IARC) are of relevance in this context: (1) a programme on the development and standardization of adequate analytical methods for the identification and quantification of chemical carcinogens in the environment; (2) the preparation of monographs on identified or suspected carcinogens giving a balanced evaluation of all epidemiological and experimental data in order to provide a basis for practical recommendations by international organizations, such as WHO and ILO, or preventive measures or legislation to be enacted by individual governments (International Agency for Research on Cancer, 1972).

Definition of chemical carcinogens

The term "chemical carcinogen" in its widely accepted sense is used to indicate a substance that is known conclusively to induce or enhance neoplasia. Induction of tumours and enhancement of tumour induction are not distinguished for present practical purposes, although it is known that there may be fundamental differences in mechanisms (Foulds, 1969). The terms "tumorigen", "oncogen" and "blastomogen" have all been used synonymously with "carcinogen".

Epidemiological evidence of human carcinogenicity

Confirmation (as well as suspicion) that a particular chemical is carcinogenic in man depends on epidemiological data that may be: (1) descriptive; (2) retrospective; or (3) prospective.

Descriptive studies can identify a cluster, or a change or difference in rates for a neoplasm in a sub-group of the population.

Retrospective studies of the histories of affected persons have revealed such occupational or iatrogenic carcinogens as shale oil, chromates, asbestos, 2-naphthylamine, benzidine, chlornaphazine,[1] Thorotrast[2] and transplacental synthetic oestrogens. Once a relationship between a chemical and human cancer is confirmed or suspected, prospective (cohort) studies can define more precisely the time relationship and the magnitude of the risk, among other aspects of cancer induction.

Prospective studies are follow-up studies. The population studied is divided into groups in accordance with the degree and duration of exposure to a suspected or known carcinogen. In case-control studies, the groups compared should, as far as possible, differ only in exposure to the agent. Follow-up studies are then carried out to determine the occurrence of cancer in the various exposure categories (from zero to heavy), and comparison

---

[1] An antineoplastic drug: N,N-bis(2-chloroethyl)-2-naphthylamine.
[2] A contrast medium containing thorium (IV) oxide, formerly used in radiology.

of the results obtained enables the magnitude of the increased risk to be assessed. The analysis will also reveal the relationship between cancer occurrence and age at first exposure, as well as the latent period. Care must be taken in the analysis to exclude the influence of variables other than the agent suspected of inducing the cancer under study (e.g., cigarette smoking in the study of lung cancer among asbestos workers).

Finally, if a specific chemical does cause cancer in man, its removal from the environment should be followed by epidemiological evidence of a decline in the frequency of the neoplasm concerned.

Validity of experimental animal data

While a limited number of individual chemicals have been shown conclusively to be associated with cancer in man, and a positive association with cancer in man has also been demonstrated for mixtures of chemicals, although no information is available on the specific components responsible, several hundred chemical substances have been shown to be carcinogenic in experimental animals. For some of them data exist that indicate the possibility of human exposure. It must be noted that, with the possible exception of arsenic, all substances for which conclusive evidence of carcinogenicity in man exists have also been proved to be carcinogenic in animals.

In many experimental carcinogenesis studies, the type of cancer seen is the same as that recorded in human studies (e.g., bladder cancer is produced in man, hamster, dog and monkey by 2-naphthylamine). In other instances, however, species variations result in the induction of different types of neoplasms at different locations by the same carcinogen (e.g., benzidine causes liver cell carcinoma in the rat and bladder carcinoma in dog and man).

Broad-spectrum chemical or physical tests to identify chemical carcinogens are not at present available, nor does it appear likely that they can be developed in the near future. This is mainly because carcinogenic chemicals constitute a varied group of agents differing widely in their level of activity, the ways in which they are activated in cells and their dosage requirements. It appears that long-term tests in experimental animals will, for a long time to come, remain the best available method of assessing the potential carcinogenicity of a chemical. All efforts should therefore be made to develop objective criteria for extrapolation from experimental data to man.

Recent developments in testing chemicals for their mutagenic properties in mammals, including host-mediated assay (see previous section) and a variety of cytogenetic methods, have opened up new possibilities of improving the criteria by which experimental animal tests can be used to assess potential hazards to man (Legator & Malling, 1971; Röhrborn, 1971).

The rapid detection of compounds that are converted into electrophilic reactants (i.e., reactants containing electron-deficient atoms) in experimental animal tissues may thus become feasible. This will be of particular value in the establishment of a reliable and rapid method for screening the ever increasing number of chemicals introduced into the environment. In fact, the large majority of chemical carcinogens need to be metabolically activated in order to exert their carcinogenic action, and all the reactive forms of chemical carcinogens appear to be strong electrophiles (Miller & Miller, 1971). Some authorities, however, do not accept these views, holding that the information so obtained is not adequate to indicate potential carcinogens.

General characteristics of environmental carcinogenic agents

Polynuclear compounds

This widespread group of substances is synthesized mainly in the combustion of organic materials; they are thus present in all kinds of soot and smoke. They occur in tobacco smoke, in smoked fish and meat, in coal and in coal tar pitch, and in the atmosphere of all urban areas, as well as in increasing quantities in rural areas, mainly as a result of the discharge of the exhaust gases from gasoline and diesel engines. Man is exposed to complex mixtures of these substances and exposure occurs under a variety of circumstances and through different routes. Some representative compounds in several of these mixtures have been identified.

Although no evidence exists to indicate that benzo[a]pyrene (BP) is either the most widespread or the most potent polynuclear carcinogen in the environment, it has been studied more than any other, and in many instances is the only one estimated.

BP has been found in the air in concentrations ranging from 0.01 to 100 μg/1000 m^3, corresponding to an annual intake of 0.05–500 μg, on the basis of 5000 m^3 of air inhaled per year per individual. Benz[c]acridine and dibenz[a,h]acridine have also been found in urban air in concentrations of 1 and 0.2 μg/1000 m^3. BP has been found in cigarette smoke at levels ranging from 2.0 to 122 μg/1000 cigarettes. Other carcinogenic poly-nuclear compounds found in tobacco smoke are dibenz[a,h]anthracene, dibenzo[a,i]pyrene, benzo[c]phenanthrene, indeno[1,2,3-c,d]pyrene, dibenz-[a,j]acridine, dibenz[a,h]acridine and 7H-dibenzo[c,g]carbazole (Shubik et al., 1970). The association between cigarette smoke and bronchial car-cinoma in man has been confirmed (US Public Health Service, 1967).

BP is a component of all kinds of soot and smoke, including wood smoke. It also occurs in coal tar and processed rubber. BP and other polynuclear compounds have been found in smoked fish, shellfish and char-coal broiled steaks. BP has also been found in other foodstuffs, e.g., in vegetables, cereals and roasted coffee.

Exposure to mixtures of polynuclear compounds has been reported to be associated with human cancer, and in particular with epitheliomas of the scrotum and other skin cancers in chimney sweeps, wax pressmen and cotton mule spinners, as well as with skin cancers in workers exposed to various mineral oils and lung cancer in gas workers (Doll, 1952; Falk, Kotin & Mehler, 1964).

Aromatic amines

For some of the compounds in this group (2-naphthylamine, benzidine) a definite association between occupational exposure and bladder cancer in man has been demonstrated (Case et al., 1954; Hueper, 1969). For others (4-aminobiphenyl, magenta, auramine, 1-naphthylamine), association with an occupational cancer risk has been reported with various degrees of uncertainty (Hueper, 1969; Goldwater, Rosso & Kleinfeld, 1965; Scott, 1952; Melick et al., 1955; Koss, Melamed & Kelly, 1969).

Exposure to aromatic amines can occur not only in industrial environments, but also through the air, foodstuffs, plastics and drinking-water. Analytical methods for the quantitative determination of carcinogenic aromatic amines have been worked out (Shubik et al., 1970).

Chlorinated hydrocarbons

Some of the compounds belonging to this group are widely used as industrial solvents, reactive intermediates, fumigants or pesticides, and are therefore widely distributed in the environment. Among them, carbon tetrachloride, chloroform and the pesticides DDT, aldrin, dieldrin, heptachlor and HCH merit special consideration. The first two may be found in industrial environments and as contaminants in food or other commodities (e.g., carbon tetrachloride in bread, chloroform in toothpaste) while some of the chlorinated pesticides (DDT, HCH) are widely distributed in the environment. Concern as to the potential hazard represented by certain chlorinated hydrocarbons, such as DDT, is based on: (*a*) their ubiquity; (*b*) their persistence in the environment; (*c*) their capacity to accumulate in living organisms, including man, and in the fetus; and (*d*) the experimental evidence of a potential carcinogenic effect (Fitzhugh & Nelson, 1947; Hayes, 1966; Innes et al., 1969; Terracini, 1967; Tomatis, 1969; US Department of Health, Education, and Welfare, 1969; Tomatis et al., 1971). There is so far no evidence, however, of DDT being harmful for man under normal circumstances of use (see pp. 205-210).

N-nitroso compounds

In recent years many compounds belonging to this group have been found to be highly carcinogenic in several animal species, in which tumours can be induced at a variety of organ sites (Magee & Barnes, 1956; Druckrey et al., 1967). There is much concern about the possibility that these compounds may represent a cancer hazard to man. They have been used as industrial solvents and chemical intermediates, but there is growing evidence that they may occur at low levels in a variety of natural products. In addition, the possibility exists that N-nitroso compounds may be formed *in vivo* through the interaction of precursors, namely nitrites and secondary amines or amides. The formation of carcinogenic N-nitroso compounds in the stomachs of rats fed with nitrite and certain secondary amines or amides has been reported (Sander, 1967; Sander & Seif, 1969; Sander & Bürkle, 1971; Montesano & Magee, 1971; Mirvish, 1971). In addition, the administration to rats and mice of nitrites and some secondary amines or amides has resulted in the induction of tumours of the same type as those induced by the corresponding N-nitroso compounds (Ivankovic & Preussmann, 1970; Greenblatt et al., 1971).

The unequivocal detection and quantification of N-nitroso compounds in biological materials is particularly difficult. However, improved analytical methods for this purpose for certain compounds have recently been developed (International Agency for Research on Cancer, 1972).

Inorganic substances

Several reports indicate an association between occupational exposure to some inorganic substances and cancer in man; examples include, in particular, the occurrence of bronchogenic carcinoma in chromium chemical manufacture (Machle & Gregorius, 1948; Bidstrup & Case, 1956), cancer of the ethmoid sinus in nickel refiners (Doll, 1958), mesothelioma in asbestos workers (Harrington et al., 1971) and skin or possibly bronchial carcinoma in workers exposed to various inorganic arsenic salts (Shubik et al., 1970; Lee & Fraumini, 1969). For other inorganic substances, evidence of carcinogenicity in experimental animals exists but human carcinogenicity has not been definitely confirmed, although it is suspected more or less strongly. This applies in particular to beryllium and beryllium salts (Hardy, Rabe & Lorch, 1967), cadmium salts, cobalt, lead salts, iron and iron(III) oxide, and selenium (Boyd et al., 1970; Shubik et al., 1970).

Naturally occurring carcinogens

The most important and most widely distributed compounds in this group are the mycotoxins, and among these the aflatoxins (Wogan, 1969). It has been shown that aflatoxin contamination can occur in virtually every food when harvesting, storage or transport conditions permit growth of spoilage moulds. A correlation between aflatoxin levels in food and liver cell carcinoma in certain population groups has been reported (Alpert et al., 1971; Shank et al., 1972a,b,c). Another mycotoxin that has been shown to occur widely in the environment and for which experimental evidence of carcinogenicity has been reported, is sterigmatocystin (Purchase &

van der Watt, 1970). Other naturally occurring substances shown to be carcinogenic in experimental animals are cycad nuts, Senecio alkaloids, bracken fern, parasorbic acid, safrole and isosafrole (Laqueur et al., 1963; Spatz & Laqueur, 1967; Pamukcu, Göksoy & Price, 1966; Pamukcu, Price & Bryan, 1970; Dickens & Jones, 1963; Long et al., 1963).

Hormonal carcinogens

Carcinogenesis in man and experimental animals can be strongly influenced by various kinds of hormonal imbalances. In addition, some synthetic hormones may possess carcinogenic properties that can be both related or unrelated to their hormonal action. Among the chemicals having hormonal effects or acting upon endocrine organs, oestrogens and goitrogens deserve attention as potential carcinogenic hazards. Oestrogenic activity is associated with a variety of chemical structures including steroids, stilbenes, flavones, and biphenols. Oestrogens of different chemical structures have produced tumours in experimental animals. Although the significance of this observation for man is not completely clear, it is relevant to note that recent reports indicate that the administration of stilboestrol to pregnant women results in a highly increased risk that their daughters will develop vaginal adenocarcinomas (Herbst et al., 1971; Greenwald et al., 1971). While this first report on transplacental carcinogenesis in man concerns exposure to stilboestrol used for medical purposes, this compound can also be found as a food contaminant and in cosmetic preparations, although in very small amounts.

Endemic goitre results from environmental factors (e.g., lack of iodine in water) and increases by a factor of about five in the incidence of thyroid carcinoma have been found in goitrous populations (Shubik et al., 1970).

Biological alkylating agents

A number of other substances belonging to a wide variety of classes of chemicals have been found to be carcinogenic in experimental animals. Among these, the most important are the biological alkylating agents, which are being introduced with increasing frequency. They are used as industrial intermediates in organic synthesis or as organic solvents, and also as chemotherapeutic agents. Examples of chemicals belonging to this group are the nitrogen and sulfur mustards, epoxides, ethyleneimines, alkyl sulfates, strained ring lactones and sulfones (Boyland & Down, 1971; Van Duuren et al., 1966; Druckrey et al., 1970).

REFERENCES

Introduction; Definition of chemical carcinogens; Validity of experimental animal data

Clayson, D. B. (1962) *Chemical carcinogenesis*, Boston, Little, Brown & Co.

Foulds, L. (1969) *Neoplastic development*, London, Academic Press, Vol. 1

Higginson, J. (1969) *Present trends in cancer epidemiology.* In: Morgan, J. F., ed., *Proceedings of the Eighth Canadian Cancer Research Conference, Honey Harbor, Ontario, 1968,* Oxford, Pergamon, pp. 40-75

International Agency for Research on Cancer (1972) *IARC monographs on the evaluation of carcinogenic risk of chemicals to man,* Lyon, Vol. I

Legator, M. S. & Malling, H. V. (1971) *The host-mediated assay, a practical procedure for evaluating potential mutagenic agents in mammals.* In: Hollaender, A., ed., *Chemical mutagens—principles and methods for their detection,* New York, Plenum, Vol. 2, pp. 569-589

Miller, J. A. & Miller, E. C. (1971) *J. nat. Cancer Inst.,* **47,** 5-24

Röhrborn, G. (1971) *Arch. Toxikol.,* **28,** 120-128

US Congress, Senate, Government Operations Committee (1971) *Chemicals and the future of man: hearings before the Subcommittee on Executive Reorganization and Government Research, 92nd Congress, 1st Session, April 6 & 7, 1971,* Washington, D.C., US Government Printing Office

US Food and Drug Administration, Advisory Committee on Protocols for Safety Evaluation, Panel on Carcinogenesis (1971) *Toxicol. appl. Pharmacol.,* **20,** 419-438

WHO Expert Committee on the Prevention of Cancer (1964) *Report,* Geneva (*Wld Hlth Org. techn. Rep. Ser.,* No. 276)

Polynuclear compounds

Doll, R. (1952) *Brit. J. industr. Med.,* **9,** 180

Falk, H. L., Kotin, P. & Mehler, A. (1964) *Arch. environm. Hlth,* **8,** 721-729

Shubik, P., Clayson, D. B. & Terracini, B., eds (1970) *The quantification of environmental carcinogens,* Geneva, International Union Against Cancer (*UICC techn. Rep. Ser.,* Vol. 4)

US Public Health Service (1967) *The health consequences of smoking: a PHS review,* Washington, D.C. (Publication No. 1696)

Aromatic amines

Case, R. A. M., Hosker, M. E., McDonald, D. B. & Pearson, J. T. (1956) *Brit. J. industr. Med.,* **11,** 75-104

Goldwater, L. J., Rosso, A. J. & Kleinfeld, M. (1965) *Arch. environm. Hlth,* **11,** 814

Hueper, W. C. (1969) *Occupational and environmental cancer of the urinary system,* New Haven & London, Yale University Press

Innes, J. R. M. et al. (1969) *J. nat. Cancer Inst.,* **42,** 1101

Koss, L. G., Melamed, M. R. & Kelly, R. W. (1969) *J. nat. Cancer Inst.,* **43,** 233

Melick, W. F., Escue, H. M., Naryka, J. J., Mezera, R. A. & Wheeler, E. R. (1955) *J. Urol. (Baltimore),* **74,** 760-766

Scott, T. S. (1952) *Brit. J. industr. Med.,* **9,** 127-132

Shubik, P., Clayson, D. B. & Terracini, B., eds (1970) *The quantification of environmental carcinogens,* Geneva, International Union Against Cancer (*UICC techn. Rep. Ser.,* Vol. 4)

Chlorinated hydrocarbons

Fitzhugh, O. G. & Nelson, A. A. (1947) *J. Pharmacol. exp. Ther.,* **89,** 18-30

Hayes, W. H., Jr (1966) *Monitoring food and people for pesticide content. Scientific aspects of pest control,* Washington, D.C. (NAS-NRC Publication No. 1402), pp. 314-322

Innes, J. R. M. et al. (1969) *J. nat. Cancer Inst.*, **42**, 1101

Terracini, B. (1967) *Tumori*, **53**, 601-618

Tomatis, L. (1969) *Studies on the potential carcinogenic hazard represented by DDT.* In: Kuroiwa, H., ed., *Proceedings of the IV International Congress of Rural Medicine, Tokyo, 1969*, Tokyo, Japanese Association of Rural Medicine, pp. 64-71

Tomatis, L., Turusov, V., Terracini, B., Day, N., Barthel, W. F., Charles, R. T., Collins, G. B. & Boiocchi, M. (1972) *Tumori*, **57**, 377-396

US Department of Health, Education, and Welfare (1969) *Secretary's Commission on Pesticides and their Relationship to Environmental Health. Report*, Washington, D.C., US Government Printing Office

N-nitroso compounds

Druckrey, H., Preussmann, R., Ivankovic, S. & Schmähl, D. (1967) *Z. Krebsforsch.*, **69**, 103

Greenblatt, M., Mirvish, S. S. & So, B. T. (1971) *J. nat. Cancer Inst.*, **46**, 1029-1034

International Agency for Research on Cancer (1972) *Analysis and formation of N-nitroso compounds*, Lyon (in press)

Ivankovic, S. & Preussmann, R. (1970) *Naturwissenschaften*, **57**, 460

Magee, P. N. & Barnes, J. M. (1956) *Brit. J. Cancer*, **10**, 114

Mirvish, S. S. (1971) *J. nat. Cancer Inst.*, **46**, 1183-1193

Montesano, R. & Magee, P. N. (1971) *Int. J. Cancer*, **7**, 249-255

Sander, J. (1967) *Arch. Hyg. (Berl.)*, **151**, 23-28

Sander, J. & Bürkle, G. (1971) *Z. Krebsforsch.*, **75**, 301-304

Sander, J. & Seif, F. (1969) *Arzneimittel-Forsch.*, **19**, 1091-1093

Inorganic substances

Bidstrup, P. L. & Case, R. A. M. (1956) *Brit. J. industr. Med.*, **13**, 260-264

Boyd, J. T., Doll, R., Faulds, J. S. & Leiper, J. (1970) *Brit. J. industr. Med.*, **27**, 97

Doll, R. (1958) *Brit. J. industr. Med.*, **15**, 217-223

Hardy, H. L., Rabe, E. W. & Lorch, S. (1967) *J. occup. Med.*, **9**, 271

Harrington, J. S., Gilson, J. C. & Wagner, J. C. (1971) *Nature (Lond.)*, **232**, 54-55

Lee, A. M. & Fraumini, J. F. J. (1969) *J. nat. Cancer Inst.*, **42**, 1045

Machle, W. & Gregorius, F. (1948) *Publ. Hlth Rep. (Wash.)*, **63**, 1114-1127

Shubik, P., Clayson, D. B. & Terracini, B., eds (1970) *The quantification of environmental carcinogens*, Geneva, International Union Against Cancer (*UICC techn. Rep. Ser.*, Vol. 4)

Naturally occurring carcinogens

Alpert, M. E., Hutt, M. S. R., Wogan, G. N. & Davidson, C. S. (1971) *Cancer*, **28**, 253

Dickens, F. & Jones, H. E. H. (1963) *Brit. J. Cancer*, **17**, 100

Laqueur, G. L., Michelson, O., Whiting, M. G. & Kurland, L. T. (1963) *J. nat. Cancer Inst.*, **31**, 919

Long, E. L., Nelson, A. A., Fitzhugh, O. G. & Jansen, W. H. (1963) *Arch. Path.*, **75**, 595

Pamukcu, A. M., Göksoy, S. K. & Price, J. M. (1966) *Cancer Res.*, **26**, 1745-1753

Pamukcu, A. M., Price, J. M. & Bryan, G. T. (1970) *Cancer Res.*, **30**, 902-905

Purchase, I. F. H. & van der Watt, J. J. (1970) *Food Cosmet. Toxicol.*, **8**, 289-297

Shank, R. C., Gordon, J. E., Wogan, G. N., Nondasuta, A. & Subhamani, B. (1972a) *Food Cosmet. Toxicol.*, **10**, 71-84

Shank, R. C., Wogan, G. N. & Gibson, J. B. (1972b) *Food Cosmet. Toxicol.*, **10**, 51-60

Shank, R. C., Wogan, G. N., Gibson, J. B. & Nondasuta, A. (1972c) *Food Cosmet. Toxicol.*, **10**, 61-69

Spatz, M. & Laqueur, G. L. (1967) *J. nat. Cancer Inst.*, **38**, 233

Wogan, G. N. (1969) *Progr. exp. Tumor Res. (Basel)*, **11**, 134

Hormonal carcinogens

Greenwald, P., Barlow, J. J., Nasca, P. C. & Burnett, W. S. (1971) *New Engl. J. Med.*, **385**, 390-392

Herbst, A. L., Ulfelder, H. & Poskanzer, D. C. (1971) *New. Engl. J. Med.*, **284**, 878-881

Shubik, P., Clayson, D. B. & Terracini, B., eds (1970) *The quantification of environmental carcinogens*, Geneva, International Union Against Cancer (*UICC techn. Rep. Ser.*, Vol. 4)

Biological alkylating agents

Boyland, E. & Down, W. H. (1971) *Europ. J. Cancer*, **7**, 495-500

Druckrey, H., Kruse, H., Preussmann, R., Ivankovic, S. & Landschütz, C. (1970) *Z. Krebsforsch.*, **74**, 241

Van Duuren, B. L., Langseth, L., Orris, L., Teebor, G., Nelson, N. & Kuschner, M. (1966) *J. nat. Cancer Inst.*, **37**, 825

C.   Teratogens

Teratology is the study of deviations occurring during prenatal development.   These deviations are roughly the same as those covered by the common term "birth defects", the only difference being that "defects" caused by obstetrical trauma are not considered developmental deviations.

The question as to just when a variation becomes a "deviation" and not a "normal variant" requires considerably more knowledge of normal development than is currently available; there is therefore some degree of arbitrariness in the very subject matter of the field itself.   It is generally agreed that variations in the offspring not compatible with normal function are not "normal" variants, although there is controversy as to what is to be regarded as normal function.   In addition, the same nosological ambiguities exist in teratology as are found in other fields, defects being sometimes named descriptively (anencephaly), sometimes etiologically ("rubella" syndrome).   All these factors underline the difficulty of achieving some degree of coherence in environmental teratology, itself a fairly new field in public health.

The emphasis here will be on post-conceptional events connected with environmental factors (in particular chemical agents), where the genotypes of the parent and the offspring are normally related but the phenotypes (individually expressed variations) are not.   Genes certainly play a crucial role in the control of development, but we shall be concerned here primarily with those instances in which this control is diverted from its normal course by additional factors.

The diversion may take several forms. At the extreme, development may cease altogether and result in the death of the conceptus. In less extreme form there may be intra-uterine growth retardation, i.e., failure to achieve normal levels of growth and development for some gestational stage. Either of these phenomena may or may not be accompanied by gross structural or functional anomaly (congenital "malformations" *per se*).

It has been estimated that over 80 % of known clinical congenital malformations and spontaneous abortions are of unknown etiology (Cohlan, 1967). Roughly 12 % can be traced to genetic factors, with a few per cent more to known "environmental insults". By contrast, it can be shown in the laboratory that a very broad range of chemical agents can produce, under the proper conditions, some type of serious developmental deviation (Cohlan, 1967). Thus substances already found to be embryopathic in animals range from highly toxic substances, such as the anti-tumour agents, to commonplace consumer items, e.g., aspirin, and completely inert materials.

As far as man is concerned, data recently collected by certain institutions on behalf of WHO contribute relatively little to knowledge of comparative frequencies, but do give some information on the average incidence of malformations in general. The outcomes of 421 181 pregnancies resulting in 426 932 post-27th-week births showed a frequency of 12.7 major malformations and 4.6 minor malformations per 1000 total births (Stevenson et al., 1966).

All agents known to be teratogenic in man, or strongly suspected of acting in this way, are also teratogenic in animals. If "potential teratogenicity" is restricted only to those cases where the agent was harmful to the embryo but not to the mother (except where, as with anti-tumour agents, the drug is supposed to be toxic to the mother), the list of teratogens is greatly reduced. Aspirin, for example, is teratogenic in rats only at doses that would be toxic to both mother and fetus (Palmer, 1969).

Despite the laboratory data indicating teratogenic "potential" for a wide variety of environmental factors in animals, only a handful have been proved or are strongly suspected to be embryopathic in man (adapted from Palmer, 1969; and Sever, 1971):

Chemical factors

Known	Strongly suspected
Methylmercury	Cortisone
Aminopterin	Vitamin A deficiency
Thalidomide	Diethylstilboestrol
Iodine deficiency (cretinism)	
Steroid hormones with androgenic activity	
Carbon monoxide (hypoxia)	

Infective micro-organisms

Known

Rubella virus
Herpesvirus
Cytomegalovirus
Toxoplasma
Treponema pallidum (syphilis)

Physical factors

Ionizing radiation
Trauma (spontaneous abortion)

The teratogenic effect of an exogenous factor varies with the stage of post-conceptual development during which it acts. These stages cover the fertilized ovum, cleavage, the blastocyst, the embryo (up to 8 weeks), the fetus (after 8 weeks), and the post-natal animal. The greatest teratological hazard is generally accepted as occurring in the embryonic period, when tissue differentiation and organogenesis occur. Thalidomide, for example, when given in the period between 6 and 8 weeks after a pregnant woman's last menstrual period can cause serious anomalies in amounts as low as 200 mg. In general, exposure in the early part of the sensitive period is associated with ear anomaly, exposure in the mid-portion with arm deformity, and exposure in the later portion with leg deformity (Fraser, 1967). In fact, the same agent can kill an embryo when given before organogenesis, cause malformation when given during organogenesis, or cause fetal distress when given late in pregnancy (Inhorn, 1967). Similar results can be obtained by varying the dosage or intensity of the agent. In addition, there appears to be a synergistic effect for certain pairs of teratogens, each at low doses, although no consistent relationship is yet apparent (Inhorn, 1967). Evidence is accumulating, moreover, to indicate that developmental deviation can also be induced by adverse influences during the entire gestational period (WHO Scientific Group on Principles for the Testing of Drugs for Teratogenicity, 1967).

Teratological investigations in laboratory animals

It is clear that single agents can cause multiple developmental deviations and that particular developmental deviations can be caused by different agents.

Choice of species

It has been possible in the mouse, rat and rabbit to demonstrate teratogenic activity by all substances that have been shown to be teratogenic in man, but it cannot be said that agents that are teratogenic in high doses in these species will necessarily produce teratogenic effects in man at environmental dose levels. There is also no absolute assurance that negative results obtained by testing chemicals in these species can be used to predict that an agent will lack teratogenic effects in man.

The choice of certain monkeys appears to be logical because of their phylogenetic proximity to man; their use is being increasingly investigated, but may not prove economically practicable in many instances. Preliminary reports suggest that the susceptibility of the monkey embryo to teratological agents resembles that of the human more closely than does the susceptibility of embryos of any other species (WHO Scientific Group on Principles for the Testing of Drugs for Teratogenicity, 1967; Wilson, 1971).

Significance of findings in animals

The predictive value of teratogenic tests is thus still open to question. One of the difficulties of interpretation is due to the constant interaction between the two different biological systems, the mother and the conceptus. Theoretically, the significance of any teratogenic activity that may be observed can be assessed by taking into account the percentage of malformations obtained, the constancy of the results in several subsequent experiments, and the dose at which the teratogenic effect has been observed. If teratogenic effects are obtained in only one of three species of animals, the probability that they will occur in man may be low.

It has been shown that the reaction of the embryo to exogenous agents depends to a large extent upon its genetic constitution. Furthermore, this reaction varies not only between different species but also within a given species from strain to strain and even between individuals of the same strain. The immediate causes of species differences in reaction to teratogenic agents are still largely unknown, but it has been suggested that they could be related to differences in metabolic pathways or possibly to the formation of noxious metabolites in some species but not in others (WHO Scientific Group on Principles for the Testing of Drugs for Teratogenicity, 1967).

Alkylating cytostatics, such as derivatives of nitrogen mustard, ethyleneimine and certain derivatives of sulfonic acid, several *N*-nitrosamines and hydrazine derivatives, as well as the natural compounds aflatoxin and cycasin and their metabolite methyl azoxymethanol, show, in addition to teratogenic activity, mutagenic and carcinogenic activity in laboratory experiments. Similar observations have been made with urethane. So far, however, no carcinogenic properties have been demonstrated for the compounds colchicine, vinblastine and such a highly teratogenic antimetabolite as 6-azauridine. Likewise, the fact that all alkylating compounds, antimetabolites and antineoplastic agents tested showed mutagenic and teratogenic properties in animal experiments does not permit the conclusion that all compounds with mutagenic effects are also capable of causing malformation in mammals. No chromosomal aberrations were found, for instance, in malformed fetuses of thalidomide-sensitive Dutch-belted rabbits.   Furthermore, hydroxyurea and L-asparaginase, which cause malformations in small rodents and rabbits, also fail to produce any mutagenic effect (Soukup et al., 1967; Adamson et al., 1970; Frohberg, 1971).

Teratogens in the environment: pesticides and defoliants

Detailed information on pesticides as teratogens has been published (US Department of Health, Education, and Welfare, 1969) and is briefly summarized below.

Organomercury compounds

Phenylmercury acetate has been reported to cause fetal malformations in mice.   A high incidence of infantile cerebral palsy (termed fetal Mina-mata disease) resulted from the consumption, by pregnant women, of methylmercury in the form of fish and shellfish contaminated by this compound.

Organochlorine compounds

Embryotoxicity in rats and dogs has been reported for organochlorine compounds, including dieldrin, chlordane and kepone.   No adverse human reproductive effects were attributed to DDT and other chlorinated hydro-carbons.

Organophosphorus compounds

It has been claimed that a number of chlolinesterase-inhibiting organo-phosphorus insecticides have been shown to be teratogenic when injected directly into the yolk sac of chick embryos or administered to mice. Evidence of the teratogenic potential of organophosphorus compounds in man has been reviewed and found inconclusive.

Chemical defoliants

Two such substances have been investigated extensively, namely 2,4,5-T (2,4,5-trichlorophenoxyacetic acid) and 2,4-D (2,4-dichlorophenoxyacetic acid).   They have definitely been shown to be teratogenic in rats and mice. Warning has also been given that they have produced teratogenic effects in man, though this has by no means been established (Robson, 1970; Aaronson, 1971; Meselson et al., 1971).

Summary

Chemical teratogenesis, like chemical mutagenesis, is a challenging new area of pharmacological investigation.   Our present understanding of mechanisms of action in this field is primitive. We do not know how any teratogen really acts. With increasing knowledge of the biochemical events in normal embryogenesis should come better understanding of teratogenesis. Eventually, therefore, as with other diseases of man, practical means may be developed for the prevention of congenital malformations (Goldstein et al., 1968).

REFERENCES

Aaronson, T. (1971) *Environment,* **13** (2), 34

Adamson, R. H., Fabro, S., Hahn, M. A., Creech, C. E. & Whang-Peng, J. (1970) *Arch. int. Pharmacodyn.,* **186,** 310-320

Cohlan, S. Q. (1967). In: Frantz, C. H., ed., *Normal and abnormal embryological development,* Washington, D.C., National Research Council (Publication No. 1497)

Fraser, F. C. (1967) *Physical and chemical agents.* In: Rubin, A., ed., *Handbook of congenital malformations,* Philadelphia & London, W. B. Saunders, pp. 365-372

Frohberg, H. (1971) *Arch. Toxikol.,* **28,** 135-148

Goldstein, A., Aronow, L. & Kalman, S. M. (1968) *Principles of drug action,* Harper & Row, New York

Inhorn, S. I. (1967) *Advanc. Terat.,* **2,** 38-99

Meselson, M. S., Westing, A. H., Constable, J. D. & Cook, R. E. (1971) *Background materials on defoliation in Vietnam: Hearing before the Subcommittee to Investigate Problems Connected with Refugees and Escapees, Committee on the Judiciary, US Senate, 92nd Congress, 1st Session, April 21, 1971,* Washington, D.C., US Government Printing Office, Appendix III

Palmer, A. J. (1969) *The relationship between screening tests for drug safety and other teratological investigations.* In: Bertelli, A. & Donati, L., eds, *Teratology, Proceedings of a Symposium Organized by the Italian Society of Experimental Teratology, Como, Italy, 21-22 Oct. 1962,* Amsterdam, Excerpta Medica Foundation, pp. 55-74

Robson, I. M. (1970) *Brit. med. Bull.,* **26,** 2212-216

Sever, J. L. (1971) *Fed. Proc.,* **30,** 114

Soukup, S., Takacs, E. & Warkany, J. (1967) *J. Embryol. exp. Morph.,* **18,** 215-226

Stevenson, A. C., Johnston, H. A., Steward, M. I. P. & Golding, D. R. (1966) *Bull. Wld Hlth Org.,* **34,** Suppl.

US Department of Health, Education, and Welfare (1969) *Secretary's Commission on Pesticides and their Relationship to Environmental Health. Report,* Washington, D.C., US Government Printing Office

WHO Scientific Group on Principles for the Testing of Drugs for Teratogenicity (1967) *Report,* Geneva *(Wld Hlth Org. techn. Rep. Ser.,* No. 364)

Wilson, J. G. (1971) *Fed. Proc.,* **30,** 104

CHAPTER 14

IONIZING RADIATION

Introduction

Naturally occurring ionizing radiation originates both from outside the body, in the form of cosmic radiation and radiation from natural radioisotopes in the environment, and from inside the body from natural radioisotopes deposited there from food, drink and air.

During the present century, mankind has been subjected to increasing levels of ionizing radiation from man-made sources, such as X-ray equipment, nuclear weapons, the nuclear fuel cycle, and artificial radioisotopes used for medical and other purposes.

Ionizing radiations may be divided into two main groups: (1) *electromagnetic radiations* (X-rays and gamma rays), which belong to the same family of electromagnetic radiations as visible light and radio waves; and (2) *corpuscular radiations*, some of which—alpha particles, beta particles (electrons), and protons—are electrically charged, whereas others (neutrons) have no electric charge. This distinction between the two groups becomes blurred, however, when their mode of absorption in materials is considered. The corpuscular types may be regarded as projectiles whose energy is greater than that binding the atoms in chemical compounds. They are therefore capable of breaking chemical bonds and dividing the electrically neutral molecules into positively and negatively charged ions. When X-rays and gamma rays are absorbed, high-energy electrons are released in the irradiated materials, and it is these electrically charged particles—which are similar to the beta particles emitted by radioisotopes—that are the effective ionizing agents. The action of neutrons is more complex. If they collide with the nuclei of hydrogen atoms, these nuclei (or protons) are set in motion, thus producing ionization. Neutrons may also enter atomic nuclei, causing such instability that the atoms disintegrate and emit radiation that, in turn, produces ionization. Thus the common characteristic of all the types of radiation referred to, whether electromagnetic or corpuscular, is that particles are responsible for the ionization they ultimately produce.

Whilst the exact nature of the biological effects of these radiations is not fully understood, they are related to the ionization that the radiations are capable of producing in living tissue. Thus, the biological effects of all ionizing radiations are essentially similar. However, the distribution of damage throughout the body may be very different according to the type, energy and penetrating power of the radiation involved. Alpha particles from radioisotopes have ranges of only about 0.001–0.007 cm in soft tissue and less in bone.

Beta particles have ranges in soft tissues of the order of several millimetres, i.e., much greater than those of alpha particles in such tissues. A beta particle therefore irradiates many more cells than an alpha particle, but the number of ions produced in each cell is much less.

For X-rays and gamma rays, depending on the energy of the radiation, penetration may amount to tens of centimetres, or even to metres, in soft tissue. As in the case of beta particles, the ion density along the tracks of the electrons ejected by X-rays and gamma rays from the medium through which they pass is much lower than for alpha particles.

Radiation units

It is necessary to distinguish, in considering radiation units, between the following three quantities of importance in radiation protection: exposure, absorbed dose and dose equivalent.

Exposure is the sum of the electrical charges of the ions of one sign produced in unit mass of air under certain defined conditions. The unit of exposure is the Röntgen, which is applicable only to electromagnetic radiation of moderate energy.

The *absorbed* dose is the radiation energy imparted to unit mass of a specified medium. The unit of absorbed dose is the rad.

For radiation protection considerations, it is necessary to introduce a modified quantity that takes into account the biological effectiveness of a given absorbed dose, depending on the type and energy of the radiation. This is done by using a quality factor. Other factors may also be introduced, such as the distribution factor, which expresses the modification in the biological effect due to the nonuniform distribution of internally deposited radionuclides. The product of the absorbed dose and the modifying factors is termed the *dose equivalent*. The unit of dose equivalent is the rem. Where the value of the quality factor is close to unity, as is true for X-rays (where it is unity), beta particles, and gamma rays, the numerical values of the absorbed dose in rads and the dose equivalent in rems are practically identical.

Biological Effects of Ionizing Radiations

Information concerning these effects has been obtained from studies of: (*a*) patients who have undergone diagnostic or therapeutic procedures with X-rays and radioisotopes; (*b*) occupationally-exposed persons (for example, pioneer medical radiologists, early workers with radioactive luminous paints, workers engaged in mining radioactive ores, persons who have been involved in accidents in or around nuclear reactors, and persons who have been exposed continuously to low radiation doses for long periods); and (c) members of general populations who have been affected by atomic bomb explosions or tests of nuclear weapons. This information has been supplemented by evidence from extensive animal experimentation. Despite these studies, there are still many gaps in our knowledge and further investigations are needed (United Nations Scientific Committee on the Effects of Atomic Radiation, 1964; Upton, 1969). The effects can be regarded as falling into two main groups, namely, somatic effects and genetic effects.

Somatic effects

These effects are observable either relatively soon after individuals have been irradiated ("early" or "short-term" effects), or after periods of a few months to several years ("late" or "long-term" effects). A dose of 1000 rad and above of total body irradiation, delivered over a short period of time, results in death within about a week. Doses of 100–1000 rad of total body irradiation delivered over a short period of time can result in damage and death in a proportion of the individuals exposed.

Acute radiation effects can be observed after irradiation of the greater part of the body. A latent period supervenes after initial symptoms of malaise, loss of appetite and fatigue. The length of this period is roughly inversely proportional to the radiation dose received. The end of the latent period is followed by the onset of the illness: early lethality, destruction of bone marrow, damage to the gastrointestinal tract associated with diarrhoea and haemorrhage, central nervous system symptoms, epilation, dermatitis, sterility. Pathological acute effects arise after exposure to doses hundreds of times greater than those likely to be received from environmental contamination, except in major accidents.

Much less is known as to the effects of small doses, e.g., up to 100 rad, received over long periods of time, yet it is these effects that are particularly important for the population at large. There are many uncertainties here—e.g., the variation of sensitivity to radiation with age and the possible reduction in effect per unit of radiation dose as compared with single large doses (over 100 rad).

It is not known whether the linear relationships between radiation dosage and the incidence of harmful effects that are sometimes observed at high dose levels also apply at low dose levels; present estimates of risk from low dose levels are based on the assumption that a linear relationship does apply and that there is no "threshold" of radiation exposure below which no effect is produced.

At low dosage levels, leukaemogenesis and carcinogenesis are at present accepted as the most serious long-term risks for the individual. There is also evidence, however, of other late effects following high doses, e.g., cataract formation, and possibly neurological damage and a general shortening of the life span. These are all examples of what are called somatic effects.

The frequency of different types of tumour has been found to be increased in irradiated populations. This is true of thyroid carcinomas in patients given X-ray therapy to the neck in childhood, carcinomas of the lung in workers engaged in mining uranium ores, haematite and fluorspar, haemangioendotheliomas of the liver in patients injected intravenously with Thorotrast, [1] and miscellaneous types of neoplasms in atomic bomb survivors and in patients subjected to radiotherapy (United Nations Scientific Committee on the Effects of Atomic Radiation, 1972).

An increased incidence of cancers occurred in workers engaged in painting watch and clock dials with luminous paints containing radium. They ingested large quantities of radium and radium daughter elements. These radionuclides, which are preferentially deposited in bone, lead in time to skeletal injury and to osteosarcoma in some victims (United Nations Scientific Committee on the Effects of Atomic Radiation, 1964).

It has only recently been possible to attempt quantitative estimates of the incidence of harmful effects (leukaemia and other forms of cancer and certain genetic effects) per unit dose of radiation, and even now the margins of uncertainty are very wide. In general, most knowledge has been gained of the effects of relatively large doses received at high intensity, notably from epidemiological studies of the survivors of Hiroshima and Nagasaki and of patients treated with radiation for ankylosing spondylitis and other disorders. Although these estimates are still imprecise, they are adequate to give a rough indication of dose-effect relationship (United States, National Council on Radiation Protection and Measurements, 1971; Upton, 1969).

Leukaemia is the malignancy whose rate of induction per rad is best known, and risk estimates are available over a fairly broad range of doses. For lung cancer and all solid cancers—the incidence of which is also clearly increased by radiation—estimates are much more uncertain, particularly as none of the surveys of irradiated people carried out so far has been pursued for a time sufficiently long to exclude the possibility that further cases of malignancies, besides those already recorded, will be observed after longer periods of observation, and because it is not known whether, some twenty years after exposure, peak incidence has yet been reached.

Despite the lack of direct, quantitative information on the sensitivity of the human embryo to irradiation, it is generally assumed that small

---

[1] A contrast medium containing thorium (IV) oxide, formerly used in radiology.

amounts of radiation may carry some risk of teratogenic effects in man, as in other species. Thus, to minimize the risk of accidentally irradiating an embryo in a particularly sensitive stage of development, the International Commission on Radiological Protection has recommended that radiological examinations of the lower abdomen and pelvis in a woman of reproductive age should be limited, as far as possible, to the ten days following the onset of menstruation; an undetected pregnancy in such a woman is most improbable at this time (International Commission on Radiological Protection, 1966b).

Because of the paucity of human data on the teratogenic effects of graded doses of radiation and the marked variation in susceptibility of animals to malformation with stage in development at the time of irradiation and with known species differences, it is not possible to estimate precisely the risks of radiation injury to the human embryo and fetus.

Likewise, studies aimed at detecting teratogenic effects associated with increased levels of environmental background radiation have given inconclusive results (Brill & Forgotson, 1964).

Data on human populations on ageing and longevity are incomplete. One of the first indications of life-shortening effects of radiation in man was the observation that radiologists in the USA have a higher age-specific death rate than medical specialists in other fields (Dublin & Spiegelman, 1948; Seltser & Sartwell, 1965). This difference implies that occupational irradiation causes a non-specific impairment of health that manifests itself in accelerated ageing. If this interpretation is correct, the lessening of the effect in recent years, during which time there has been increasing attention to radiation safety standards, suggests that the hazard may not be detectable under present working conditions. This is also suggested by the absence of increased mortality in British radiologists (Court Brown & Doll, 1958).

Genetic effects

Genetic effects are the results of gene mutations or chromosome anomalies that, arising in the *germ cells* of the irradiated individuals, may become apparent in their descendants, sometimes generations removed from the irradiated ancestor. Genetic effects are generally detrimental but may have various degrees of severity, from prenatal death to major malformations or mental dysfunctions, to mild impairments of an individual's reproductive performance or of his viability. Because they occur among the descendants of irradiated persons, they are of greater concern to the population than to the individuals actually exposed to radiation. Clear evidence of genetic damage in the offspring of irradiated human subjects is so meagre that the genetic harm cannot be quantitatively expressed in terms of the social burden to which a given dose of radiation will eventually give rise. However, the possibility that genetic damage, once induced, may persist for generations must be constantly borne in mind when exposing individuals or populations to new sources of radiation (WHO Expert Committee on Radiation, 1959; United Nations Scientific Committee on the Effects of Atomic Radiation, 1966).

Critical organs

For the development of radiation protection guides, the identification of the particular organs or tissues that are critical because of the damage they may suffer is the essential simplifying step. For example, in the case of radioisotopes of iodine, the critical organ is the thyroid, since the concentration of such isotopes in it, and therefore the dose received, is far greater than for any other organ. Since radioiodine is widely used in medicine and may also be of importance in nuclear energy, the thyroid may often be the critical organ, especially among children (United States, National Council on Radiation Protection and Measurements, 1971).

In general, for irradiation from internally deposited sources, whether alone or combined with external irradiation, the critical organ is determined more by the metabolic pathways of nuclides, their concentration in organs, and their effective residence times, than by inherent sensitivity factors. Depending on the individual radionuclide under consideration, the critical organ may be the gastrointestinal tract, lung, bone, thyroid, kidney, spleen, pancreas, muscle or fatty tissue.

For general irradiation of the whole body, the critical organs and tissues are the gonads (fertility, hereditary effects), the haematopoietic organs, or more specifically the bone marrow (leukaemia), and the eye (cataracts).

The relation between choice of a critical organ and the development of radiation protection guides is not always evident. The position has been summarized as follows:

"The dose to the critical organ from any particular mode of radiation exposure does not define the overall risk which will always be greater than this to the extent to which other organs are irradiated. The concept of critical organ is administratively convenient and in some circumstances logically justifiable, but it does not allow summation of risks according to the relative radiosensitivities of the irradiated tissues" (International Commission on Radiological Protection, 1969b).

Radiation Protection Standards

The concept of "tolerance dose"

The radiation protection measures first adopted were not based on any strict quantitative determination of ionizing radiation, but rather mainly on the dose in Röntgens that would produce skin erythema. This was considered to be 6 R per month or about 0.2 R per day. This figure and the concept of tolerance dose were adopted in 1931 by the US Committee on X-ray and Radium Protection, and then in 1934 by the International Commission on Radiological Protection (ICRP).

The concepts of "maximum permissible dose" and "dose limit"

The maximum permissible dose was originally regarded as one that, in the light of the knowledge available at the time, was not expected to cause appreciable bodily injury to any occupationally-exposed person at any time during his life. The phrase "appreciable bodily injury" was defined as "any bodily injury or effect that a person would regard as being objectionable and/or competent medical authorities would regard as being deleterious to the health and well-being of the individual" (International Commission on Radiological Protection, 1955).

TABLE 1

ESTIMATED RISK OF CANCER FROM EXPOSURE TO 1 RAD[1]

Type of cancer	Estimated no. of cases per 10^6 persons exposed [2]	Order of risk to the individual
Fatal neoplasms:		
Leukaemia [3]	40	5th
Others	100	5th
Thyroid carcinoma [4]	40	5th

Data derived from United Nations Scientific Committee on the Effects of Atomic Radiation (1972).

[1] A linear dose-response relationship is assumed.

[2] Effects would be experienced over a number of years.

[3] Risk may be much higher if the fetus is exposed.

[4] Estimate derived from observations for 25 years after exposure. No allowance made for the possibility of further cases appearing subsequently.

The ICRP has subsequently paid increasing attention to the concept of maximum permissible dose. In the absence of any definite information to the contrary, the Commission believes that the policy of assuming a risk of injury even at the lowest dose levels is the most reasonable basis for radiation protection. This represents a radical change from the "tolerance dose" philosophy. The Commission recognizes that its recommendations as to the levels of maximum permissible doses for occupationally-exposed persons involve a "considerable element of judgement" with regard to the degree of risk that can be considered acceptable when balanced against the benefits derived from the many uses of ionizing radiations. At the present time, in the absence of any proved relationship between dose and effect, the ICRP has estimated the magnitude of the risk of various types of cancer from the exposure of 1 million persons to 1 rad per capita, on the assumption that there is a linear dose/effect relationship. The figures are given in Table 1 (United Nations Scientific Committee on the Effects of Atomic Radiation, 1972); the reference cited should be consulted for information about the various studies on which the estimates are based. Since almost all the evidence is for irradiation by X-rays or gamma rays, the absorbed dose in rads is unlikely to be significantly different from the dose equivalent in rems.

So as not to convey "an unwarranted impression of accuracy", the Commission suggests that effects should be described only in terms of the ranges of probability of their occurrence. For example, a fifth order risk would imply that the probability of an injury to any individual is in the range 1×10^{-5} to 10×10^{-5}, equivalent to about 10–100 injuries per million persons exposed (International Commission on Radiological Protection, 1966a).

The ICRP retains the term "maximum permissible dose" for the exposure of radiation workers. By monitoring the doses received by individual workers and by controlling their environment it is possible to ensure that the maximum permissible doses are not exceeded, except in the case of accidents. It is not possible, however, to determine the doses received by members of the public. It is therefore necessary to control the sources giving rise to exposure and to assess the average dose received by a specific group or an entire population, both by means of sampling procedures in the environment and, in appropriate cases, checks on the doses received by a few individuals in the group or population involved. The ICRP believes that the term "maximum permissible dose" is seldom meaningful in relation to individual members of the public and has recommended that, in their case, the term "dose limit" should be used.

ICRP radiation protection standards

The current values of the maximum permissible doses and dose limits for specified organs and tissues, as recommended by the ICRP, are given in Table 2.

The ICRP has recommended that the *genetic dose limit for a whole population* should not exceed 5 rem from all sources, in addition to the dose from natural background radiation and from medical procedures. The genetic dose should be kept to the minimum, and the additional contribution to the genetic dose from medical procedures should also be kept to the minimum, consistent with medical requirements. The genetic dose limit of 5 rem is based on a mean age of child-bearing of 30 years. The limit, as stated by the ICRP, is equivalent to about 0.15 rem per year.

The ICRP has not given a value for the *somatic dose limit for a whole population*. It expects that the setting of dose limits for individuals will ensure that the number of somatic injuries that could occur in a population will be low. If a population were to receive a mean annual dose to the red bone marrow of 0.5 rem, i.e., the value given in Table 2 as the dose limit for members of the public, it is estimated that the increased incidence of leukaemia and other neoplasms would amount to 6–12 cases a year per million persons according to ICRP Publication 14 (International Commission on Radiological Protection, 1969b).

TABLE 2

MAXIMUM PERMISSIBLE DOSES AND DOSE LIMITS [1]

Organ or tissue	Maximum permissible dose for adults exposed in the course of their work[2]	Dose limits for members of the public (average for groups of individuals)
Whole body (in case of uniform irradiation), gonads and red bone marrow	5 rem in a year	0.5 rem in a year
Skin, bone and thyroid	30 rem in a year	3 rem in a year[3]
Other single organs	15 rem in a year	1.5 rem in a year
Hands and forearms; feet and ankles	75 rem in a year	7.5 rem in a year

[1] As recommended by the International Commission on Radiological Protection (1966b).
[2] In any period of a quarter of a year, up to one half of the annual permissible dose may be accumulated.
[3] For children up to 16 years of age, the dose limit to the thyroid is 1.5 rem in a year.

The primary standards in radiation protection are the maximum permissible doses and dose limits to the whole body and to various body organs; these doses and limits should not be exceeded either by individual isotopes or by the sum of the dose from multiple isotopes, if used. In the case of radioisotopes, a number of secondary standards have also been established. These are given in various ICRP publications.

Components of Environmental Radiation

Environmental radiation can be divided into two types: (1) naturally-occurring radiation ("natural background radiation"); and (2) man-made radiation. These can themselves be further sub-divided into a number of components.

Natural background radiation

This has three components: (1) cosmic radiation originating in outer space and reaching the earth's surface after reacting with, and being partially absorbed by, the earth's atmosphere; (2) terrestrial radiation coming from natural radioisotopes present in the earth's crust; and (3) radiation from natural radioisotopes that have been accumulated in the body as a result of the consumption of food and water and the inhalation of air containing such radioisotopes.

The average values of the dose rates of these three components of environmental radiation lead to a total of about 90 mrad per year to gonodal tissue and bone marrow.

Man-made radiation

The evaluation of the radiation exposure of the population presented here applies only to highly developed countries; it refers to the genetic dose [1] received by a whole population, rather than to the exposure of individuals or groups. In many countries, the frequency with which radiation is used is much less than in the highly developed countries; the methods applied and the radiation protection measures adopted are, however, sometimes such that the radiation exposure *per capita* per application is greater. It is impossible, therefore, to give an accurate estimate of the mean genetic dose to the whole world population. The figures quoted will, however, provide an idea of the order of magnitude to be expected (United Nations Scientific Committee on the Effects of Atomic Radiation, 1972; Mole & Ardran, 1971).

The contributions to the total dose from man-made radiation will be considered under the following headings:

(1) radiation to patients from the medical uses of radiation;

(2) radiation to occupationally exposed persons;

(3) radiation from "fallout" from nuclear tests;

(4) radiation from other forms of radioactive contamination; and

(5) radiation from radioactive consumer goods and from electronic devices.

---

[1] This ICRP defines the genetic dose to a whole population as the annual genetically significant dose multiplied by the mean age of child-bearing, which is taken to be 30 years. The annual genetically significant dose to a population is the average of the individual gonad doses, each weighted for the expected number of children conceived subsequent to the exposure.

Radiation to patients from medical uses of radiation

The doses received by patients from X-ray diagnostic procedures, from the treatment of malignant and non-malignant conditions, and from diagnostic and therapeutic uses of unsealed radioisotopes have been assessed (Committee on Radiological Hazards to Patients, 1960; International Atomic Energy Agency, 1969; International Commission on Radiological Protection, 1970b, 1971b). The main factors in medical exposure are the region of the body examined or treated and the technique used. This explains the wide differences in the estimates of the average genetic dose to the population resulting from medical applications. It is clear from all the investigations that the major part of medical radiation exposure comes from the use of X-rays in diagnosis. Whilst the range is still wide— 7–55 mrem per year—most of the values seem to the about 20 mrem per year or less. The contribution from the use of unsealed radioisotopes is only about 0.2 mrem per year, and can therefore be ignored. As regards therapeutic procedures, genetic exposure is largely the result of the treatment of non-malignant conditions, and averages about 4 mrem per year. The exposure resulting from the treatment of patients with malignant tumours cannot be evaluated, owing to the uncertainty as to the weighting factors to be used for the expectation of life and to the fact that many such patients will not have children (International Commission on Radiological Protection, 1971a; International Atomic Energy Agency, 1969).

The average genetic dose to the whole population in some of the highly developed countries amounts, therefore, to about 25 mrem per year (United Nations Scientific Committee on the Effects of Atomic Radiation, 1962).

Radiation to occupationally exposed persons

The radiation exposure of the majority of persons professionally engaged in handling radiation sources and radioactive substances is less than about 1 rem per year, or less than one fifth of the maximum permissible dose allowed for radiation exposure of the gonads. A number of countries have reported that the genetic dose to the whole population arising from the dose received by occupationally exposed persons, who constitute only a small fraction of the total population, is about 0.1–0.2 mrem per year. Although the data may be incomplete, the population dose due to occupational exposure does not exceed 1% of the natural background radiation, even after allowing for an increased use of nuclear energy (United Nations Scientific Committee on the Effects of Atomic Radiation, 1962).

Radiation from fallout from nuclear tests

Nuclear tests caused large quantities of radioactive substances to be injected into the stratosphere, from where they have continued to fall back to earth until the present time. Those substances that decay rapidly (i.e., have a short half-life) have largely vanished, but radioisotopes with a long half-life, such as ^{90}Sr and ^{137}Cs, are still falling today in small quantities.

Radioactive fallout can affect man in two main ways: (i) by radiation from fallout deposited on the ground; and (ii) by radiation from the radioactive substances that man has taken into his body by ingestion (particularly of food) and by inhalation. The last comprehensive estimates by UNSCEAR of the "dose commitments" up to the year 2000 from fallout from nuclear tests carried out before 1971 indicate that the contributions to the gonadal dose from external radiation from ^{137}Cs and from short-lived fission products amount to 124 mrem for the North Temperate Zone, and to 35 mrem for the South Temperate Zone. The contributions from internal radiation from ^{137}Cs and ^{14}C are 26 mrem and 12 mrem respectively for the North Temperate Zone, and 7 mrem and 12 mrem respectively for the South Temperate Zone.

For this dose commitment, it is estimated that more than half the external dose had already been delivered by the end of 1967, and two thirds of that from internally deposited ^{137}Cs. In contrast, only one tenth of the internal dose due to ^{14}C will have been delivered by the year 2000. It is not possible to quote an average exposure per year derived from this dose commitment. However, the average dose received by the population in any one year can be calculated. Thus in 1970 the average gonad dose per caput received by the populations of the northern and southern hemispheres amounted to less than 10 mrem and about 5 mrem respectively.

If atmospheric nuclear tests are discontinued, the yearly exposure from this source of radiation will decrease over subsequent years unlike exposure to radiation from some other man-made sources which will tend to increase with time.

Radiation from radioactive contamination by other sources

Compared with the fallout from nuclear tests, all other sources of radioactive contamination of the environment are negligible at the present time (International Atomic Energy Agency, 1969). However, four main groups of uses might, in the future, be considered as sources of environmental contamination, namely: (i) nuclear power reactors and other reactors; (ii) reprocessing plants and "hot" laboratories; (iii) medical applications of radioisotopes; and (iv) industrial and research applications of radioisotopes. Of these sources, nuclear reactors and reprocessing plants are the most important. Medical applications involve mainly short-lived isotopes; their extent is limited by the amounts of radioactivity acceptable to patients, and by the number of applications, which in turn depends on the number of potential patients. These applications will not, therefore, have a serious impact on the environment. The remaining applications, i.e., those referred to in (iv) above, are too limited in scope at the present time to constitute an environmental problem; their further development should, however, be kept under review.

Radiation from radioactive consumer goods and from electronic devices

"Small sources" of radiation that are more or less widespread throughout the population include the luminous dials of wrist watches and alarm clocks, shoe-fitting X-ray fluoroscopes, television sets, and the continually increasing number of applications of radioactive substances, e.g., in fluorescent lamps and electronic components of various devices. Singly, they produce only small gonadal doses, but their total contribution should be kept under observation. In some cases, somatic doses may be higher. For example, the local exposure of the skin of the wrist from radium luminized watches was found some years ago to be about 1–30 R per year. This has since been considerably reduce by: (*a*) restricting the amount of radioactive material on the dials; and (*b*) introducing low-energy beta-particle emitters, such as tritium and ^{147}Pm, instead of the penetrating gamma-ray emitter ^{226}Ra. Beta particles cause no radiation exposure of the gonads, so that the earlier value of the genetic dose to the whole population, which was about 1 % of the natural background, has therefore been substantially reduced.

The main hazard from shoe-fitting fluoroscopes is to the feet. The dose to the foot of a child can reach about 10 rad in a year, if fluoroscopy is carried out repeatedly. The gonadal doses to customers and shop assistants, however, are small, and the genetic dose to the population is estimated to be less than 0.1 % of the natural background.

Occasionally, imperfections in the design of colour television sets lead to the escape of narrow beams of X-rays. The voltage regulator is the main source of such radiation, which can easily be eliminated by shielding this component. Radiation also escapes through the viewing screen and reaches viewers, and the ICRP has recommended a maximum value for the dose rate near the screen. This is so small that the genetic dose to a viewing population is less than 1 % of the natural background.

For other consumer goods containing radioactive substances, the genetic dose to the population at the present time is believed to be insignificant.

Thus, for all the sources mentioned here there is good reason to believe that altogether they contribute not more than 1–2 % of the natural background radiation (WHO Expert Committee on Radiation, 1962, 1963, 1965).

Dose rate from man-made radiations

The contributions to the genetic dose to the whole population from the various components are:

(1) 25 mrem per year from the medical exposure of patients (this applies to the highly developed countries);

(2) less than 1 mrem per year from the exposure of persons professionally engaged in dealing with radiation and radioactive substances;

(3) 4 mrem in 1970 from fallout from nuclear tests;

(4) a still quite small contribution from radioactive contamination from other sources; and

(5) 1–2 mrem per year from radioactive consumer goods and from electronic devices that emit ionizing radiations.

This gives a total of about 30 mrem per year, which is about one-third of the natural background radiation.

The specific environmental hazards of ionizing radiation still need attention, although at the present time they are under reasonable control in most countries. The increasing use of nuclear power, stratospheric flights, the application of radioactive isotopes for many purposes, and the medical applications of radiation, particularly for diagnosis and in preventive medicine, will probably result in an increased population exposure that—in the future—may exceed the unavoidable variations in the natural background radiation. Accurate quantitative assessment of the total risk to individuals as well as communities thus requires increased and continuous attention.

REFERENCES

Brill, A. B. & Forgotson, E. H. (1964) *Amer. J. Obstet. Gynec.*, **90**, 1149-1168

Committee on Radiological Hazards to Patients (1960) *Second report*, London, HM Stationery Office

Court Brown, W. M. & Doll, R. (1958) *Brit. med. J.*, **2**, 181-187

Dublin, L. I. & Spiegelman, U. (1948) *J. Amer. med. Ass.*, **137**, 1519-1524

International Atomic Energy Agency (1969) *Environmental contamination by radioactive materials*, Vienna

International Commission on Radiological Protection (1955) *Recommendations of the ...*, Brit. J. Radiol., Supplement No. 6

International Commission on Radiological Protection (1966a) *The evaluation of risks from radiation*, Oxford, Pergamon Press (*ICRP Publication 8*)

International Commission on Radiological Protection (1966b) *Recommendations of the International Commission on Radiation Protection*, Oxford, Pergamon Press (*ICRP Publicatin 9*)

International Commission on Radiological Protection (1969a) *General principles of monitoring for radiation protection of workers*, Oxford, Pergamon Press (*ICRP Publication 12*)

International Commission on Radiological Protection (1969b) *Radiosensitivity and spatial distribution of dose,* Oxford, Pergamon Press (*ICRP Publication* 14)

International Commission on Radiological Protection (1970a) *Protection against ionizing radiation from external sources,* Oxford, Pergamon Press (*ICRP Publication* 15)

International Commission on Radiological Protection (1970b) *Protection of the patient in X-ray diagnosis,* Oxford, Pergamon Press (*ICRP Publication* 16)

International Commission on Radiological Protection (1971a) *The assessment of internal contamination resulting from recurrent or prolonged uptakes,* Oxford, Pergamon Press (*ICRP Publication* 10A)

International Commission on Radiological Protection (1971b) *Protection of the patient in radionuclide investigations,* Oxford, Pergamon Press (*ICRP Publication* 17)

Mole, R. H. & Ardran, G. M. (1971) *Mod. Med.,* May

Seltser, R. & Sartwell, P. E. (1965) *Amer. J. Epidem.,* **91,** 2-22

United Nations Scientific Committee on the Effects of Atomic Radiation (1962) *Report...,* New York, United Nations (Official Records of the General Assembly, Seventeenth Session, Supplement No. 16 (A/5216))

United Nations Scientific Committee on the Effects of Atomic Radiation (1964) *Report...,* New York, United Nations (Official Records of the General Assembly, Nineteenth Session, Supplement No. 14 (A/5814))

United Nations Scientific Committee on the Effects of Atomic Radiation (1966) *Report...,* New York, United Nations (Official Records of the General Assembly, Twenty-first Session, Supplement No. 14 (A/6314))

United Nations Scientific Committee on the Effects of Atomic Radiation (1972) *Ionizing Radiation: Levels and Effects,* Vols I and II, New York, United Nations (E.72.IX.17 and E.72.IX.18)

United States, National Council on Radiation Protection and Measurements (1971) *Basic radiation protection criteria,* Washington, D.C. (*NCRP Report* No. 39)

Upton, A. C. (1969) *Radiation injury,* Chicago, University of Chicago Press

WHO Expert Committee on Radiation (1959) *First report. Effect of radiation on human heredity: investigation of areas of high natural radiation,* Geneva (*Wld Hlth Org. techn. Rep. Ser.,* No. 166)

WHO Expert Committee on Radiation (1962) *Third report. Radiation hazards in perspective,* Geneva (*Wld Hlth Org. techn. Rep. Ser.,* No. 248)

WHO Expert Committee on Radiation (1963) *Fourth report. Public health responsibilities in radiation protection,* Geneva (*Wld Hlth Org. techn. Rep. Ser.,* No. 254)

WHO Expert Committee on Radiation (1965) *Fifth report. Public health and the medical use of ionizing radiation,* Geneva (*Wld Hlth Org. techn. Rep. Ser.,* No. 306)

Williams, K. D., Cooper, J. F., Moore, R. T. & Hilberg, A. W., eds (1967) *Reduction of radiation exposure in nuclear medicine,* Rockville, Md, National Center for Radiological Health

CHAPTER 15

NON-IONIZING RADIATION AND ULTRASONIC WAVES

Non-ionizing radiation includes all those forms of radiation whose primary mode of interaction with matter, in their passage through it, does not involve the production of ion-pairs, whether directly or indirectly. These radiations are a part of the continuum of the electromagnetic spectrum. The non-ionizing portion of the electromagnetic spectrum extends from the low-energy region up to a photon energy of about 100 electron volts. It includes the high-frequency radiations used in communications and broadcasting; the microwave radiations used in radar, television transmissions, and industrial applications; the infrared radiation used in heat-lamps, and the visible light used in some lasers; and the ultraviolet radiation used in germicidal and "black" lights.

Non-ionizing radiation may be produced by a variety of electronic devices, such as microwave ovens, lasers, ultraviolet lamps, and medical diathermy equipment. These devices have been available in significant quantities only in recent years, but the electronic products industry is expanding and both the number of manufacturing plants and the variety of products are increasing. Although these products offer certain benefits to the public, they may also create potential hazards to health through uncontrolled or excessive radiation emissions.

Research into the biological effects of non-ionizing radiation—and the subsequent formulation of health criteria—has lagged behind research into and development of their technology. The different end effects of these radiations have also confused the picture. For example, in the microwave frequencies, some researchers have looked only at the pathological changes that result from the more obvious "thermal" effects of the radiation, while others have looked only at the subtle behavioural effects. Information on the long-term and genetic effects, and on the synergistic effects with other environmental insults, is lacking or very limited at best. Excessive exposures of large population groups have fortunately not occurred, but this also means that the data available on which to base criteria are limited. The existing protection criteria, guides and standards are apt, therefore, to be both arbitrary and contradictory.

Because the information pertaining to the uses, trends and biological effects of the various devices emitting non-ionizing radiation is basically different for the different types of both devices and emitted radiation, it will be dealt with under separate headings. The population at risk is the public in general, including occupational groups, but the magnitude and extent of exposure have not been systematically evaluated. Some estimates, in the USA for example, suggest that at least half the population is exposed to measurable levels of microwave radiation (US Department of Health, Education and Welfare, 1970). Sources of non-ionizing radiation include, but are not limited to:

(1) those used in the home, such as microwave ovens;

(2) those used in commerce and industry, such as lasers and microwave communication devices;

(3) those used in medicine for diagnosis and therapy, such as diathermy equipment;

(4) special devices used for educational, research and defence purposes, such as radar.

In addition to the non-ionizing radiation discussed above, some consideration will be given in this chapter to ultrasonic waves and their effects.

Microwave Radiation

Uses and trends

Microwave radiations are electromagnetic radiations in the frequency range of 30–300 000 megahertz (MHz) (Gilbert, 1970). Microwave radiation is emitted from a variety of electronic devices including diathermy units, ovens, heating devices, television receivers, and communications and radar units. It is impossible, at present, to assess the extent to which such devices are used in the world as a whole, but estimates are available of the use of various selected devices in certain countries (Harris, 1970; US Public Health Service, 1970a). The numbers of devices generating microwave radiation is expected to increase by 50–100 % over the period 1969-1973 (Harris, 1970). However, of the various industries using microwave processes, the one in which widespread application seems most probable is the food industry.

Biological effects

Biological effects depend on factors such as the frequency of the radiation, intensity of the beam, length of exposure, dielectric constant and thermal conductivity of the irradiated tissue and its ability to dissipate heat, and the size of the object in which absorption takes place.

Absorption of microwave radiation by body tissues results in an increase in temperature. Until recently, the generation of heat was considered as the principal cause of biological damage from microwave radiations. It was observed that, if sufficient energy was absorbed, burns could be produced, often by a local hot spot caused by disturbances in the field. The skin, eyes and testicles were found to be most sensitive to the thermal effects, with cataracts being the most common manifestation of excessive exposure (Moore, 1968). Recently, however, a number of other effects have been recorded in the absence of any demonstrable increase in the temperature of the body or the media concerned. These apparent non-thermal effects due to the microwave radiation itself may occur at low intensities, and include changes in the cardiovascular, central and peripheral nervous systems (Cleary, 1970). Some genetic effects have also been suspected (Michaelson, 1971). It seems that some kind of cumulative effect can be produced. In the lens of the eye repeated small doses may produce clinical effects (Faber, 1971).

The greatest need today in the assessment of the biological effects of microwave exposure is to determine the mechanisms by which cell damage is produced, the biological tolerance of the most susceptible tissues, the cumulative effects of repeated small doses, and the safe levels of radiation intensity. In view of the many uncertainties, research is required on the non-thermal effects, both at the molecular and cellular levels and at that of the organism as a whole; this should include observations on man (occupational or other exposure).

Existing exposure guidelines, criteria, and standards

A review (Gilbert, 1970; Michaelson, 1971; Swanson et al., 1970) of microwave exposure criteria for workers used in the USA and other western countries in the past ten years shows that, on the basis of the risk of cataract formation, there is a general acceptance of an occupational exposure limit in terms of power density of 10 milliwatts per square centimetre (mW/cm^2) for limited periods. The permissible levels specified in the USSR and Poland range from power densities of 10 microwatts per square centimetre ($\mu W/cm^2$) for a working day to 1000 $\mu W/cm^2$ for 15 minutes exposure daily. (For the general population, the permissible power density for frequencies from 300 MHz to 300 000 MHz is 1 $\mu W/cm^2$.) These differences by a factor of up to 1000 may be due to the use of different biological effects, such as the thermal effects in the western countries as opposed to the non-thermal effects in eastern Europe, as the basis for the criteria.

Laser Radiation

Uses and trends

Lasers emit a beam of coherent electromagnetic radiation of wavelengths in the range 0.3–10 micrometres (Faber, 1971), depending on the nature of the material emitting the beam. They are used for welding and cutting, surveying, communications, and in different measuring devices.   In medicine they are used in bloodless surgical operations, e.g., re-attaching the retina to the choroid, where advantage is taken of their high precision and combined cutting and coagulant effect.

Biological effects

The main biological effects of laser radiation are due to heating of the tissues and are essentially local.   There may also be non-thermal effects, such as erythema of the skin due to photochemical reactions.   Non-thermal effects occur mainly with high power density, pulsed lasers.   No genetic effects or late effects, such as skin cancer, have been reported (van Daatselaar & van der Werf, 1971).

The primary hazard from laser radiation is exposure of the eye.   Eye damage can range from mild retinal burns, with little or no loss of visual acuity, to severe lesions with loss of central vision, and ultimately to gross over-exposure with total loss of the eye (Bartleson, 1968; Burnett, 1969; Ham, 1970; Mellerio, 1967; Moore, 1970; Van Pelt et al., 1970).

The other organ of concern, besides the eye, is the skin.   It is not as sensitive as the eye, and if damaged, is usually more easily repaired.   However, it may be also subject to severe damage from laser impact when energy densities approach several joules per square centimetre (J/cm^2).   Laser damage to the skin may range from a mild erythema to a surface charring, and ultimately to a deep hole literally burned and blown into the skin.

Under certain circumstances, the organ of concern may also be the blood vessels or the underlying organs.   Blood vessels may be easily occluded or cauterized by a laser hit.

Existing exposure guidelines

For laser radiation, the levels that constitute a hazard are difficult to establish because of the existence of different types of laser and variations in relevant biological factors.   Different wavelengths, intensity levels, exposure times, pulse durations and pulse repetition rates all directly affect the possibility of tissue damage.   Because of the large number of such factors, it is impractical to establish a single threshold value for biological damage for all types of laser systems and conditions of operation.   Current guides are therefore based on the minimum dose required to produce a visible lesion (Carpenter et al., 1970; Flood, 1967; Mendoza, 1967; Peppers & Hammond, 1969; Powell et al., 1970; Vassiliadis et al., 1970).

At present, threshold values (in J/cm^2 on the retina) for visible lesions produced on the critical organ, the eye, are approximately as follows:

Q-switched ruby laser	0.07
Pulsed ruby laser	0.8
Continuous white light	6.0
CO_2 laser	0.2

Other Electromagnetic Radiations

Ultraviolet radiation is that part of the electromagnetic spectrum lying between visible light and the soft X-rays. It is present in normal solar radiation, and is produced by arcs and incandescent sources operating at high temperatures. Population exposure results from the use of a wide range of apparatus in homes, industries, places of entertainment, health clubs and scientific and medical establishments. Typical apparatus emitting ultraviolet radiation includes cosmetic and therapeutic sun lamps, equipment for disinfection and sterilization, and analytical instruments.

The biological effects of ultraviolet radiation depend on the absorbed dose, and on the wavelength and intensity of the radiation. They are due mainly to the absorption of energy by the proteins and nucleic acids of the exposed organism. There are also indirect effects, such as those resulting from exposure to ozone, which is produced in air by the radiation. The extent of penetration by ultraviolet radiation is usually slight, except for such tissues as the lens and humours of the eye, so that the critical organs are usually the skin and eyes. Exposure of the surface layer of the skin to such radiation may result in erythema, skin cancer (after repeated exposures), rapid skin ageing and photo-sensitization. In the case of the eye, the radiation is absorbed primarily in the cornea and may produce lesions that could lead to blindness. Some portions of the ultraviolet spectrum are mutagenic and may be lethal to cells (Leach, 1970).

Visible light may present a hazard to the eye. This is primarily dependent on factors such as the intensity of the light, pupil dilation, and length of exposure. If these factors are controlled so as to keep the absorbed energy below the threshold for thermal burning (reported to be between 40 to 50 calories/cm^2 per minute), no visible lesions should develop in the eye, although damage or injury might still result.

Electromagnetic Interference

Electromagnetic interference has been studied and reported in some detail since implanted cardiac pacemakers were first developed (Ruggera & Elder, 1971). Most of the published information concerns such devices and the frequency ranges that are most likely to be encountered in normal daily life. Implanted pacemaker dysfunction has been observed near electrocautery and diathermy apparatus, radar and communications systems, electric shavers, spark coils and gasoline engine ignition systems.

Ultrasonic Waves

Uses and trends

The term "ultrasound" denotes mechanical vibrations at frequencies above the limit of human audibility, i.e., from about 16 KHz up to about

10 MHz. Although ultrasound is a relatively new energy source, its versatility has led to its widespread use in various industrial, medical, scientific and consumer applications. Industrial ultrasound is used for cleaning and welding plastics, drying fine powders, emulsification, detecting flaws in materials, and non-destructive testing. The use of ultrasonic devices in medicine includes both therapy (surgery) and diagnosis (detection of tumours). It is also being used in obstetrics, cardiology, neurology and ophthalmology.

Biological effects

The interactions of ultrasonic waves may involve complex properties of the propagating media and the nature of the waves. The waves may be focused, dispersed, reflected, transmitted, refracted or absorbed.

The interactions of ultrasound in tissue have been studied (Goldstein 1969), but because such interactions are very complex, much further study is needed. It is suspected that the biological effects of ultrasonic waves are related to the local generation of heat. Whether any cellular destruction is associated with cavity formation in tissues is not known for certain (Faber, 1971). Hearing loss and effects on the heart and blood vessels, such as vasoconstriction, that may affect the adrenal cortical function have been observed (van den Eijk, 1971). Observations of the mother and fetus in the course of several thousand obstetric procedures did not indicate any hazard (Hellman et al., 1970). However, no long-term follow-up studies have been done on those receiving ultrasound therapy in medicine (Aldes, 1957). Experimental biological studies at reasonably low exposure intensities (as opposed to clinical studies) suggest strongly that undetected biological damage is associated with diagnostic exposure (Hill, 1971). This may be caused by one of the biophysical mechanisms of interaction, namely, heating, cavitation, or the "direct" effect.

Where ultrasound passes into the air, as in certain industrial applications, the probability of tissue damage is lower than in the case of direct contact, since the coupling obtained between ultrasonic transducers and air is very poor. The dangers of airborne hearing damage, systemic effects, and psychological effects necessitate caution even in the case of airborne ultrasound. Such airborne ultrasound is sometimes emitted by certain machines, so that surveillance based on appropriate measurements is necessary.

No exposure guidelines are available at present for ultrasound.

Instrumentation and Survey Methodology

One of the problems associated with the control of non-ionizing radiation is the lack of suitable survey or monitoring instruments that will enable the public health control specialist or the manufacturer to determine accurately the magnitude of the exposure to radiation from a particular source (Moore, 1970; Swicord, 1971; US Public Health Service, 1970b). The radiation biologist has an equally difficult task in measuring the amount of energy that is absorbed in the biological system under investigation. In the past, therefore, many experiments were conducted by calculating the energy that was expected to be absorbed in the system. This may account for some of the inconsistencies in the reported results of biological experiments.

For those types of radiation, such as microwave radiation, for which survey instruments are available, extreme care must be taken in interpreting the readings. Until recently, microwave instruments were designed for measuring the "far field" at some distance from the source. The use of these far-field instruments close to the source ("near field") will result in incorrect readings. Microwave instruments are also energy- and direction-dependent. There are also parts of the electromagnetic spectrum for which no survey instruments are available. Some effort has been made recently to overcome these problems, but until commercial instruments are readily available, public health workers will be limited in their ability to control these radiations.

REFERENCES

Aldes, J. K. (1957) *The indications and contraindications for ultrasound therapy in medicine.* In: Kelly, E., ed., *Ultrasound in biology and medicine*, Washington, American Institute of Biological Sciences, pp. 66-68

Bartleson, C. J. (1968) *Amer. industr. Hyg. Ass. J.*, **29**, 415-424

Burnett, W. D. (1969) *Amer. industr. Hyg. Ass. J.*, **30**, 582-587

Carpenter, J. A., Lehmiller, D. J. & Tredici, T. J. (1970) *Arch. environm. Hlth*, **20**, 171-176

Cleary, S. F. (1970) *Amer. industr. Hyg. Ass. J.*, **31**, 52-59

Faber, M. (1971) *The health effects on personnel of ionizing radiation and other physical factors*, Copenhagen, World Health Organization (Unpublished document EURO 4701/7)

Flood, J. M. (1967) *Ann. occup. Hyg.*, **10**, Suppl., 47-53

Gilbert, H. (1970) *Amer. industr. Hyg. Ass. J.*, **31**, 772-778

Goldstein, N. (1969) *Health hazard from ultrasonic energy*, Cambridge, Mass., Massachusetts Institute of Technology (Document PB 185963)

Ham, W. T. (1970) *Arch. environm. Hlth*, **20**, 156-160

Harris, J. Y. (1970) *Electronic product inventory study*, Rockville, Md, US Department of Health, Education, and Welfare (Document BRH/DEP 70-29)

Hellman, L. M., Duffus, G. M., Donald, I. & Sunden, B. (1970) *Lancet*, **1**, 1133-1135

Hill, C. R. (1971) *Occupational hazards from radiation generated by ultrasonic devices*, Copenhagen, World Health Organization (Unpublished document EURO 4701/8)

Leach, W. (1970) *Biological aspects of ultraviolet radiation, a review of hazards*, Rockville, Md, US Department of Health, Education, and Welfare (Document BRH/DBE 70-3)

Mellerio, J. (1967) *Ann. occup. Hyg.*, **10**, Suppl., 31-41

Mendoza, A. (1967) *Ann. occup. Hyg.*, **10**, Suppl., 43-46

Michaelson, S. M. (1971) *Amer. industr. Hyg. Ass. J.*, **32**, 338-345

Moore, R. T. (1970) *Arch. environm. Hlth*, **20**, 203-206

Moore, W. (1968) *Biological aspects of microwave radiation, a review of hazards*, Rockville, Md, US Department of Health, Education, and Welfare (Document TSB 4)

Peppers, N. A. & Hammond, A. H. (1969) *Amer. industr. Hyg. Ass. J.*, **30**, 218-225

Powell, C. H., Bell, H. E., Rose, V. E., Goldman, L. & Wilkinson, T. K. (1970) *Amer. industr. Hyg. Ass. J.*, **31**, 485-491

Ruggera, P. S. & Elder, R. L. (1971) *Electromagnetic radiation interference with cardiac pacemakers*, Rockville, Md, US Department of Health, Education, and Welfare (Document BRH/DEP 71-5)

Swanson, J. R., Rose, V. E. & Powell, C. H. (1970) *Amer. industr. Hyg. Ass. J.*, **31**, 623-629

Swicord, M. L. (1971) *Microwave measurements and new types of detectors for evaluation of health hazards*, Rockville, Md, US Department of Health, Education, and Welfare (Document BRH/DEP 71-1)

US Department of Health, Education and Welfare (1970) *Man's health and the environment—some research needs*, Washington, D.C., US Government Printing Office

US Public Health Service (1970a) *Survey of selected industrial applications of microwave energy*, Rockville, Md, US Department of Health, Education, and Welfare (Document BRH/DEP 70-10)

US Public Health Service (1970b) *The effects of instrument averaging time on microwave power density measurements*, Rockville, Md, US Department of Health, Education, and Welfare (Document BRH/DEP 70-12)

van Daatselaar, C. J. & van der Werf, B. (1971) *The occupational hazards from non-ionizing radiation generated by coherent electromagnetic devices, the consequent biological effects on personnel and the respective rules and regulations which have been developed in Europe*, Copenhagen, World Health Organization (Unpublished document EURO 4701/5)

van den Eijk, J. (1971) *Occupational hazards from sound and light*, Copenhagen, World Health Organization (Unpublished document EURO 4701/6

Van Pelt, W. F., Stewart, H. F., Peterson, R. W., Roberts, A. M. & Worst, J. K. (1970) *Laser fundamentals and experiments*, Rockville, Md, US Department of Health, Education, and Welfare (Document BRH/SWRHL 70-1)

Vassiliadis, A., Zweng, H. C., Peppers, N. A., Peabody, R. R. & Honey, R. C. (1970) *Arch. environm. Hlth*, **20**, 161-170

CHAPTER 16

NOISE

General Considerations

Noise is generally defined as a sound without agreeable musical quality, or as un unwanted or undesirable sound.

The word "sound" denotes a periodic mechanical disturbance in gases, fluids or solids. With airborne sound, the vibratory movement of molecules of the atmospheric gases sets up small variations in atmospheric pressure, known as "sound pressure". The latter can be expressed in microbars or as dynes per square centimetre (Bell, 1966).

Noise is a normal feature of life and provides one of the most effective alarm systems in man's physical environment. It is an accompaniment to most human activity and as such may constitute a hazard or a stimulant. Very low sound levels, as encountered in a soundproof chamber, for example, lead to temporospatial disorientation, while high or continuous levels may cause permanent loss of hearing. Hearing cannot be "switched off" at will, and man is thus unavoidably exposed to the environmental noise produced by modern society.

The structure and function of the auditory system are both of great neurophysiological complexity; the system is linked, in addition, with a whole series of other systems, such as those of balance, vision, circulation, and level of general activity. These are themselves interdependent, stratified and integrated before they reach the auditory cortex. The sense of hearing can therefore never be considered in isolation, and always, although to varying degrees, involves other functions. In man, in particular, there is a special interrelationship between hearing and phonation, regarded as a means of communication (Wisner, 1967). Furthermore, individuals differ widely in their reactions to noise, depending on age, sex and socio-cultural background.

Attention was focused initially on the most obvious effects of noise on hearing and those most amenable to objective analysis, namely impairment and loss of hearing, mainly from occupational causes. This pathological effect is fairly well understood. So also is the "masking" effect, particularly with respect to conversation, which is susceptible to reasonably straight-forward assessment. In contrast, although their importance is generally recognized, the physiological, psychophysiological and psychosocial effects of noise and their impact on health and behaviour are more difficult to assess objectively as a result, *inter alia*, of the variety and complexity of their manifestations. The nature and distribution of noise in different human environments is shown in the accompanying table, although no precise dividing line exists between such environments as regards sound level.

SOUND LEVELS OF SOME NOISE SOURCES FOUND IN DIFFERENT ENVIRONMENTS [1]

Overall level in dB [2]		Industrial and military	Community (outdoor)	Home (indoor)
140 –		Carrier deck jet operation (140 dB)		
	Painfully loud	Oxygen torch (126 dB)		
130 –		Pneumatic chipper (122 dB)		
120 –		Pavement breaker (115 dB)		Discotheque (120 dB)
	Uncomfortably loud	Textile loom (112 dB)		
		Cut-off saw (106 dB)		
110 –		Farm tractor (103 dB)	Jet aircraft flyover at	
		Newspaper press (101 dB)	300 m (110 dB)	
			Power mower (103 dB)	
100 –			Excavation rock drill	
		Bench lathe (95 dB)	at 15 m (100 dB)	
	Very loud	Milling machine (90 dB)	Motorcycle at 8 m (96 dB)	Food blender (90 dB)
90 –		Bed press (86 dB)	Heavy truck at 15 m (93 dB)	Alarm clock (85 dB)
		Key-punch machine (82 dB)	Train whistle at 150 m (90 dB)	Garbage disposal (83 dB)
				Clothes washer (82 dB)
80 –			Passenger car, 100 km/h	Living room music (78 dB)
			at 15 m (76 dB)	Dishwasher (76 dB)
	Moderately loud		Church bells at 50 m (70 dB)	TV-audio (73 dB)
70 –			Light traffic at 30 m (66 dB)	Vacuum cleaner (72 dB)
				Toilet flush (65 dB)
60 –				Conversation (60 dB)
50 –	Quiet			
40 –				
30 –				
	Very quiet			
20 –				
10 –	Just audible			
0 –	Threshold of hearing			

[1] After Cohen (1969).
[2] Reference sound pressure level: 0.0002 microbar.

Perception of Noise

The response of the ear to noise depends on the physical parameters of the sound concerned. The intensity of the response is related to sound pressure and increases logarithmically with the degree of stimulus. The unit of measurement is the "decibel" (dB), which is a relative unit of gradation; to say that a sound is 60 dB means that it is 60 dB more intense than a sound standardized as the reference level. In making physical measurements, we use as a base a sound pressure of 0.0002 microbar, the weakest sound pressure detectable by the keen young human ear under very quiet conditions (Bell, 1966).

However, for a given sound pressure, the intensity of the response varies with frequency, maximum sensitivity occurring between 1000 and 4000 cycles per second or Hertz (Hz) (Bell, 1966).

With regard to frequencies, the auditory field extends from 20 to 20 000 Hz. The threshold of differentiation between two sounds varies with frequency, and each frequency has specific maximum and minimum audibility thresholds. The differential threshold varies very little between 1000 and 4000 Hz, which is the zone of maximum sensitivity to intensity. The audibility threshold is at its minimum at 4000 Hz and at this frequency is located the zone of impairment of the perception of high pitched tones that occurs in the early stages of hearing loss (Grognot, 1965).

To make allowance for the variation in response with frequency when making measurements of the sound spectrum, the high and low frequency components are filtered out so that the measured values are roughly proportional to the subjective effects of noise. For noise of average intensity, the "A weighting" of the noise-measuring instrument is generally used (Bell, 1966).

Other parameters also need to be considered, such as the duration, frequency distribution, number of transient frequencies and variations in energy, unexpectedness, association with vibration, and the significance of the noise.

The mechanism known as the acoustic reflex, protects the ear from noise. The simultaneous contraction of the stapedius and tensor tympani muscles reduces the amount of energy transmitted to the sound receptors of the inner ear: the basilar membrane and the hair cells. There is a limit, however, to the protection afforded, due both to the delay in the response (approximately 10 milliseconds, so that it is ineffective against very sudden noise) and to fatigue in the muscles concerned. Finally, the ear tends to adapt or acclimatize itself to exposure to continued noise, from its onset, whatever the sound level. Adaptation increases with sound level, but disappears rapidly when the noise stops.

Physiological Effects of Noise

Such effects include both specific auditory responses and non-specific non-auditory responses.

Auditory fatigue and the masking effect are the most important direct physiological effects.

Auditory fatigue is manifested by a temporary threshold shift, measured at least two minutes after exposure has ceased. It appears in the 90dB region and is greatest at 4000 Hz. Auditory fatigue increases with the intensity of the sound, in which case it may be associated with side effects such as diplacousis and whistling and buzzing in the ears. Recovery may be slow if the threshold has risen by more than 50 dB (Wisner, 1967).

Pure tones are more damaging than broadband noise, but intermittent, sudden or unexpected sounds are more harmful than continuous noise. This must be taken into account when assessing sound levels, particularly as such intermittent noise is common in industry (Wisner, 1967; Mery, 1968).

The *masking effect* refers to the decrease in the perceptibility or intelligibility of a sound when other noise is present. This masking noise causes a shift in the audibility threshold of the sound masked, and the effect becomes more noticeable as the frequencies of masked and masking noise come closer together. As the masking noise increases in intensity, its effect extends progressively to the higher frequencies. The extent of the masking effect is measured by its SIL (Speech Interference Level), and for good speech intelligibility it is considered that the speech sound level must exceed the SIL by approximately 12 dB. If the level of speech is 10 dB lower than the masking noise, syllable intelligibility falls to 5%. The masking effect has important repercussions in industry, where it may interfere with speech communication and even endanger safety. In everyday life, the frequencies causing most disturbance to speech communication lie in the 300 to 500 Hz range. Such frequencies are commonly present in noise produced by road and air traffic (Wisner, 1967; Mery, 1968; Kryter, 1970).

One of the direct responses to noise that should be mentioned is the startle reaction, produced by a sudden high intensity pulse of sound. Apart from the various effects that it may have on the autonomic nervous system, the startle reaction may also affect psychomotor performance.

As a long-term effect, *impairment of hearing acuity* with age (presbycousis), cannot be entirely dissociated from the noise occurring in modern society. Indeed, even though it is an accepted fact that hearing acuity generally decreases with age, there is no proof that this condition is of exclusively physiological origin since exposure to noise is becoming increasingly common. Presbycousis appears from the age of 30 onwards and becomes noticeable after the age of 40. It is more marked in men than in women and generally affects the higher frequencies, the "sensitive" frequencies mentioned earlier of the order of 4000 Hz being the first to become involved. Presbycousis is the more marked and rapid in its onset the greater the amount of exposure to noise, but in this context individual reactions vary widely and some persons are particularly sensitive to noise for reasons that are not fully understood (Bell, 1966; Hinchcliffe, 1958).

Noise has a wide variety of *non-specific physiological effects* that are not always the same and whose significance is not fully understood.

With regard to the *cardiovascular system*, noise may affect the rate of heart beat, but may either increase or decrease it, depending on the type of noise (Mery, 1968). Sudden changes in sound level or sound spectrum also modify heart rates. Noise generally causes heart output to decrease,

as well as an increase or fluctuations in arterial blood pressure and vasoconstriction of peripheral blood vessels (Mery, 1968; Kryter, 1970).

The *respiratory system* reacts with apnoea to impulsive noise. Changes
in breathing amplitude have been reported (Kryter, 1970), indicating a
state of alarm or a feeling of discomfort (Mery, 1968).

Observed effects on the *eye* include pupillary dilatation, narrowing of
the visual field, decrease in the rate of colour perception and impairment
of night vision (Mery, 1968; Lang & Jansen, 1970).

Galvanic skin responses, which are a sign of activity in the reticular zone
of the brain stem, reflect a decrease in the electrical resistance of the skin
(Mery, 1968; Kryter, 1970).

Changes in the *blood and other body fluids* have also been reported, such
as eosinophilia, hypokalaemia, hyperglycaemia, hypoglycaemia and effects
on the endocrine system (Kryter, 1970; Grognot, 1965).

Generally speaking, the variety and variability of these non-specific
responses show that they reflect the intensity of the reactions of the autonomic nervous system to noise intensity and band width.

Psychophysiological Effects of Noise

At the psychophysiological level, noise mainly affects sleep and work
performance; at the psychosocial level, it causes annoyance and irritation.

Noise may lead to sleep disturbance or awakening. *Sleep disturbance,*
even though it may not lead to full awakening, is frequently cited as the main
cause of annoyance. Electro-encephalography provides a means of study-
ing the effect of noise on sleep. Depth of sleep is affected by noise, and
periods of very deep sleep may be reduced in length by impulsive noise of
very short duration, whose intensity is 20 dB greater than that of the background noise. Above 70 dB, sound of no more than 300 milliseconds duration can interrupt deep sleep, and acoustic stimuli (white noise) of short
duration cause EEG changes. In the same way, when individuals sleeping
naturally are subjected to continuous noise of 70 dB, periods of deep sleep
may be appreciably reduced in length. The probability that an individual
will be *awakened* by pulse levels of 40 dB (A) is 5 %, and this rises to 30 % for
pulse levels of 70 dB (A). Apparently, noise not only affects depth of sleep
but also the type of sleep. When the mean sound level is low, an individual
will take longer to go to sleep the greater the number of sound pulses.
Noise-induced deprivation of sleep in the early part of the night appears
to be compensated by a longer period of deep sleep in the second half of the
night (Kryter, 1970; Lang & Jansen, 1970; OECD Consultative Group on
Transportation Research, 1971; Metz & Mery, 1967). Here again, however, such responses show wide individual variation; some people are
awakened by sounds of 40 dB (A) while others are roused only by sounds
of over 70 dB (A). The significance of the noise is undoubtedly an important factor.

Noise may affect the performance of *psychomotor tasks*, although the results of the investigations carried out in industry seem, at first sight, to be contradictory. Two factors are involved: the type of work involved and the characteristics of the noise concerned.

Depending on its intensity, duration, frequency distribution, intermittence and significance, noise has been shown both to improve and to reduce work performance, and both to increase and decrease reaction times. Nevertheless, the occurrence of any intense unexpected noise always interferes with the performance of work, whether mental or physical, and temporarily reduces the efficiency with which it is carried out.

Work demanding a high degree of skill is particularly affected by noise (Lang & Jansen, 1970; Metz & Mery, 1967; Meyer-Schwertz et al., 1968). There is some evidence that the frequency of noise occurrence and its sound level are not the only important factors, and that the rise time, i.e., the time taken by a sound to reach its maximum intensity, also plays a part (Mery, 1968). These parameters would seem to be of importance since they also affect the autonomic nervous system, causing, as has been seen, an overall alarm response, which, together with the startle reaction, may affect the performance of psychomotor tasks.

Noise may cause feelings of *annoyance* and *irritation*; these are now receiving increasing attention, at both the individual and the collective level. It is always very difficult to correlate attitudes and feelings, such as discomfort or irritation, with factors such as the masking effect, sleep disturbance, changes in the autonomic nervous system or the physical parameters of noise. It is rare for any of these various factors to be linked directly in any way. In spite of the fact that some degree of adaptation to noisy environments does occur and that individual reactions vary widely, research has shown that social contacts are disturbed in such environments, e.g., in industry, in towns and cities, and near airports. In contrast to its occasional positive effect on mental activity, mentioned above, noise is here a negative influence. The significance of the noise and the attitude of the individual to it undoubtedly play a part in the feeling of annoyance experienced (Jonsson & Sorenson, 1967).

Pathological Effects of Noise

Although there is no doubt that noise causes annoyance and may adversely affect well-being, there is as yet no clear epidemiological proof that the various physiological and psychophysiological responses to noise will, in the long term, lead to pathological changes. Long-term comparative studies are needed in order to gain a fuller understanding of this problem.

Deafness is, of course, the major hazard involved in exposure to noise that is too intense or too prolonged.

Deafness may occur suddenly due to acoustic trauma following exposure to very high intensity noise, but more usually appears gradually as a result of repeated exposure to noise. The most typical case is that of *occupational deafness*, in the early stages of which hearing impairment, as determined by audiometric methods, occurs in the 3000–6000 Hz octave bands. The individual concerned is in most cases unaware of this impairment. Damage then becomes more serious and its extent increases; it becomes particularly troublesome when the voice frequencies are affected. Impairment progresses in an irregular manner towards severe deafness, associated with very high levels of mean hearing loss (see figure).

AUDIOGRAMS SHOWING DIFFERENT STAGES OF NOISE-INDUCED HEARING LOSS

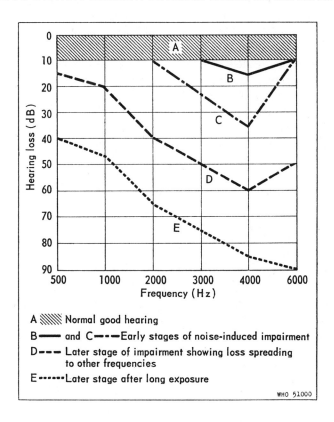

Although there are some similarities between effects such as temporary threshold shift, auditory fatigue and acoustic trauma, no conclusive evidence exists of any definite relationship between them.

Noisy environments

There is no clear-cut dividing line between the various types of noise, and noise from different sources can be combined and added together (see table, p. 258). It is nevertheless convenient to consider *industrial noise* separately, since it is the major source of high sound levels and prolonged noise exposure; as a result, it is associated with the most serious health hazard from noise, i.e., deafness. A complex of many factors is involved, including: individual susceptibility; age; the total energy content of the noise; its spectrum; its continuity or intermittence: and the length of exposure (temporary, daily and total) (National Safety Council, 1971). This explains why it is so difficult to define limits of exposure. While it has been estimated that six million workers in the USA are exposed to noise hazards (Jones & Cohen, 1968), little is known of the possible non-auditory effects of noise on the worker and his work. Further research is needed to determine what effects, if any, noise may have on the cardio-vascular system, absenteeism or even the possible synergistic effects of vibration when associated with noise. More information is also needed on noise as a cause of disturbance during work.

Control of industrial noise comprises:

(1) definition of permissible sound levels;

(2) measurement of noise and its components, including measurement of background noise, measurement of noise at the workplace and measurement of noise at source;

(3) reduction of noise at source;

(4) acoustic zoning to prevent airborne propagation of noise or propagation of noise through solids;

(5) sound-proofing; and

(6) provision, where necessary, of personal protection devices.

In communities, particularly in towns and cities, traffic constitutes the major noise nuisance. Possible effects of noise, as yet lacking long-term confirmation, may include acceleration of the presbycousis process and disorders due, in particular, to prolonged disturbance of sleep (OECD Consultative Group on Transportation Research, 1971; Orlova, 1958; Goromosov, 1968). Sleep disturbance, together with speech interference, are the major annoyances most frequently mentioned in sociological surveys (OECD Consultative Group on Transportation Research, 1971). Despite the many parameters to be considered, such surveys show that the noise indices are related to annoyance scales (OECD Consultative Group on Transportation Research, 1971). This relationship is most marked in the case of noise associated with airports (Kryter, 1970).

Noise generated in the home by communal or personal equipment (radio, television, games, etc.) may also, depending on the construction of the building, constitute a nuisance to be added to other sources of noise exposure. As a result, it is now increasingly difficult to ignore such sources of noise when examining the relationship between noise and health.

Noise from various forms of transport and its transmission into the home may be reduced:

(1) at the source, i.e., by controlling the *emission* of noise;

(2) by means of town and country planning and traffic engineering, i.e., by controlling the *transmission* of noise;

(3) in the home, i.e., by controlling the *reception* of noise by the occupants.

REFERENCES

Bell, A. (1966) *Noise. An occupational hazard and public nuisance*, Geneva, World Health Organization (*Publ. Hlth Pap.*, No. 30)

Cohen, A. (1969) *Sound and vibration*, Bethesda, Md, National Library of Medicine

Goromosov, M. S. (1968) *The physiological basis for health standards for dwellings*, Geneva, World Health Organization (*Publ. Hlth Pap.*, No. 33)

Grognot, P. (1965) *Horiz. méd.*, Nos 120-125

Hinchcliffe, R. (1958) *Gerontologia*, **2**, 311

Jones, H. H. & Cohen, A. (1968) *Publ. Hlth Rep. (Wash.)*, **83**, 7

Jonsson, E. & Sorenson, S. (1967) *Nord. Hyg. T.*, **48**, 35-45

Kryter, K. D. (1970) *The effects of noise on man*, New York, Academic Press

Lang, J. & Jansen, G. (1970) *The environmental health aspects of noise research and noise control*, Copenhagen, World Health Organization (Unpublished document EURO 2631)

Mery, J. C. (1968) *Caractère, effets et évaluations des bruits intermittents dans l'industrie et l'habitat*, Strasbourg, Centre de Biologie climatique du CNRS

Metz, B. & Mery, J. C. (1967) *Présentation d'une recherche expérimentale sur les effets du bruit au cours du travail et au cours du sommeil. Caractéristiques des bruits étudiés: banc d'essai de moteurs et grosse chaudronnerie au cours du travail. Décollages d'avions de transport à réaction au cours du sommeil.* In: *Actes du 4ème Congres de la Société d'Ergonomie de Langue Française, Octobre 1966, Marseille*, Paris, *Travail hum.*, No. 1-2

Meyer-Schwertz, M. T., Geber, M. & Marbach, G. (1968) *Arch. Sci. physiol.*, **22**, 195-228

National Safety Council (1971) *Fundamentals of industrial hygiene*, Chicago, Ill.

OECD Consultative Group on Transportation Research (1971) *Urban traffic noise. Strategy for an improved environment*, Paris, Organisation for Economic Co-operation and Development

Orlova, T. A. (1958) [*Some neurodynamic effects of sound stimuli of various intensities*]. In: [*Noise prevention and the action of noise on the organism*], Leningrad, No. 11

Wisner, A. (1967) *Audition et bruits.* In: Scherrer, J., ed., *Physiologie du travail*, Vol. 2, Paris, Masson, pp. 3-72

PART III

SURVEILLANCE AND MONITORING

CHAPTER 17

DEFINITIONS AND SCOPE

According to standard dictionaries, the terms *monitoring* and *surveillance* are almost synonymous, but in public health practice during the past 20 years they have taken on rather specific and somewhat different meanings. As related to human health and for the purposes of this publication, the following definitions are proposed:

Monitoring is the making of routine observations on health and environmental parameters, and the recording and transmission of these data.

Health surveillance is the collation and interpretation of data collected from monitoring programmes and from any other available sources, with a view to the detection of changes in health status of populations.

According to these definitions, monitoring becomes one specific and essential part of the broader concept embraced by surveillance. Monitoring requires careful planning and the use of standardized procedures and methods of data collection, but can then be carried out over extended periods of time by technicians and automated instrumentation. Surveillance, in contrast, requires professional analysis and sophisticated judgement of data leading to recommendations for control actions.

For operational purposes in surveillance and monitoring, the human environment is considered here as consisting of the physical, chemical, biological, and social processes and influences that directly or indirectly have a *significant* and *detectable* effect on the health and wellbeing of the individual or of communities.

It is entirely beyond the resources of health authorities to attempt to compile and digest information on *all* the factors in the human environment. Such an approach would not only be impracticable but also exceedingly wasteful. Since the systematic study of environmental effects on man is a relatively new field of science, care must be taken in deciding which variables are to be studied intensively. Furthermore, even when environmental factors are known to have an effect or are strongly suspected of so doing, the relative importance to health may differ widely, since the nature of the effect can vary from minor irritation to acute toxicity or potent carcinogenicity. Consequently, a careful selection needs to be made and the programme restricted so as to include only those factors likely to have a significant impact, good or bad, on the health of man.

Because a large part of the current international concern with environmental degradation appears to be directed towards the detection of changes in the external environment, it should be emphasized that one of the key indicators of deleterious environmental influences, and certainly the most pertinent, is the status of human health itself. A change in the health status of populations, whether it be local and sudden, or global and gradual, is a strong indication that the human environment is causally involved. Parameters of health status, such as mortality and morbidity by age, sex, and cause of death or illness, and the epidemiological indices to be discussed below, are of crucial importance in the assessment of the health effects of the environment.

CHAPTER 18

ENVIRONMENTAL PARAMETERS

Before the problems connected with direct observations for determining changes in the health status of populations are discussed, it is useful to consider briefly those aspects of surveillance and monitoring of the environment that are not usually the functions of health authorities but for which data are required for integration with health information; this is necessary both to increase our knowledge of environmental effects on human health and to provide information that would contribute to an early-warning system. Within governments and at the international level, information on such environmental parameters is dealt with by various agencies and organizations.

For illustrative purposes, the following discussion will be limited to the international level, where the activities and resources of WHO would be involved jointly with those of other international organizations, and with regional and national efforts. The major categories of information and data required, and the activities involved, are:

Physical

Meteorological and geographical (with WMO and other agencies)
Radiation (with IAEA and FAO)
    Emphasis on background, incorporated (food chains), and human tissue levels.

Chemical and biological

Food (with FAO)
    Emphasis on chemical contaminants, especially mercury, lead, cadmium, and pesticides.
Drinking-water (with national health authorities)
    Emphasis on microbial and chemical contaminants.
Surface waters (with FAO, UNESCO, United Nations, and other agencies)
    Emphasis on indicators of general pollution in rivers, lakes, coastal waters, and estuaries.
Air pollution (with regional and national authorities, WHO reference centres, and WMO)
    Emphasis on particulate matter, sulfur dioxide, hydrocarbons, oxidants, carbon monoxide, lead, and special industrial emissions.
Soil (with FAO, UNESCO, and national authorities)
    Emphasis on pollutants.
Vectors and other biota (with national authorities, FAO, and UNESCO)
    Emphasis on domestic animals, wildlife, and insects.
Natural disasters and catastrophes (with WMO, International Red Cross, and national authorities)
    Emphasis on earthquakes and floods.

The relationships between many of the above categories and human health are considered elsewhere in this publication, and have recently been summarized from the standpoint of the requirements for global environmental monitoring (International Council of Scientific Unions, Scientific Committee on Problems of the Environment, 1971). They will not be discussed further here.

Chapters 19-31 will be concerned primarily with surveillance and monitoring of health status, but accurate measures of exposure to environmental influence are essential to obtain meaningful correlations between environmental conditions and health effects. Much of the needed information on environmental parameters may be obtained through monitoring systems designed for purposes other than health surveillance. However, such data will often have to be supplemented by information obtained from specifically designed systems closely associated with epidemiological and other health studies.

A good illustration of the systematic monitoring of environmental parameters and its use in assessing possible health effects is provided in the following chapter on environmental radiation (Chapter 19), which is one of the few parameters for which considerable experience has accumulated over many years and on a worldwide scale.

REFERENCE

International Council of Scientific Unions, Scientific Committee on Problems of the Environment (1971) *Global environmental monitoring*, Stockholm

ENVIRONMENTAL RADIATION

Environmental radiation monitoring systems were first organized in a number of countries to obtain information on the possible harmful effects on populations of radioactive fallout from nuclear weapon tests. At a later stage, systems were developed to monitor the surroundings of nuclear installations, nuclear power stations, research reactors, fuel processing plants, and the like. Originally, these systems were the responsibility of national atomic energy commissions, and it was only later that public health authorities in some countries became involved in the monitoring of radioactivity levels in the environment.

At the present time, responsibility is divided: monitoring is carried out both by producers and users of radioactive substances, and by public health authorities concerned with preventing the radioactive contamination of the population. Monitoring is of two types: (1) global or national monitoring; and (2) monitoring of the controlled zone surrounding nuclear installations, Samples of air, water, soil, food and biological tissues are collected in different places and analysed for their content of ^{90}Sr, ^{137}Cs, radioiodine, tritium, etc. Monthly or quarterly reports are published by the national authorities with the aim of informing the public and government of the level of radioactivity in the country (National Institute of Radiological Science, 1971; Zykova et al., 1968).

Global and/or regional surveillance of radioactive fallout in air and water is also carried out by some national authorities, e.g., the Health and Safety Laboratory of the US Atomic Energy Commission determines monthly fallout deposition rates for ^{90}Sr for 36 sites in the USA and 103 locations in other countries (*Radiol. Hlth Data*, 1971). The United Kingdom has 8 monitoring sites within the country and a further 20 overseas.

The regional system of Euratom consisted in 1970 of 94 sampling stations for air, 55 for water, and 20 for milk (*Radioactivité ambiante dans les pays de la Communauté*, 1970). The Pan American Milk Sampling Program (Pan American Health Organization and US Environmental Protection Agency) has 5 sampling stations, and the Pan American Air Sampling Program (Pan American Health Organization and US Public Health Service) has 12 sampling stations (*Radiol. Hlth Data*, 1971).

Radioactivity in the human body is measured in occupational groups and, in some countries, in the general public by whole-body radioactivity monitors. For this purpose, 230 monitors are used in 31 countries (International Atomic Energy Agency, 1970).

Environmental monitoring in radiation accidents has caused some national and international problems because of the possibility of the spread of radioactivity across national borders. To unify and promote the methods of handling of radiation accidents, a special manual was published jointly by IAEA, ILO, FAO, and WHO in 1969 (International Atomic Energy Agency, 1969a), and a system of mutual emergency assistance for countries in the event of radiation accidents was established by the same organizations in order to arrange for the provision of essential services, including monitoring and preventive measures to protect the general public from radioactive contamination (International Atomic Energy Agency, 1971a).

Evaluation of radiation doses received by the population should also include the irradiation resulting from the use of certain types of equipment, e.g., medical X-ray equipment (Committee on Radiological Hazards to Patients, 1960) and colour television receivers (Bureau of Radiological Health, 1970). In some countries, the users and producers are responsible for the control of such irradiation, and at the same time public health authorities inspect the sources and installations with the aim of reducing external radiation exposure of the general public as far as possible. This dual control system is supplemented by the practice of licensing personnel, equipment and the installation, as well as by the creation of codes of good practice for the use of different sources of radiation.

The evaluation of present and potential hazards to the population from different sources of radiation is based on accepted international standards and norms; these are enforced by national systems of surveillance of global and local radioactive inspection, and for the control of the emissions from consumer goods, industrial and medical sources of radiation, nuclear installations, etc. The development of international standards plays an important part in this process by providing guidelines for the creation of national legislation and the organization of radiation protection.

International evaluations of the results of surveys and measurements, together with assessments of the risks arising from any increase in the level of radiation and radioactivity, are made by the United Nations Scientific Committee on the Effects of Atomic Radiation (UNSCEAR), which requests and collects information obtained by the national monitoring programmes of different countries. Reports on the world-wide level of environmental radioactivity and the risk to populations are published every two or three years (United Nations Scientific Committee on the Effects of Atomic Radiation, 1969b).

UNSCEAR was created by the United Nations in response to worldwide concern for radioactive fallout from nuclear tests, but its task has from the beginning involved assessing the risk to populations from all sources of radiation, including medical and industrial equipment.

A common problem in the evaluation of the data obtained from national monitoring systems is their incomparability, a difficulty caused by the use of different methods of measurement and of interpreting results. To overcome this difficulty, programmes of intercomparison measurements of environmental samples in different countries have been initiated by the International Atomic Energy Agency and WHO. At the request of UNSCEAR, WHO has developed a programme for the measurement of ^{90}Sr in bones obtained from 12 tropical countries (US Atomic Energy Commission, 1971). Measurements are made in a single central laboratory, and additional information for UNSCEAR is thus obtained on the contamination by environmental radioactivity of populations in these areas. Incomparability of results is avoided since a standard method is used in the central laboratory. The second part of this programme is designed to compare the methods of measurement in different countries by sending standard samples of bone ashes for measurement to laboratories in the countries that supplied information on ^{90}Sr in bone to UNSCEAR.

A WHO Reference Centre for Environmental Radiation has been set up to promote uniformity of measurement techniques and comparative studies of radioactivity in environmental samples in different countries.

The risk to populations cannot be evaluated by physical monitoring alone, and further research on the biological effects of low levels of radiation and radioisotopes on human beings is required. Biological studies are largely based on the evaluation of the genetic, carcinogenic and other somatic effects of radiation on populations. (For the genetic effects, see: United Nations, 1962.)

UNSCEAR continuously evaluates biological data on the effects of radiation on human beings. WHO and the International Atomic Energy Agency support these activities by collecting new information (International Atomic Energy Agency, 1969b), as well as by carrying out a limited research programme to evaluate the significance of some biological changes for the assessment of the biological effects of radiation and the risk to populations. The search for suitable biological parameters and indicators that could be used in epidemiological studies should be continued because available information on this subject is scanty (International Atomic Energy Agency, 1971b).

One of the most promising methods in this field is the study of chromosome aberration rates in population groups exposed to different environmental factors, including radiation. Some evidence suggests that chromosome aberrations in somatic cells are significant in the development of certain late somatic effects, such as cancer and leukaemia, and possibly other manifestations of radiation damage (United Nations Scientific Committee on the Effects of Atomic Radiation, 1969b).

A relatively complete system for the international evaluation of radiation hazards to the public has thus been established. The international activities in which WHO participates at different levels are briefly as follows:

(1) *The United Nations Scientific Committee on the Effects of Atomic Radiation* (UNSCEAR) deals with the evaluation of new scientific findings on the biological effects of radiation, dose-effects relationships and the evaluation of risks for the population from all sources of radiation (United Nations Scientific Committee on the Effects of Atomic Radiation, 1969b).

(2) *The International Commission on Radiation Units and Measurements* (ICRU) is responsible for the establishment of recommendations on international systems of radiation units, dosimetry and measurements.

(3) *The International Commission on Radiological Protection* (ICRP) is responsible for the establishment of international radiation standards (maximum permissible doses and derived levels) for persons occupationally exposed to radiation and for individual members of the public. These standards, recommended by ICRP, provide the basis for national legislation and international guides and manuals (International Commission on Radiological Protection, 1966a,b, 1971).

(4) *WHO, the International Atomic Energy Agency* (IAEA), and other international organizations publish guides and manuals for the practical implementation of radiation protection norms and ICRU and ICRP recommendations (World Health Organization, 1966, 1968). The periodic collection of information on the biological and other effects of environmental radiation on man, and the discussion of the main findings at WHO/IAEA international scientific meetings, have played an important part in the creation of mutual understanding amongst scientists from different countries as a first step in the establishment, acceptance and revision of international norms and standards (World Health Organization, 1957: International Atomic Energy Agency, 1969c).

During the last few years the risk of an increase in global radioactive fallout has diminished; local monitoring of radioactivity has become more important, however, in connexion with the development of nuclear power stations, fuel processing plants and other peaceful uses of atomic energy.

The tendency towards an increase in radioactivity at the global level must be closely watched; this is particularly important in connexion with the disposal of radioactive wastes into the sea, and the peaceful use of nuclear explosions.

REFERENCES

Bureau of Radiological Health (1970) *Present federal control of health hazards from electronic product radiation and other types of ionizing radiation (as of November 1969)*, Rockville, Md.

Committee on Radiological Hazards to Patients (1960) *Second report*, London, HM Stationery Office

International Atomic Energy Agency (1969a) *Planning for the handling of radiation accidents*, Vienna (*Safety Series*, No. 32)

International Atomic Energy Agency (1969b) *Radiation-induced cancer, Proceedings of a Symposium, Athens, 29 April - 2 May, 1969*, Vienna

International Atomic Energy Agency (1969c) *Environmental contamination by radioactive materials, Proceedings of a Seminar, Vienna, 24 - 28 March 1969*, Vienna

International Atomic Energy Agency (1970) *Directory of whole-body radioactivity monitors, 1970 edition*, Vienna

International Atomic Energy Agency (1971a) *Mutual emergency assistance for radiation accidents*, 3rd ed., Vienna

International Atomic Energy Agency (1971b) *Biochemical indicators of radiation injury in man*, Vienna

International Commission on Radiological Protection (1966a) *The evaluation of risks from radiation*, London, Pergamon Press (*ICRP Publication 8*)

International Commission on Radiological Protection (1966b) *Radiation protection*, London, Pergamon Press (*ICRP Publication 9*)

International Commission on Radiological Protection (1971) *The assessment of internal contamination resulting from recurrent or prolonged uptakes*, London, Pergamon Press (*ICRP Publication* 10A)

International Commission on Radiation Units and Measurements (1971) *Radiation quantities and units*, Washington, D.C. (*ICRU Report* 19)

National Institute of Radiological Sciences (1971) *Radioactivity survey data in Japan*, Chiba (No. 32, August 1971)

Radioactivité ambiante dans les pays de la Communauté, 1970, Luxembourg, Direction Générale des Affaires Sociales, Commission des Communautés Européennes (*Bulletin trimestriel*, No. 3/70)

Radiol. Hlth Data, 1971, **12**, 52-56

Rangarajan, C., Gopalakrishnan, S., Sadasivan, S. & Chitale, P. V. (1965) *Measurements of airborne radioactive fallout in India*, Bombay, Government of India Atomic Energy Commission

United Nations (1962) *The use of vital and health statistics for genetic and radiation studies. Proceedings of the Seminar sponsored by the United Nations and the World Health Organization*, New York

United Nations Scientific Committee on the Effects of Atomic Radiation (1969b) *Report...*, New York, United Nations (Official Records of the General Assembly, Twenty-fourth Session, Supplement No. 13 (A/7613))

US Atomic Energy Commission (1971) *Fallout program, quarterly report summary, Health and Safety Laboratory*, New York

WHO Expert Committee on Radiation (1962) *Third Report. Radiation hazards in perspective*, Geneva (*Wld Hlth Org. techn. Rep. Ser.*, No. 248)

World Health Organization (1957) *Effect of radiation on human heredity*, Geneva

World Health Organization (1966) *Methods of radiochemical analysis*, Geneva

World Health Organization (1968) *Routine surveillance for radionuclides in air and water*, Geneva

Zykova, A. S., Teluškina, E. L., Rublevskij, V. P., Efremova, G. P. & Kuznecova, G. A. (1968) *Soderžanie stronci-90 i cezi-137 v nekotoryh ob"ektah vnešnei sred i v organizme ljudei v 1958-1967 gg.* [*Strontium-90 and caesium-137 content in some items of the external environment and in the human body, 1958-1967*], Moscow, (information submitted to UNSCEAR by the USSR Scientific Committee for the Utilization of Atomic Energy)

CHAPTER 20

ROLE OF EPIDEMIOLOGY AND HEALTH INDICES IN THE EVALUATION OF ENVIRONMENTAL HAZARDS

Epidemiology

Epidemiology is the systematic study of states of health in population groups and of the factors that influence them. In epidemiological research, the variables that affect health cannot be controlled as they can in experimental types of research. Epidemiological methods take them into account, however, and the population is classified with respect to the variables under study. Naturally occurring variables, such as age, time after exposure, and climate, also need to be identified and classified so that their effects on the population groups being studied can be separated or combined.

Epidemiological research can be carried out with the health and other data already available, or special studies may be undertaken in which both exposure data and health data are collected primarily for the purpose of answering some important question.

While epidemiological research in communicable or chronic diseases usually starts from a disease and looks for possible associated or causal factors, many epidemiological studies of environmental hazards start from a given exposure and look for possible health effects. Not all of these are necessarily the onset of identifiable diseases; other health effects of importance are impairments of physical or physiological capacity, production of new symptoms, aggravation of pre-existing illness, or non-specific effects on morbidity or mortality.

The types of hazard on which epidemiological studies can provide essential information include those with long-term, complex, or non-specific effects. Thus the health effects of community air pollution in the United Kingdom were not fully appreciated until epidemiological studies of excess mortality during episodes of pollution were reported. This, plus the epidemiological finding that pollution was one of the causal factors in chronic bronchitis, provided a strong basis for the Clean Air Act of 1956

(Royal College of Physicians of London, 1970) and its implementation. Similarly, in the USA, epidemiological studies provided an important justification for the control of motor vehicle exhaust (Goldsmith, 1969; Goldsmith & Cohen, 1969; US National Air Pollution Control Administration, 1970a, b; Wright, 1969).

An important and valuable feature of epidemiological research is that it can suggest the end effects of an environmental control strategy even if the mechanisms whereby these effects are produced are not known. This was true for the health benefit resulting from the control of particulate air pollution in the United Kingdom: the Royal College of Physicians reported that "the overall improvement in the cleanliness of the air—with the absence of peaks of pollution and decrease of sulfur dioxide—has been greater than was expected. This abatement in pollution has been associated with some decrease in morbidity" (Royal College of Physicians of London, 1970).

With many occupational respiratory diseases, such as pneumoconiosis (black lung disease), and the increased risk of lung cancer due to occupational exposure to radon gas (in uranium mining) or to asbestos, epidemiological research is required to indicate the nature and magnitude of the effect (Lundin et al., 1969; Selikoff et al., 1968; US Department of Health, Education, and Welfare, 1972).

Where environmental agents have prompt, irritating, or other obvious effects, epidemiological studies for the evaluation of these effects may not appear to be required or justified, but some agents that produce such effects also produce long-term or more complex effects.

A major reason for conducting epidemiological studies of the effects of environmental agents is to determine whether effects suggested by animal experimentation also occur in human populations. Active exchange of hypotheses and data between experimental research and epidemiological research increases the usefulness of both disciplines.

In general, epidemiological research is most important when it is necessary to evaluate environmental hazards that have either complex or delayed reactions, or when protection against the hazard is likely to require costly or disruptive measures (e.g., a change in patterns of fuel usage, methods of mining, or of the design of motor vehicles).

Epidemiology can also contribute, however, to environmental health monitoring ,which can make it possible to determine whether some newly introduced agent constitutes a potential health hazard or could cause any adverse effect on health. All epidemiological work depends on the recognition of differences in health status between groups differentially exposed to hazards in time or space: the most direct way of determining whether a suspected environmental factor needs to be taken seriously is therefore to examine background monitoring data for recent unfavourable trends in health in areas where the suspected factor is present.

Health Indices

In order to carry out the monitoring function mentioned in the previous section, indices of community health that can be collected systematically must be available. The indices that can be collected will depend both on the nature and extent of the organization of health services and on cultural characteristics.

Currently available mortality and morbidity statistics

Many countries publish routine mortality and morbidity statistics collected from established sources. Mortality statistics based on death registration, statistics on notifiable diseases, and hospital patient statistics, are the most widely available. For the purpose of environmental monitoring and surveillance, however, they suffer from various defects because of under-reporting, incomplete geographical coverage, unreliable diagnosis, insufficient breakdown, publication delays, etc.

In spite of their limitations, routine statistics provide data useful for the study of historical series with respect to the correlation between exposure and health hazard. Statistics on the same population group may be suitable for analysis as a time series, provided that the amount of bias and other defects remain at the same level over some period of time, as can often be assumed.

For environmental monitoring and surveillance, three criteria need to be satisfied, as follows:

(1) statistics should be compiled promptly;

(2) the breakdown should be in terms of small population groups; and

(3) the period covered by statistics should be short—i.e., they should be prepared on a daily, weekly, or monthly basis.

These criteria have often received inadequate attention in traditional data collection and processing, but it should be possible to make improvements in this regard once the need for them is appreciated by national and local authorities.

The achievement of an overall improvement in the quality of the existing source data will obviously be a long process, since these statistics form an integral part of a long-established tradition, associated with considerable organizational complexity. Mortality and morbidity statistics should therefore be supplemented by data collected from *ad hoc* inquiries on a sampling basis.

Social suitability of indices

Health and epidemiological indices that are otherwise acceptable will not be useful unless they can be applied to a substantial fraction of the population to be studied. At the present time this is true only for birth rates, death rates, and the incidence of certain communicable diseases, and then only in a very few countries.

This does not mean that all good epidemiology must be based on the study of a large fraction of a national population. For health monitoring purposes, background knowledge is needed on the health and other related characteristics of a substantial fraction of the population of any region or population sub-class that it is desired to study. Since it cannot be known in advance which region or population sub-class will be the focus of interest, data are needed for as high a proportion as possible of the population as a whole.

The collection in the near future and on a comprehensive scale of the type of data that could constitute sensitive epidemiological indicators of many of the effects, for example, of environmental pollution, seems unlikely. Such data will have to be found among the alternative indices already mentioned, and will have to be gathered either from socially organized groups (such as infants at welfare clinics, schoolchildren, expectant mothers attending antenatal clinics, or workers required to attend regularly at factory clinics) or from volunteers among the general population attending specially established health clinics.

All the sources suggested constitute selected fractions of the total population, but this in itself is not necessarily undesirable, provided that sensitive indices can be devised that are capable of detecting environmental effects and are appropriate to the population fractions represented.

It is important for the success of any monitoring programme based on such sources of health indices, however, that the groups should be as stable as possible in composition. The country in which such groups are studied must have an accepted, active, and co-operative school medical service, antenatal service, or industrial medical service. If voluntary health clinics are to be instituted, members of the public must be sufficiently motivated to attend such clinics regularly.

Some of these conditions may obtain in certain areas of intensive industrial or agricultural activity in developing countries, but they will be satisfied to any large extent only in some of the developed countries. This should not be a deterrent to the setting up of a surveillance and monitoring programme, any more than should the need to monitor selected fractions of the population. Although the pollution pattern, for example, is naturally complex in a developed country, it should be possible to disentangle its essential features. Furthermore, the chance of demonstrating otherwise unsuspected interactions between environmental factors would be greater than in a developing country.

In addition, studies carried out in such relatively heavily polluted regions as exist in some developed countries would be exceedingly useful preliminaries to the extension of surveillance and monitoring programmes to developing countries, since they would give much better guidance than is at present available for the determination of priorities in such programmes.

Utility of Health and Epidemiological Indices

Discrete indices [1] depend on the occurrence of step changes of state in individuals (alive/dead, well/ill), and indicate the terminal event in a chain that may have been affected by environmental factors at more than one point. For this reason, overall death rates or death rates for any form of chronic disease will be of value mainly for historical purposes and where it is necessary to establish long-term trends. Infant death rates and maternal mortality rates are more likely to be affected by relatively recent events, and therefore by current as well as by less recent environmental factors. Crude mortality data reported day by day, so that excess mortality can be determined by comparison with the data for previous years, will reveal the action of current lethal agents.

Continuous indices [1] measure average values of individual attributes (e.g., nutritional status), so that measurements made in a comparable manner from month to month or year to year can always be used to determine current trends. Continuous indices, in general, can be used in the same way as excess mortality.

The kinds of index available can therefore also be classified as follows:
(1) historical (indicating the operation of past influences);
(2) intermediate (affected to an indeterminate degree by past events);
(3) real time (determined mainly by recent events).

For the purposes of an early-warning system, the real time indices are of prime importance, but the intermediate and historical indices are also needed. It is through them that any long-term trend not detected by the early-warning system will be discovered. They are also essential as a means of checking the efficacy and comprehensiveness of the early-warning system.

Sensitivity and *specificity* are the most valuable properties of an epidemiological index that is to be used for early warning of possible environmental hazard. For a discrete index, the sensitivity depends on the frequency of the event taken as the basis of the index. For instance, primary liver cancer has a frequency of one per 100 000 per annum in the USA. The smallest group in which it could be established that a doubling of this frequency was not due to chance has been estimated to be 6 000 000 people. If one wished to detect a 25 % increase, a population of about 60 000 000 would have to be considered, and it is extremely unlikely that such a large population would be subjected even approximately uniformly to a new environmental hazard. In contrast, in many countries, death rates are in the region of one per 100 per annum. The corresponding minimum size of population necessary to establish that a 25 % increase was not a matter

---

[1] These indices also incorporate stochastic (chance or random) events.

of chance would be about 10 000. It follows that events likely to occur in a population with a frequency not much less than 1 % per annum should be chosen for this sort of index.

For indices based on continuously variable parameters, however, sensitivity depends on something that cannot be determined before measurements have been made, namely the extent of spread of individual values around the average. The greater the normal spread of these values, the larger the population needed to be confident that a change of average value is not a matter of chance.

The following health and epidemiological data would be valuable for an environmental health monitoring system providing verifiable early warning of environmental health hazards:

Real time indices and data

Indices of physiological status: height, weight, strength, reaction time, blood chemistry, karyotype, and chromosomal abnormalities.

Broad demographic data: short-term data on mortality rates, and all available specific morbidity rates, including those for communicable diseases and respiratory and nervous disorders.

Accidents, poisonings: comprehensive data on a short-term basis on casualty admissions to clinics and hospitals, and on deaths due to accident.

Intermediate indices and data

Complications of pregnancy, childbirth and the puerperium, and infancy: antenatal, perinatal, infant, and maternal mortality rates, and rates for congenital abnormalities and aberrations.

Historical indices and data

Cause-specific mortality and (where possible) morbidity rates under the following headings:
(a) neoplasms: particularly of lungs, stomach, liver, bladder, and bone marrow (leukaemias);
(b) neurological, mental, and behavioural disorders, including alcoholism and drug dependence;
(c) circulatory disorders, particularly ischaemic heart disease, arteriosclerosis, and pulmonary hypertension;
(d) respiratory diseases, particularly asthma, bronchitis, emphysema, and pneumonia;
(e) diseases of the digestive system, particularly cirrhosis of the liver;
(f) renal diseases, particularly nephritis and nephrosis.

The following chapters contain a discussion of some of the special indices mentioned above; these are being developed further for incorporation into the first stage of a WHO environmental health surveillance and monitoring system, some of whose ongoing operations are also described.

REFERENCES

Goldsmith, J. R. (1969) *J. Air Pollut. Control Ass.*, **19**, 714-719

Goldsmith, J. R. & Cohen, S. I. (1969) *J. Air Pollut. Control Ass.*, **19**, 704-713

Lundin, F. E., Jr, Lloyd, J. W., Smith, E. M., Archer, V. E. & Holaday, D. A. (1969) *Hlth Phys.*, **16**, 571-578

Royal College of Physicians of London (1970) *Air pollution and health: A report for the Royal College of Physicians of London*, London, Pitman

Selikoff, I. J., Hammond, E. C. & Churg, J. (1968) *J. Amer. med. Ass.*, **204**, 106-112

US Department of Health, Education, and Welfare (1972) *The health consequences of smoking: A report to the Surgeon-General: 1971*, Washington, D.C. (*Publication* No. (HSM) 71-7513)

US National Air Pollution Control Administration (1970a) *Air quality criteria for carbon monoxide*, Washington, D.C. (*Publication* No. AP-62)

US National Air Pollution Control Administration (1970b) *Air quality criteria for photochemical oxidants*, Washington, D.C. (*Publication* No. AP-63)

Wright, G. W. (1969) *J. Air Pollut. Control Ass.*, **19**, 714-719

CHAPTER 21

COMMUNICABLE DISEASES

Physical environmental components play major roles in almost all parasitic diseases, as well as in tuberculosis, infectious hepatitis, rabies, trachoma, bacterial meningitis, and many other communicable diseases. The modification of the physical environment by a single undertaking, such as the construction of a dam, can affect the flora and fauna of large geographical areas with a resultant profound impact on vector-borne diseases, such as malaria, schistosomiasis, and onchocerciasis. Conversely, fluctuations in a single disease, such as syphilis, reflect a complex of many psychosocial elements. Hence surveillance and monitoring of communicable diseases is an indispensable part of any early-warning system with regard to environmental hazards to human health.

The World Health Organization is charged with the major responsibility for international surveillance of communicable diseases. WHO has access to a large amount of information from Member States, provided partly by national health authorities in accordance with formal agreements, and partly on a voluntary basis. The Organization attempts to consolidate all relevant information and to disseminate it by appropriate means through its headquarters and regional offices. Networks of WHO reference centres and collaborating laboratories in all parts of the world for viral, bacterial, and parasitic diseases play a crucial role in international surveillance of these diseases.

The International Health Regulations constitute a formal international agreement to which most Member States of WHO are bound without reservation. They stipulate that each health administration shall notify the Organization of the occurrence of diseases subject to the Regulations (plague, cholera, yellow fever, and smallpox). Even individual cases of these diseases must be reported to the Organization by the speediest possible means.

Another group of diseases subject to international surveillance comprises viral influenza, paralytic poliomyelitis, louse-borne typhus, relapsing fever, and malaria. The obligation of Member States to report these diseases to WHO is governed by World Health Assembly resolutions, but only outbreaks have to be reported.

WHO is currently publishing in the *Weekly Epidemiological Record* a series of technical guides on systems of surveillance for specific diseases. The guides issued so far cover influenza, poliomyelitis, louse-borne typhus, malaria, cholera, yellow fever, and African trypanosomiasis. [1]

In addition to these formally established means of international surveillance, a number of more or less informal sources of information are available to the Organization. These include the network of WHO-sponsored reference and collaboratoring laboratories mentioned above, and three WHO serum reference banks, which contain collections of freeze-dried human sera of different population groups taken at various time intervals. Such sera can be used for studies of changing patterns of communicable and other diseases. WHO-assisted projects, in particular those aimed at strengthening national health services and those related to epidemiology and health laboratory services, provide a large amount of current information. Morbidity and mortality statistics, despite their deficiencies, are valuable for the study of long-term trends in major communicable diseases. Many other sources of information are available, e.g., WHO consultants, personal contacts with key personnel in the national health administrations, diplomatic channels, and the mass media (newspapers, radio, and television).

Present activities in surveillance and monitoring for *Salmonella* provide an illustration of the usefulness of such procedures as sources of information that can identify environmental factors as possible health hazards.

Salmonella, a common cause of food poisoning, is a pathogen for both man and lower animals, and poses an international problem because of the large volume of international trade in food products, animals, and animal feeds, a considerable proportion of which is contaminated. In addition, the host-adapted human strains (*S. typhi* and *S. paratyphi, A, B,* and *C*) play a role in international travel. As a first phase in a global programme, WHO is co-ordinating surveillance activities for *Salmonella* in co-operation with some European countries that are participating on a voluntary basis.

An international programme in surveillance of communicable diseases, including salmonellosis, always entails certain difficulties over and above those encountered in national surveillance, e.g., owing to differences between countries in the methodology applied in the laboratory, the varying geographical coverage within each country, and the intensity of field investigations. Another obstacle is the scarcity of epidemiological information that can be related to laboratory findings, and this, in turn, makes the evaluation of the reported data very difficult.

Regular examinations for contamination with *Salmonella* of food, food products, animal feeds, surface water, and sewage are practised by some countries in Europe. The extent of environmental contamination, how-

---

[1] Reprints are available on request from Epidemiological Surveillance of Communicable Diseases, WHO, 1211 Geneva 27, Switzerland.

ever, is difficult to assess on a comparative international basis because of the differences between countries in priorities given to individual items selected for examination, and the lack of comparable sampling procedures for any one item.

Examination of sewage, not surprisingly, seems to provide a good indication of the commonest *Salmonella* serotypes afflicting man in a particular region or country, and is used for this purpose in Austria, the Federal Republic of Germany, Romania, and Finland. Samples from abattoir meat, bone meal, sausages, and animal feeds are also indicative of human infections in a particular country (*Wkly epidem. Rec.*, 1971).

Although contamination of the environment with *Salmonella* constitutes a health hazard to man, the extent of the problem cannot readily be ascertained, partly because of the unsystematic and often biased sampling methods used. The need for the introduction of common practices in the monitoring of the environment is evident. Furthermore, the results of the monitoring of raw materials for food preparation must be evaluated in relation to the great variety of methods of food processing used, such as heat treatment, and the storage of food products before consumption.

It is clear from this account that data obtained from the surveillance and monitoring of communicable diseases, while in themselves of great value as indicators of environmental hazards, must be integrated with data derived from other sources, notably those reflecting environmental factors and other changes in health status. As experience and data accumulate and are subjected to integration and analysis, correlations and interrelationships between environmental factors and disease should emerge, thus facilitating the short-term and long-term predictions that are very much needed.

REFERENCE

Wkly epidem. Rec., 1971, **46**, 437-445

CHAPTER 22

INDICES OF NUTRITIONAL STATUS

Improper and insufficient nutrition still contributes to disease, disability, and death in a high proportion of the world's population. Poor nutrition is a major factor in ill health, especially in the developing countries (World Health Organization, 1963), and reflects environmental influences such as availability of food, cultural practices, and economic level. It is estimated that possibly 3 % of pre-school children in developing countries suffer from severe protein-calorie malnutrition (PCM) and 40 % have moderate signs of malnutrition.

The possible antecedents to malnutrition and its sequelae are numerous and often complex. In general, they include, in various combinations, imbalances between a population and its food supply, improper selection or preparation of foodstuffs, and inadequate means with which to purchase available foods. The nutritional status of a population is therefore the product of several concurrently operating "sub-systems", such as health, education, economics, agriculture, and meteorology. The health component reflects the relative contribution that poor nutrition makes in lowering the health status of the community, but it is clear that this information is inadequate for the formulation of an optimum corrective strategy because the level of poverty and lack of resources are not under the control of the health sector.

The main available indices of nutritional status, in order of usefulness and practicality, are age-specific mortality rates, disease-specific mortality rates, anthropometric measurements, morbidity, selected clinical signs, and laboratory measurements (Jelliffe, 1966).

Infant Mortality Rate, 1–4-year Mortality Rate

The high frequency of malnutrition as soon as breast milk is no longer adequate as the sole source of food, combined with the synergism of this malnutrition with the infections to which the child is heavily exposed, make the postneonatal and infant mortality rate (2–12-month mortality rate) and second-year death rate the most direct reflectors of nutritional status in this vulnerable age group. However, both these indices are difficult to determine, so that it is generally necessary, in practice, to use the infant mortality rate and 1–4-year mortality rate, since these are the most readily available in national records (Scrimshaw, 1964; Jelliffe, 1966).

Neonatal mortality is less directly involved with nutritional status than mortality during the remainder of the first year, and the influence of malnutrition becomes gradually less after the third year of life. Thus it has been estimated that 15 % of the world's population lives in areas having infant mortality rates (IMR) of between 15 and 30 per 1000 live births, with another 7 % in areas having an IMR of about 40. For the rest, IMRs vary between 60 and 150 or more, and 50 % of all deaths are in children less than 5 years old (cited in World Health Organization, 1963). The IMR in prosperous countries, as compared with those less well developed economically, may thus be lower by a factor of as much as 10. In contrast, 1–4-year mortality rates for these same countries may differ by a factor of 30–40 or more (DeMaeyer & Bengoa, 1971). For example, in 1966, the mortality rate (per 1000) of 1–4-year-olds was 0.7 in Sweden, 17 in Ecuador, and 29.5 in Guatemala. Many authors (see, for example, Gordon et al., 1967 and Ascoli et al., 1967) cite evidence to show that the wider gap between 1–4-year mortality rates in the developed countries and the developing countries, as compared with the differences between infant mortality rates for these same areas, is due to combined nutritional, infective and, in some societies, psychological stress in the older age group.

Disease-specific Mortality

Except where modified by immunization programmes, disease-specific mortality rates for the common communicable diseases of childhood are good practical measures of the effect of malnutrition on resistance to these infections. Chickenpox and measles are examples of diseases to which children are almost universally exposed. Measles, in particular, is an easily recognized disease, often with a specific local name, facilitating field surveys or searches of hospital records. In 1966, the fatality rate from measles in Guatemala was 66.6 per 100 000 inhabitants as compared with 0.1 in the USA (Pan American Health Organization, 1970). In fact, in Central and West Africa, measles fatality rates are so high (10–15 % of hospitalized cases) that the disease ranks second only to malaria as a cause of death in children (Millar, 1970). There is little evidence, however, of any variation in the virulence of the measles virus, so that nutritional state must be largely responsible for such case-mortality differences.

Anthropometric Measurements

Differences in nutrition in a child population are manifested in corresponding differences in growth rates, so that improvements in nutritional status are accompanied by increased growth. Standards drawn from lower socio-economic groups in developing countries are inadequate in that the groups themselves are usually undernourished and not in the optimum state of health (Dean & Jelliffe, 1960). It has therefore been suggested that children of the educated, prosperous élite in a community, excluding those with serious illness or congenital anomalies, should be used as the standard.

In many cases local standards will be impossible to obtain, and general standards, based on measurements on well-nourished Caucasians in the USA and western Europe, can then be used. Ford (1964) has shown that well-nourished children of different genetic backgrounds conform to these standards very closely, and has found them useful in assessing malnutrition.

The most common anthropometric measurement is that of weight. In the early pre-school years, weight-for-age compared with a standard weight is a convenient measure; protein-calorie malnutrition results in weight deficiencies in all age groups. Weight-for-height compared with standard height at any age indicates the degree of fatness or leanness. In both cases the Baldwin-Wood (1923) standards may be used. Bengoa (1972) has proposed height at age 7, the usual age of school entry in developing countries, as a good indicator of the cumulative effects of malnutrition and infection in the preceding years. It is a good basis for comparing the relative nutritional status of pre-school child populations. Head circumference is also reduced by early malnutrition, and can therefore be used as a nutritional index (Stock & Smythe, 1968).

Morbidity

A number of recent studies have indicated that overall morbidity, morbidity from diarrhoeal disease, and morbidity from respiratory disease are also sensitive indicators of changes in nutritional status among pre-school children (Scrimshaw et al., 1968; Gordon et al., 1968). The difficulty lies in the fact that the data must be specially and properly collected through weekly or bi-weekly contacts with the family by a trained and supervised observer; this makes the use of such indicators impracticable for most purposes.

Selected Clinical Signs

Physical examination for nutritional status is almost useless because of the non-specificity and subjective nature of most of the signs. In the special case where a specific nutritional disease is known to be present in a population, a rapid clinical survey to detect a particular sign associated with the disease may give a rough indication of its prevalence. Age must be taken into account, since clinical signs caused by specific nutrient lacks may differ in different age groups.

Some typical examples are:

(1) presence of oedema in pre-school children as an indicator of protein-calorie malnutrition of the kwashiorkor type;

(2) absence of knee or ankle reflexes as an indicator of beri-beri;

(3) palpation and classification of the size of the thyroid gland as an indicator of endemic goitre;

(4) inspection of the skin of the arms and neck for the dermatosis of pellagra.

Unless there is good evidence that the disease already exists to a significant extent in the population, however, such methods of ascertainment are likely to be inefficient and uninformative.

Laboratory Measurements

The general requirement of easy collection of data limits the use of laboratory tests for large-scale surveys, particularly in rural areas.

Nutritional anaemias involving iron, folic acid, and vitamin B_{12} can be estimated by determination of haemoglobin or haematocrit, while the specific identification of iron deficiency anaemia can be effected either by direct examination of smears, determination of the mean cell volume, or measurement of the serum iron or iron binding capacity.

The use of urine or serum vitamin levels is sometimes helpful in estimating the likelihood or relative degree of risk in a population, but is not sufficient to indicate the frequency of clinical deficiency.

REFERENCES

Ascoli, W., Guzman, M. A., Scrimshaw, N. S. & Gordon, J. E. (1967) *Arch. environm. Hlth*, **15**, 439

Baldwin, B. T. & Wood, T. D. (1923) *Mother and Child*, July 23rd, Supplement

Bengoa, J. M. (1972) *Significance of malnutrition and priorities for its prevention.* In: *Proceedings of an International Conference on Nutrition, National Development and Planning, Cambridge, Massachusetts, 19-21 October 1971*, Cambridge, Mass., M.I.T. Press (in press)

Dean, R. F. A. & Jelliffe, D. B. (1960) *Courrier*, **10**, 249

DeMaeyer, E. M. & Bengoa, J. M. (1971) *Mortality and morbidity in nutritional disorders.* In: *Proceedings of an International Conference on Amino Acid Fortification of Protein Foods, Cambridge, Massachusetts, 16-18 September 1969*, Cambridge, Mass., M.I.T. Press

Ford, F. J. (1964) *J. trop. Pediat.*, **10**, 47

Gordon, J. E., Wyon, J. B. & Ascoli, W. (1967) *Amer. J. med. Sci.*, **254**, 357

Gordon, J. E., Ascoli, W., Mata, L. J., Guzman, M. A. & Scrimshaw, N. S. (1968) *Arch. environm. Hlth*, **16**, 424

Jelliffe, D. B. (1966) *The assessment of the nutritional status of the community*, Genève, World Health Organization (*Monograph Series*, No. 53)

Millar, J. D. (1970) *Seminar on smallpox eradication and measles control*, Washington, US Public Health Service (*SEP Report* Vol. IV, No. 2)

Pan American Health Organization (1970) *Health conditions in the Americas, 1965-1968*, Washington, (*Scientific publication* No. 207)

Scrimshaw, N. S. (1964) *Amer. J. clin. Nutr.*, **14**, 112

Scrimshaw, N. S., Guzman, M. A., Flores, M. & Gordon, J. E. (1968) *Arch. environm. Hlth*, **16**, 223

Stock, M. B. & Smythe, P. M. (1968) *Undernutrition during infancy, and subsequent brain growth and intellectual development.* In: *Malnutrition, learning and behavior*, Cambridge, Mass., M.I.T. Press, pp. 278-289

World Health Organization (1963) *Malnutrition and disease*, Geneva (*Freedom From Hunger Campaign Basic Study* No. 12)

CHAPTER 23

INDICES OF DISEASE VECTORS

A vector is capable of transmitting disease among human populations only if it is present in sufficient numbers. It is therefore possible, for certain diseases, to work out indices that can be used both to give warning of an impending disease outbreak and to assess the effectiveness of the various control methods available.

This approach was first adopted in the case of malaria. It was reported by Russell & Rao (1942), for example, that in a highly malarious area of India more than 15 *Anopheles* vectors could be collected per man-hour of effort in houses in this area during the four months of the main transmission season. The corresponding value of this index in a neighbouring non-malarious area was always less than 15. Similarly, the larval population of the non-malarious locality never exceeded 1 per man-hour of collecting, while that for the malarious locality always exceeded 2 per man-hour.

A world-wide malaria eradication programme was inaugurated in 1956 with the aim of interrupting the transmission of the disease by using residual insecticides to reduce the vector population. The index used in assessing the effectiveness of these insecticides is the number of bites per man per night. A residual insecticide for use in malaria eradication should be capable of reducing the mosquito population to such an extent that, for a number of months after its application, the value of this index does not exceed unity. The persistence of the insecticide is also important; this is expressed in terms of the bio-assay mortality (WHO Expert Committee on Insecticides, 1970), which should not fall to less than 70 % during the post-application period.

Whereas malaria is essentially a problem of country villages, Bancroftian filariasis is a problem of rapidly-growing towns and cities of the tropics. Here, plentiful supplies of standing water heavily polluted with human wastes provide a breeding ground for large numbers of the tropical house mosquito, *Culex pipiens fatigans*, the vector of the filarian *Wuchereria bancrofti*. In populated centres where filariasis has become endemic, about 0.1 % of these mosquitos carry the infectious microfilariae. In Rangoon, Burma, where transmission rates are particularly high just after the monsoon, it was found (de Meillon et al., 1967) that the biting rates of this *Culex* at sunset rise to an average of 8 per man-hour indoors and

15 outdoors, from corresponding values of 2 and 5, respectively, in the immediately preceding period.   The threat of the vector to the community can be expressed by a "risk of infection" index.   This is the product of three factors: (i) the biting density (number of bites per man-hour); (ii) the proportion parous to total biting (usually about 0.5 %); and (iii) the proportion infective to total parous.

Of the many arthropod-borne viruses (arboviruses) that cause human disease, the most important is that of yellow fever, endemic in tropical West Africa.   The mosquito *Aedes aegypti* is predominant as the vector of this disease because it has adapted its habits most closely to those of man, breeding in his domestic water-storage vessels and in the discarded containers and tyres around his houses.   By a systematic campaign, *Ae. aegypti* has been eradicated from most of Central and South America, and has completely disappeared from the Mediterranean area, although it persists in the Caribbean.

The following three indices have been used to measure the abundance of *Aedes aegypti*, based on the frequency with which the larvae are found: (i) the house index (percentage of houses infested); (ii) the container index (percentage of water-filled containers infested); and (iii) the Breteau index (number of *Ae. aegypti*-positive containers per 100 houses).   Of these, the Breteau index is the most useful.   From the experience gained in an epidemic of yellow fever in Senegal (Chambon et al., 1967), it can be concluded provisionally (Pichon et al., 1968) that the disease will not be transmitted if the Breteau index is less than 5, and that hazardous areas are characterized by an index of over 50.   On the average, where the Breteau index is about 50, the house index will be about 40 and the container index about 20.

As far as the virus itself is concerned, the indications are that, in epidemic areas, not more than 0.1 % of mosquitos are positive.   It follows that assessments of the virus content of "pools" of 50 or more mosquitos that consistently prove negative may not be a completely reliable indication of the absence of the virus.

Ae. aegypti is also a vector of dengue fever.   This is not a fatal disease, but was formerly an unpleasant hazard in the Mediterranean, as it still is in the Caribbean.   In south-east Asia, outbreaks of a variant of this disease, known as dengue haemorrhagic fever (DHF), have frequently reached epidemic proportions; the disease is not infrequently fatal, and is considered to be due to infection with more than one of the four known types of dengue virus.   This would not be surprising, in view of the fact that, in certain countries in the area, e.g., Thailand and the Philippines, it is common to find Breteau indices exceeding 200, house indices exceeding 75, and container indices exceeding 40.   This situation is the consequence of the habit of storing domestic water in large jars that cannot be completely emptied.

Indices for the vectors of plague concern essentially those species of fleas, among the many found on rodents, that are efficient carriers of the bacterium *Pasteurella pestis*; the most important is the oriental rat flea, *Xenopsylla cheopis*. If infection is active in an area, there is considered to be a risk of an epidemic of plague in man if the average number of *X. cheopis* per rat is greater than 1.0, or if more than 30 % of rats are infested with the flea, or if *X. cheopis* constitutes more than 25 % of the flea species on rats (Pollitzer, 1954). Rough estimates of the size of the rat population can be based on the number of rat-runs, on the amounts of droppings and gnawings, or on the amount of experimentally exposed bait that is found to have been eaten.

Prominent among vectors in houses are the triatomid bugs belonging to the genera *Triatoma*, *Panstrongylus*, and *Rhodnius*, which in South America transmit trypanosomiasis to man. In this region, therefore, their presence in any number implies a serious hazard to health. Although these bugs can live in the surrounding vegetation, their continuing presence in houses is determined mainly by the type of construction used, since crevices in the walls allow them to lurk there between their nocturnal blood-meals.

Other vectors characteristic of buildings, particularly decrepit stone houses and walls, are sandflies of the genus *Phlebotomus*, which transmit leishmaniasis to man, as well as the virus of sandfly fever. It has been found in the Mediterranean and Near East that, once malaria has been eradicated by annual DDT applications, infestation by *Phlebotomus* has recurred. The index specified on grounds of comfort, e.g., 1 bite per man-night, since sandfly bites are painful, might also be such as to ensure a level where transmission becomes very rare.

Two groups of vectors are creatures of the open air and bite by day. These are the *Glossina* tsetse-flies, which transmit trypanosomiasis, and the *Simulium* black-flies, which transmit onchocerciasis. The tsetse-flies, found only on the African continent, are primarily pests of game animals, and transmit *Trypanosoma brucei* from them to domestic livestock, thus causing nagana disease. The flies also attack man, and may transmit *T. gambiense* or *T. rhodesiense* to cause the human trypanosomiasis known as sleeping-sickness. At present, the criterion used to assess measures to protect man is the same as that used to assess measures to protect his livestock.

The *Simulium* black-flies develop their larval stage in the rapids of streams and rivers. In tropical Africa and Central America, they transmit the microfilariae of *Onchocerca volvulus* that cause onchocerciasis in man. Whereas *Simulium* can be extremely abundant in the holarctic region, with landing-rates exceeding 500 per man-hour, personal comfort is alone involved since the flies do not transmit *Onchocerca*. In the African tropics, however, an index as low as 1 per man-hour is considered not free of risk, since commonly 5–10 % of the flies carry the infection in onchocerciasis areas (Lewis, 1956). In control programmes based on insecticidal treatment of the streams, an index of 0.5 bites per man-hour is accepted as a rough criterion of success (Crosskey, 1958).

REFERENCES

Chambon, L. et al. (1967) *Bull. Wld Hlth Org.*, **36,** 113-150

Crosskey, R. W. (1958) *Bull. ent. Res.*, **49,** 715-735

de Meillon, B., Grab, B. & Sebastian, A. (1967) *Bull. Wld Hlth Org.*, **36,** 91-100

Lewis, D. J. (1956) *Ann. trop. Med. Parasit.*, **50,** 299-313

Pichon, G., Hamon, J. & Mouchet, J. (1968) *Cah. O.R.S.T.O.M. Ent. méd.*, **7,** 39-50

Pollitzer, R. (1954) *Plague*, Geneva, World Health Organization (*Monograph Series*, No. 22)

Russell, P. F. & Rao, T. R. (1942) *Amer. J. trop. Med.*, **22,** 535-538

WHO Expert Committee on Insecticides (1970) *Seventeenth report. Insecticide resistance and vector control*, Geneva (*Wld Hlth Org. techn. Rep. Ser.*, No. 443)

CHAPTER 24

CONGENITAL MALFORMATIONS, CHROMOSOME ABERRATIONS, BIOCHEMICAL PROFILES

This chapter will be devoted to a brief consideration of indicators that could provide evidence of certain adverse environmental effects on human beings in an early-warning system.

Work in these fields is now under way in several countries, but the stage has not been reached as yet where operational requirements can be fulfilled. They are mentioned here because they are examples of possible monitoring techniques that merit further research and development.

Congenital Malformations

The closer to the etiological event that teratogenesis is detected, the greater the protection of the as yet unexposed, and the greater the chance that the etiology can be discovered. For this reason, the examination of fetal wastes from spontaneous abortions has been suggested as a valuable procedure capable of revealing a large number of malformations. This is a great advantage from the statistical standpoint, since it increases both detectability and reliability. However, collection of fetal wastes from spontaneous aborters is notoriously incomplete, and heavily skewed toward the later aborters. Therapeutic abortions are less suitable, both because the rate of malformation is much lower, and because the specimens obtained in this way are usually too macerated to permit any conclusions as to developmental deviation.

The recording of major malformations in full-term infants eliminates some of these problems, although it is further removed from the etiological event. Existing systems of vital statistics permit "rough and ready" monitoring, provided that the sampling is done frequently enough (at monthly, not yearly, intervals). It has been shown that retrospective studies based on birth and still-birth records were capable of detecting the effects of the rubella epidemics of the last decade, and of the thalidomide disaster. Another example involves an unrecognized epidemic of anencephaly and spina bifida that occurred between 1920 and 1949 (MacMahon & Yen, 1971). Delivery-room logs kept by staff at two New England hospitals were examined as far back as 1832 in one instance and 1885 in the other for records of delivery of infants with neural-tube defects. While this epidemic was detected in a retrospective study, it would have been detectable within a few years of onset by very simple statistical analysis following collection of the reports. Unfortunately, detection of an event of this type does not mean that the agent or cause can be identified. No adequate explanation has been advanced for the epidemic discovered by MacMahon and Yen.

Improving and upgrading systems of registering vital events to ensure that developmental deviations are noted and the results sampled at appropriate intervals would seem to be the most practical type of monitoring system at present. This might be coupled with examination of fetal wastes in selected areas.

Minor malformations, that is, those with neither clinical nor cosmetic significance for the patient, might be used as markers for possible environmental events that alter morphogenesis. It is known that infants with multiple minor malformations have a much higher incidence of major deformity than the general population, and further that the major pathology is frequently occult abnormality of the central nervous system and cardiovascular system (Hook, 1970). The multi-factorial, non-specific origin of the minor malformations is a drawback, although this might be tolerated if these markers are used only in an alerting system. Screening can be done quickly and without disturbing the infant. It has also been claimed that the work can be done easily by semi-skilled personnel. In a pilot study, two clinically inexperienced technicians were given a two-month training period after which they were able to agree 99 % of the time on what constituted a minor anomaly in the newborns that they screened (Hook, 1970). Again, the high rate of incidence of minor malformation (palpebral folds, extra digits, etc.) allows a small increase in incidence to be detected more reliably and with a smaller sample than with major malformations, where the rate is far lower.

Chromosome Aberrations

Chromosome aberrations are microscopically visible changes in the number or structure of the chromosome set. They are only one of the possible types of damage to an organism's genetic apparatus (see Chapter 13). However, the damage they cause is so severe that the resulting cells are for the most part incompatible with the production of viable offspring, and the changes are therefore not inherited. Nevertheless, gross cytogenetic changes of this kind can be viewed as one extreme of a process that may produce lesser changes in the genetic mechanism. There appears to be a high degree of correlation between the severe, grossly visible types of damage to the genetic material and the more subtle forms of impairment

(Crowe, 1970). Consequently, it is reasonable to assume that agents that cause one type of effect probably cause others as well. Any change in the genetic material may therefore be regarded as an indication of danger.

Cytogenetic screening for chromosome aberrations can be done on the somatic or germ cells of adults, newborns, or fetuses. At the present time, the use of fetuses from spontaneous abortions appears to hold out certain advantages. Cytogenetic analyses of unselected spontaneous abortions showed that the yield of chromosome abberrations from this population was considerably higher than normal (Carr, 1971). This is an advantage in screening because base-line rates and deviations from the base-line are then more easily and more reliably detected. In addition, detection is closer to the mutagenic (or abortogenic) event, so that the likelihood of uncovering the etiology by retrospective analysis is increased. A study has been instituted to collect certain types of epidemiological data on all patients admitted to hospital with the diagnosis of abortion (Carr, 1971). All fixed material received from these cases in the pathology department is investigated; this includes embryos, fetuses, and chorionic sacs. However, there is still a good deal of uncertainty in ascertainment resulting from, e.g., the large number of undiagnosed early abortions lost in the home, as well as unknown biases caused, among other things, by a heavier contribution from habitual aborters, and possible biases in the source material (e.g., a predominance of women involved in pre-natal care programmes).

The use of cord blood from newborns or blood specimens from adults is another possibility, but the considerably lower expected yield of chromosome defects would necessitate the expenditure of an enormous number of cytogeneticist man-hours. Automated cytogenetic screening by computer may be achieved in the future but is not yet possible.

Germinal mutations are detected most reliably from the appearance of a variant human phenotype, but this is an inefficient and expensive procedure (Crowe, 1971). The emphasis on somatic mutation, therefore, has a practical basis.

Biochemical Profiles

The introduction of automated multiple channel analysers for human body fluids has stimulated interest in routine determination of biochemical profiles on a population basis as a screening test for disease states. The devices have reached the stage of development where it is now cheaper to perform a standard batch of tests (comprising 12, 15, or as many as 21 tests) than any specially selected subset of them.

The measurement of a large number of variables in this manner poses some questions, however. If a "normal" result is defined by the central 95 % of results from a large sample, then with 12 tests the chance that any particular individual will have no test result outside this range is 0.95^{12}, or

0.54; this means that 46 % of the population will have at least one abnormal test result out of twelve. With 20 tests, the chance that the results will all be "normal" falls to 36 %, and with 100 tests there is only a 0.6 % chance that a randomly selected individual from the population under consideration will have a "profile" entirely within the normal range.

From the standpoint of immediate benefit to the population at risk, the most rational procedure at the present time would be to apply only those routine screening tests that are pathognomonic for selected environmental hazards, e.g., blood lead determinations. Careful selection of a few such tests chosen for their pertinence to prevalent disease states is likely to be the most efficient procedure.

For the purposes of monitoring and surveillance of new or undetected environmental hazards, longitudinal and cross-sectional studies of certain sub-populations might be considered. Occupational groups, groups living in certain geographical areas (e.g., residents of industrial or rural areas), or certain age categories (e.g., the elderly or young adults) might be used as the basis for detecting certain trends or differences in particular variables. This is not the same procedure as screening individuals *per se*. What is being studied here is the occurrence of abnormal results among a number of individuals rather than in a single individual. With respect to the latter, new criteria of "normality" are necessary. This would involve the use of a specially selected and fixed set of tests, capable of being automated, about which joint-probability distributions could be determined. No such data exist at present, although the technological means to initiate such a scheme are available.

Automated techniques have also been suggested as a means of carrying out systematic surveillance for possible genetic effects. Again there are problems. Although it is possible to determine quantitative differences in body chemistry, their genetic correlates are difficult to pinpoint. In most cases, the degree of quantitative variance that is indicative of a qualitative change is unknown. There are a few exceptions as, for example, when a particular entity is completely absent. Here the quantitative change indicates a qualitative change. Thus in the genetic disorder phenylketonuria (PKU), the enzyme phenylalanine hydroxylase, normally synthesized in the liver, is absent. This metabolic defect entails a number of clinical signs and symptoms in newborns suffering from it, one of which is mental retardation. Low blood tyrosine levels or the presence of phenylpyruvic acid in the blood or urine are considered good indications of PKU, although false negatives and false positives do occur. The pros and cons of screening for PKU have been widely discussed (Bessman & Swazey, 1971), but the example illustrates that it is at least possible to envisage automated testing as an alerting system for an increase in particular genetic events.

In this connexion, it has been remarked that the ideal system would detect variations in protein synthesis, since this is "close to the gene". For example, the determination of amino-acid sequences in human proteins such as a haemoglobin might be a way to detect increasing incidences of "point mutations." Unfortunately, electrophoresis, although feasible as far as automation is concerned, is not sensitive enough in this regard and no other suitable automated techniques for this purpose exist at present.

The great importance of the monitoring of biochemical profiles is that it should be capable of detecting the trivial departures from health that occur much more frequently than specifically diagnosed disease. This is precisely what is required by a monitoring system, namely, indicators that make their appearance frequently and early: frequently, because the index is then sensitive, so that significant changes can be detected without the use of prohibitively large numbers of test subjects; and early, for the obvious reason that a good monitoring system must be an early-warning system.

REFERENCES

Bessman, S. & Swazey, J. (1971) *PKU: a study of biomedical legislation.* In: Mendelsohn, E., Swazey, J. & Taviss, I., ed., *Human aspects of biomedical innovation,* Cambridge, Mass., Harvard University Press

Carr, D. H. (1971) *Fed. Proc.,* **30,** 102-103

Crowe, J. (1971)   In: Hollaender, A., ed., *Chemical mutagens, principles and methods for their detection,* New York, Plenum Press

Hook, (1970) *Proceedings of the Albany Conference on Monitoring for Birth Defects, October 1970*

MacMahon, B. & Yen, S. (1971) *Lancet,* **1,** 31-33

CHAPTER 25

ADVERSE REACTIONS TO DRUGS

Pharmacologists and toxicologists accumulate a large amount of information on drugs while these are being tested prior to marketing, but information about the clinical effects (whether beneficial or adverse) of drugs on the market is usually scarce.

The increase in number and potency of new therapeutic preparations has been followed in recent years by several tragic episodes that indicated clearly the inadequacy of existing test procedures and knowledge of drug metabolism. The long period of time that elapsed before it was recognized that certain undesired effects had occurred shows how difficult it was to relate them to the administration of a specific drug.

In general, unless a given effect has a high incidence or unless special observation procedures are set up to look for it, its stochastic distribution over large segments of the population is such that it will pass unnoticed by both individual practitioners and hospital doctors. Many retrospective studies have shown the extent and complexity of adverse drug reactions and the difficulty of detecting them. This is illustrated by the examples given below.

The thalidomide episode is an example of an unexpected effect of a drug that affected populations in different countries. An unusual syndrome (phocomelia), previously of extreme rarity, was repeatedly observed in various university paediatric clinics from 1959 onwards; within three years numerous cases had been noticed, typical cumulative incidence figures (Taussig, 1962) being as follows:

	1949-1958	1959-1961
Bonn	0	71
Munich	3	60
Liverpool	0	33

In a study of 46 mothers delivered of deformed babies, it was established with certainty that 41 had taken thalidomide in early pregnancy, while in a control series of 300 mothers delivered of normal babies, none had taken thalidomide (Wade, 1970). Experiments with animals confirmed that thalidomide was teratogenic and if given in early pregnancy might cause limit abnormalities of the fetus (Mellin & Katzenstein, 1962).

Another example of an adverse drug reaction is the induction of small-bowel stenosis by enteric-coated tablets of potassium chloride (Baker et al., 1964). The attention of the authors was arrested by the fact that, up to June 1963, there was no record of the disease in their hospital, while during the following period of 15 months 11 cases were recorded.

The problems produced by the adverse effects of drugs that are self-administered and available without medical prescription are well demonstrated by the occurrence in Japan of several thousand cases of sub-acute myelo-optico-neuropathy (SMON) associated with various preparations containing clioquinol (Kono, 1971).

Inman & Adelstein (1969) made a retrospective study of the number of deaths that occurred in England and Wales between 1959 and 1969 following treatment of bronchial asthma by means of sympathomimetic amines in aerosol form. This study involved about 3500 deaths, but the phenomenon had previously been detected by McManis (1964), who observed only 3 unexpected deaths. The effect of the drug was thus rediscovered in the United Kingdom, where it took between two to three years to make a definite assessment.

Certain adverse effects of drugs, such as photosensitivity, have been shown to be linked to environmental factors. Another example is provided by the use of monoamine oxidase inhibitors in the treatment of depression. If cheese is eaten by patients taking these drugs, hypertensive attacks are induced that, in a number of cases, have resulted in cardiac failures and intracerebral haemorrhage (Blackwell et al., 1967).

In all these cases, an "unusual" or "rare" event (i.e., one seen as such by some individual doctor) prompted an inquiry that ended in the demonstration of the existence of an adverse drug reaction. Such events, however, like many health hazards due to environmental factors, have to occur in rather large numbers in order to be considered significant. In general, the medical profession has no way of integrating an increasing number of individual "feelings of surprise" originating from practitioners who do not communicate among themselves. Thus, in all the cases mentioned above the discovery of the adverse effect took several years, during which time the drug concerned caused serious damage to health.

Drug monitoring and surveillance systems provide a partial solution to this problem (WHO Meeting on International Drug Monitoring: The Role of National Centres, 1972). They are based on information consistently and systematically collected and evaluated at various levels of statistical significance (e.g., for hospital patients, or national or international populations). These systems are able to accumulate evidence pointing to a change in the incidence of a new health event.

Following the thalidomide experience, national drug monitoring systems were established in a number of countries, and in recognition of the need for the surveillance of large populations the World Health Assembly in

1966 undertook the establishment of an international system for monitoring adverse reactions to drugs (Royall, 1971).

The WHO drug monitoring system, now located in Geneva, Switzerland, receives each month approximately 1500 reports of suspected adverse reactions to drugs from national collecting centres in twelve countries. Up to the end of 1971, a total of 49 825 reports had been received, of which 30 557 were selected for entry into the computer files. These reports cover 5577 different drug names representing 1926 different active therapeutic substances. Surveys are periodically carried out to determine the rate of increase in reporting, and special searches in the files can be made immediately on request.

The various trends that constitute the main output of the present monitoring system raise many delicate problems of interpretation. It was the aim of the Organization to study the methods by which all Member States could be provided with relevant information that might be derived from data accumulated in the project. In this regard, the partially unevaluated character of the reports collected as a result of the efforts of national centres presented initial problems of interpretation and use. In almost every instance, the information did not normally lead to definitive conclusions until verification studies had been carried out. Detailed medical, pharmacological, and epidemiological studies were necessary to confirm and scientifically demonstrate a cause-and-effect relationship between a drug and an adverse effect (WHO Meeting on the Role of the Hospital in International Drug Monitoring, 1969).

For example, a sudden observed increase in the number of reports of a given reaction may have a variety of causes, as follows:

(1) an increase in the level of reporting. The incidence of the effect may not vary, but the medical profession, warned of a possible effect, pays more attention to it, e.g., an increase from 150 to 800 reports a month is mentioned by Doll (1969) after a letter of warning was sent to the British medical profession;

(2) an increase in the use of a drug. In order to eliminate this factor, figures for drug consumption are necessary;

(3) genetic factors. Drugs may affect in different ways patients with different genetic backgrounds (Jick et al., 1969);

(4) environmental factors, such as alcohol, tobacco, nutrition, climate, occupation, household hazards, industrial hazards, and cultural practices.

To be of use in drug monitoring, certain vital statistics need to be improved in various ways, e.g., they need be made available more frequently and without delay, and the information integrated with previous data. This is now possible by the use of computer technology. A retrospective study of the effect of the sympathomimetic bronchodilators on asthmatics showed that the increase in the number of deaths from asthma could have been observed after 6 months, instead of 3 years, the delay being mainly due to defects in the health statistics system.

The WHO drug monitoring system is an example of the application of computer technology to a classical field resulting in further extensions of the methods previously used. The same type of system, with the same international procedures and the same technology, can be used for the monitoring and surveillance of many other health hazards. The data derived from drug monitoring systems provide useful information needed by an early-warning system for environmental hazards to human health.

REFERENCES

Baker, D. R., Schrader, W. H. & Hitchcock, C. R., (1964) *J. Amer. med. Ass.*, **190**, 586

Blackwell, B., Marley, E., Price, J. & Taylor, D. (1967) *Brit. J. Psychiat.*, **113**, 349

Doll, R. (1969) *Brit. med. J.*, **2**, 69-76

Jick, H. et al. (1969) *Lancet*, **1**, 539

Kono, R. (1971) *Jap. J. med. Sci. Biol.*, **24**, 195-215

Inman, W. H. W. & Adelstein, A. M. (1969) *Lancet*, **2**, 279-285

McManis, A. G. (1964) *Med. J. Aust.*, **2**, 76

Mellin, G. W. & Katzenstein, M. (1962) *New Engl. J. Med.*, **267**, 1184

Royall, B. W. (1971) *Biometrics*, **27**, 689-698

Taussig, H. B. (1962) *J. Amer. med. Ass.*, **180**, 1106-1114

Wade, O. L. (1970) *Adverse reactions to drugs*, London, Heinemann

WHO Meeting on International Drug Monitoring: The Role of National Centres (1972) *Report*, Geneva (*Wld Hlth Org. techn. Rep. Ser.*, No. 498)

WHO Meeting on the Role of the Hospital in International Drug Monitoring (1969) *Report*, Geneva (*Wld Hlth Org. techn. Rep. Ser.*, No. 425)

CHAPTER 26

CANCER

Cancer monitoring may be considered as one of a number of methods for the detection of carcinogenic risks to man. It is clearly impossible to test each of the hundreds of possible carcinogenic agents in man's environment by means of separate prospective studies involving the measurement of individual exposures followed by that of cancer incidence, over a prolonged period, in those exposed. Under certain circumstances, however, the systematic operation of a cancer monitoring system could provide a feasible method for screening for carcinogens. This could be expected to lead to hypotheses that would have to be tested by other methods.

A monitoring system would require data both on exposure to specific environmental factors and on subsequent cancer incidence. The system would depend to a large extent on data collected for other purposes but retrievable at reasonable cost for use in monitoring. The inferences possible will depend on whether such data are available for individuals or only for general populations, as discussed below.

Latent Period of Cancer in Relation to Priorities for Monitoring

Unlike communicable diseases, a basic biological characteristic of most cancers is the long interval (commonly 20–40 years) between exposure to an agent and the diagnosis of cancer. Priority must therefore be given, when the introduction of cancer monitoring is being considered, to those cancers where the latent period may be relatively short. Latent periods may be shorter, for example, with cancers in children and young persons, as has been demonstrated for those due to maternal irradiation (MacMahon, 1962) and the transplacental effects of drugs, e.g., diethylstilboestrol, given during pregnancy (Herbst et al., 1971). In many cases of cancer arising from high exposures in industry, the latent period may also be relatively short (Hueper & Conway, 1964). Although this group forms only a small proportion of human cancers, the agents concerned are often more widely distributed in the environment, and hence may be associated with cancers in larger populations. Thus the demonstration of the risk to workers in shipyards from asbestos may have oncogenic significance for the population at large, which is exposed to significantly lesser amounts of this material (*Lancet*, 1968).

Linking Exposure to Environmental Factors and Cancer

A cancer monitoring system would attempt to discover associations between:

(*a*) exposure to a suspected environmental factor; and

(*b*) a change in the frequency of a specific cancer at a later date.

Exposure might be documented in special registers based on retrievable data, particularly in groups with high exposures.   An estimate of the risk of cancer in such groups might be provided by subsequent record linkage with cancer registries covering the same population.

A change in cancer frequency *per se* could lead to the investigation of previous exposure to environmental factors, although there are many difficulties with such an approach owing to the lack of easily retrievable specific data on previous exposures, e.g., on occupational history.

Exposure registration

Data on exposure to environmental factors may be available for a general population, or for individuals.   General population data may include, for example, measurements of air pollution or of the amounts of a chemical added to or present in the water supply.   Data on individual exposure may be available in routine medical records (drug dosage, radiation) and in industry (work in processes involving specific chemicals).

Exposure of general population

A major disadvantage of data representative of general populations is that it may be difficult, if not impossible, to estimate from such data the variation in individual exposure.   Thus a series of stations for monitoring atmospheric pollution may provide data from which the overall situation in a city can be assessed, but give little information on the range of individual exposures; similarly, data on the consumption of specified foods by populations is of no use in determining individual diets.   There are also considerable differences in the exposure of populations as a whole, not only between countries in different stages of industrialization, but also between the different geographical regions of a country or continent.   For example, urban-rural differences in cancer incidence are significant.

It is likely that a large number of environmental factors may be inter-related in such a way that populations with high exposure to one such factor may have a high exposure to others, thus rendering analyses very difficult. Such general population exposures may be only weakly carcinogenic, which still further increases the difficulties of evaluation.

Data on variation in the exposure of general populations might be useful in providing evidence for the absence of a carcinogenic effect. It might conceivably be shown that, despite continued differences between a number of populations in exposure to a suspected environmental factor, there were no differences in the incidence of specific cancers.

Under exceptional circumstances it may be possible to estimate the variation in individual exposure in a general population and to relate this to subsequent variation in cancer incidence. This could occur in relation to an episode of exposure to ionizing radiation, as in the case of an atomic explosion (Miller, 1969). Such events are rare and do not in themselves justify the monitoring of the exposure of general populations.

Individual exposure

The search continues for markers or stigmata of previous individual exposure; for example, the observation of DDT in fat tissue is being used as a measure of previous exposure. A distinction should be made between compounds that are rapidly metabolized and those that are slowly metabolized. Although results so far have been disappointing, the approach has been poorly explored (International Agency for Research on Cancer, 1968).

For use in a monitoring system, data on individual exposure should be recorded and retrievable. Priority should be given, as already mentioned, to exposures, such as *in utero* and industrial exposure, that give rise to cancers with shorter latent periods. The selection of environmental factors to be registered will be influenced by the cost of data retrieval, the duration of exposure, the presence or absence of interfering exposure variables, and the possibility of subsequent measurement of cancer occurrence, both in those exposed and in suitable groups of non-exposed controls.

1. *Exposure to drugs or chemicals in pregnancy*

The recent demonstration (Herbst et al., 1971) that diethylstilboestrol administered during pregnancy may result in vaginal adenocarcinoma in the offspring some 15–20 years later suggests the possibility that other tumours in the young may be due to *in utero* exposure to drugs or environmental factors (Miller, 1971a).

Data on exposure may be retrievable from three main sources. Firstly, certain centres (e.g., Northern Ireland, Livingstone New Town in Scotland) are collaborating in the WHO Drug Monitoring Programme and have computer records of the dosages of all drugs administered, including those given during pregnancy.   A number of studies of the incidence of congenital abnormalities, in which all drugs taken by a large group of pregnant women are recorded, are in progress.

Secondly, where data on exposure to all drugs are not easily retrievable, priority should be given to exposures of women to selected drugs during pregnancy.   Drugs should be selected on the basis of their suspected carcinogenic risk.   For example, in countries with a national health service, it should be possible to identify all women who have had prescriptions filled, e.g., for phenytoin,[1] and to identify the offspring of such women, either through national record linkage systems, birth registers, or hospital records.   The cost of retrieving data for such an exposure register would be considerable, and this procedure may be feasible only in certain countries.

Thirdly, it may be possible in some countries to keep registers of the offspring of women in certain industrial occupations who continued to work during part or all of a pregnancy.   The numbers thus registered might be small, so that pooling of data in international studies would be useful. Similar groups might be constituted by pregnant women exposed accidentally to poisons, e.g., parathion.

The risk of cancer in persons with recorded *in utero* exposure would be assessed by periodic record linkage with cancer registries.   The methodology would be similar to that used to study the effects on the offspring of smoking during pregnancy (Neutel & Buck, 1971).   The diagnosis of cancer in the young is likely to be more accurate, and interfering variables, such as occupational factors and smoking, may be less important in this age group.   It would also be desirable to assess cancer incidence in the mothers, since they too will have had their exposure registered.

2.   *Occupational exposure*

A knowledge of industrial processes may make it possible to identify and register persons exposed or not exposed to a potential carcinogenic agent, such as a chemical.   For example, Case et al. (1954) obtained lists of all men who had been employed in certain sections of the chemical industry.   These were divided into groups according to whether or not they were likely to have been exposed to 1- and 2-naphthylamine, benzidine, aniline, and other chemicals.   Men in these groups who had died from cancer of the bladder were found by scrutiny of death certificates.   Mortality rates for the various groups were then calculated and compared with the national mortality experience.

In monitoring industrial exposures, it is desirable to select industries in which the processes used have remained the same over fairly long periods, and workers who have not changed jobs frequently.   Owing to the specialized nature of much of modern technology, and its high productivity,

---

[1] An anticonvulsant (5,5-diphenylimidazolidin-2,4-dione).

relatively few persons may have been industrially exposed to a specific chemical in any single country. Evaluation of carcinogenic risk may then be possible only with pooled data from a number of countries, collected through an international organization such as the International Agency for Research on Cancer.

The risk of cancer would be assessed by means of record linkage between exposure registers and, preferably, cancer incidence registries. Data from cancer incidence registries are likely to provide an earlier and more sensitive indication of carcinogenic risk than mortality data. However, mortality data have been shown to be useful, and in many areas in which exposure registers could be established, cancer incidence registries do not exist.

Cancer registration

The measurement of cancer incidence by means of cancer incidence registries is an important requirement of any cancer monitoring system. Cancer mortality data are derived from death certificates and, apart from any inaccuracies in diagnoses, may seriously underestimate cancer incidence. The extent to which incidence is underestimated will vary with the type of cancer and its case fatality rate.

Cancer registries should cover the population whose exposure is registered. Although national cancer registries may be too large to ensure a uniformly high standard of registration, restriction of coverage to a limited area may weaken record linkage between exposure and cancer, as a result of internal migration.

Registries should cover countries in different stages of industrial development. Registration should be continued for prolonged periods, to permit both the identification of time trends and the evaluation of the risk to those persons included in exposure registers for whom the latent period may not be relatively short.

Changes in the incidence of certain cancers might be detected by the examination of cancer incidence registry data alone. This would be possible with unusual histological types of tumours, such as the asbestos-linked mesothelioma of the pleura. Where occupational histories are registered, it may be possible to demonstrate an association between an occupation and a specific cancer, but such histories are generally not reported in adequate detail.

Cancer registries are increasingly recording the histological type of cancer, thus making possible the more specific evaluation of possible environmental carcinogenic factors (International Union Against Cancer, 1970).

The International Agency for Research on Cancer is now receiving information from approximately 60 cancer incidence registries around the world. Seven registries, covering widely different environments, are collaborating in a pilot study of time trends and other variations in cancer incidence.

Persons with congenital abnormalities

Evidence from experiments on animals shows that certain chemicals may be teratogenic at one stage in fetal life, and carcinogenic at another, It has been shown in man that certain congenital abnormalities are associated with specific cancers (Miller, 1971b).

Discovery of an association between a cancer and a congenital abnormality might lead to the identification of exposure to a hitherto unsuspected carcinogen during pregnancy.

Registers of persons with congenital abnormalities have existed in a number of countries for many years; many of these are national registers, whereas others are limited to a particular region, or to the outcome of a series of, say, 20000 pregnancies. It would be relatively easy to measure the cancer risk in such persons in areas where incidence registries exist. In some countries it would be possible to identify only those reported as having died from cancer.

Summary

Cancer monitoring as a method for drawing attention to possible environmental carcinogens is most likely to succeed:

(1) where changes in cancer risk can be related to exposure to an environmental factor that is both variable and identifiable, particularly in relation to individuals;

(2) where data on exposure can subsequently be linked to cancer incidence data;

(3) where exposures are high, and/or where the latent period between exposure and cancer detection is relatively short;

(4) where cancer registries record tumour morphology and previous occupation;

(5) where exposure results in an unusual histological type of tumour.

The establishment of a cancer monitoring system will depend to a large extent on whether the retrieval at reasonable cost of data collected primarily for another purpose is possible.

REFERENCES

Case, R. A. M., Hosker, M. E., McDonald, D. B. & Pearson, J. T. (1954) *Brit. J. industr. Med.*, **11**, 75

Herbst, A. L., Ulfelder, H. & Poskanzer, D. C. (1971) *New Engl. J. Med.*, **284**, 878

Hueper, W. G. & Conway, W. D. (1964) *Chemical carcinogenesis and cancers*, Springfield, Ill., Thomas

International Agency for Research on Cancer (1968) *Annual report*, Lyon

International Union Against Cancer (1970) *Cancer incidence in five continents*, Vol. 2, Berlin, Springer

Lancet, 1968, **1**, 32

MacMahon, B. (1962) *J. nat. Cancer Inst.*, **28**, 1173

Miller, R. W. (1969) *Science*, **166**, 569

Miller, R. W. (1971a) *J. nat. Cancer Inst.*, **47**, 1169

Miller, R. W. (1971b) *Israel J. med. Sci.*, 7, 1461

Neutel, C. I. & Buck, C. (1971) *J. nat. Cancer Inst.*, **47**, 59

CHAPTER 27

INDICES OF MENTAL DISORDERS

There has been much controversy about what should be included in the category of mental illnesses. Many consider that normality, neurosis, and psychosis are different points on a continuum that represents degrees of severity of behaviour disturbance. Reported prevalence rates for mental disorders have shown wide variations between studies, depending on the definition of a "case". Thus, both the type and the severity of disorder included will affect the rates. Lin (1953), for example, found a prevalence rate of mental disorder of 10.8 per thousand population, the count including mental retardation, psychoneuroses, epilepsy, psychopathy, and alcoholism. On the other hand, when a much wider range of psychiatric symptoms was included, in a study in the USA, it was found that 81.5 % of the respondents had such symptoms (Srole et al., 1962).

Several studies have subdivided cases according to the severity of psychiatric impairment (Rennie et al., 1957; Leighton, A. M. et al., 1963; Leighton, D. C. et al., 1963). In one study "impairment" was considered in terms of interference with work, with family duties, and with community and wider social roles, and was divided into minimal, mild, moderate, and severe: a lifetime prevalence of 1 % of severe total impairment caused by psychiatric disorders was found in the population investigated.

There is much less variation between survey findings on rates for psychoses than on rates for total mental disorders. According to an unpublished WHO review, prepared in 1964, of 50 surveys carried out in various countries, psychosis rates of 2–20 per 1000 population were found in 46 of the surveys. However, in 4 of the surveys, psychosis rates of 28.7–80.5 per 1000 population were found, the higher rates being accounted for probably by the greater intensity of the search among the total population surveyed and the fact that, in 2 cases, lifetime prevalence was measured. In the same 50 surveys, prevalence rates for schizophrenia varied from 0.9 to 10.0 per 1000 population. Mischler & Scotch (1963), reviewing studies on schizophrenia, suggested that about 1 % of any population is likely to develop schizophrenia at some point during life.

Careful surveys indicate that 1–3 % are likely to be mentally retarded. Those classed as moderately, severely, or profoundly retarded comprise about 4 per 1000 in the age-range 10–14 years, when cases are most easily identified and studied (WHO Expert Committee on Mental Health, 1968; Gruenberg, 1964).

In recent years, the relationship between the prevalence of mental retardation and poverty has aroused considerable interest, since poor school performance may depend not only on poor intellectual capacity but also on environmental understimulation.

Rates for the prevalence of alcoholism in communities will, of course, depend on the criteria used to define a case, but Jellinek (1960) has done much to clarify these and his concepts are widely used. Liver cirrhosis is an important indicator used for measuring the prevalence of alcoholism; other, probably less reliable, indicators used in various studies are: arrests for drunkenness, deaths from alcoholism, and deaths from alcohol poisoning. Lint & Schmidt (1971) point to the value of data on alcohol consumption averages for estimating the prevalence of alcoholism.

There has also been much controversy about the reliability of reported suicide rates and their value, particularly for comparative purposes (World Health Organization, 1968). Responses to a WHO questionnaire on this topic indicate that differences in procedures may be such as to cast considerable doubt on the validity of comparisons, at least between data for different countries. However, Sainsbury (1968) studied suicide rates among immigrants in the USA and compared them with the rates in their countries of origin; he also compared the rates in different metropolitan boroughs of London (Sainsbury, 1955). He concluded that the evidence supported the view that differences in rates are due to social phenomena (see also Bagley, 1968). Changes in suicide rates among young people in Japan were related to the changing social and economic conditions (Lin, 1967). In general, a particularly high risk of suicide has been found among persons suffering from depressive disorders, alcoholics, persons who have previously attempted suicide, and the socially isolated (World Health Organization, 1968).

Rates for attempted suicide show far greater variation than those for suicide, and are no doubt much less reliable. However, data on trends in the same geographic area can be valuable for research on the effects of psychosocial changes (Kessel, 1966). Efforts are now being made to record suicide attempts nationally (Czechoslovakia, Institute for Health Statistics, 1968).

In considering the possible relationship between crime and mental morbidity, it should be realized that only a small proportion of the information collected on crime and delinquency is analysed and published. Methods and practices with regard to detection and arrest as well as notification also vary widely and affect statistics. Crime "is what the law says it is". In a review covering many countries, it was noted that a large percentage of juevnile delinquents showed no obvious signs of mental illness, but a number were labelled "constitutional psychopaths"—a term about which there is much controversy (Bovet, 1951).

Some studies of populations have shown that the rates for possible indicators of mental morbidity (such as dependence on alcohol and other drugs, suicide, attempted suicide, homicide, divorce, applications for divorce, and separation) are associated with those for criminal offences of certain types—e.g., sexual offences and drunkenness.   Relatively high rates for several of these indicators have been found in association in certain geographically defined populations as compared with others—e.g., in the centres of old cities and in socially disorganized areas, such as shanty towns. Where such high rates are found in association they are likely to be prognostic of high rates of mental disorder in the next generation (Faris & Dunham, 1939; Hare & Wing, 1970; Hollingshead & Redich, 1958).

It is apparent that there are many problems involved in measuring levels of mental morbidity.   These problems have been reviewed concisely by Reid (1960) and expanded by several authors during a symposium on the definition and measurement of mental health (Sells, 1968).

Critical reviews of epidemiological studies of mental disorders have been made by, among others, Lin & Standley (1962), [1] who point out that carefully planned and conducted longitudinal studies of mental disorder in total populations would undoubtedly provide the most useful epidemiological information, but that the cost in money and manpower would be enormous.   Many studies are limited to information concerning patients receiving psychiatric attention, and the results are inevitably affected by the level of psychiatric facilities available.

Initially such information was confined largely to data concerning persons in mental hospitals.   Although mental hospital statistics taken alone cannot be used for measuring morbidity in a population, trends in resident patient rates, combined with data on the ages of patients and their length of stay, will indicate whether the long-term patient population is being reduced, as is now possible with existing therapeutic measures. In most countries where modern mental health services have been developed, marked reductions are being noted in the numbers of long-term patients in mental hospitals, although large increases have occurred in admissions and short-term care: in the USA, for instance, total admissions to public mental hospitals rose by 52 % in the 7 years 1955–1962 (US Department of Health, Education and Welfare, 1963) and a similar increase was seen in Great Britain (Brooke, 1963).

In many countries an increasing number of mental patients are being cared for in general hospitals, partly in an attempt not to dissociate them

---

[1] See also Plunkett & Gordon, 1960; Primrose, 1962; Taylor & Chave, 1964).

from their own community. About 1 per 1000 of the total population are being treated annually for mental disorders in general hospitals in the United Kingdom and the USA (Brooke, 1960). [1]

Many mental patients are now being treated without being admitted to residential hospital care, through day hospitals and psychiatric out-patient clinics (WHO Regional Office for Europe, 1971a). Others are treated by psychiatrists in private practice.

The movement towards developing comprehensive psychiatric services geared to the needs of the community (WHO Regional Office for Europe, 1971b) is accompanied by efforts to co-ordinate the collection of statistics from the network of services. Such statistics are beginning to give a clearer picture of the extent, variety, and duration of mental disorders and their repercussions on the patient, family, and community.

In a few areas of the world, psychiatric case registers have been set up to obtain counts of all persons in a geographically defined area who receive psychiatric care (e.g., Wing et al., 1968). This material can be particularly valuable for research purposes.

Some information on psychiatric morbidity may be obtainable from statistics on sickness benefit claims in national insurance systems, hospital insurance plans, and social welfare funds (Densen et al., 1960).

As pointed out by Kramer in a chapter on data collection and analyses for programme planning and evaluation (American Public Health Association, 1962): "No health agency has developed a mechanism for the systematic collection of morbidity data on the mental disorders that can be used to provide reliable, current estimates of the total incidence, prevalence and duration of these disorders". However, in many countries data are now collected systematically on the mentally ill under care in various psychiatric facilities. Studies are being carried out on means of achieving comparability of the data collected, as in the "model reporting areas" in the USA. A publication of a "joint information service" in the USA (Kanno, 1971) sets out 11 indices as an aid in reviewing State and local mental health and hospital programmes. It brings together information on public and private psychiatric hospitals and on out-patient clinics and mental health centres. When properly collated and analysed, such data can be of great value for indicating trends in the frequency of various types of mental disorder and the possible effects of environmental factors. Examples would be the changes in the prevalence of pellagra psychosis with the advent of knowledge of the underlying cause, and changes in the chronicity of certain mental disorders following the widespread introduction of psychotropic drugs and other therapeutic measures.

Reviews have been made of applications of mental health statistics (Kramer, 1969) and of the place of psychiatric morbidity statistics in a

---

[1] Referred to also by the late President John F. Kennedy in his "Special message on mental illness and mental retardation", delivered from the White House, Washington, D.C., on 5 February 1963.

mental health information system (Brooke, in press). A WHO programme in the European Region is stimulating governments to utilize such statistics (WHO Regional Office for Europe, 1971c) and courses are being held to train staff in methods of collecting and analysing the data.

Many attempts are being made to improve the standardization of diagnostic procedures and the classification of mental disorders. Several committees have been trying to establish uniform classifications within national boundaries and a series of annual WHO seminars has been devoted to the international standardization of psychiatric diagnosis, classification, and statistics (Shepherd et al., 1968; Rutter et al., 1969; Astrup & Ødegaard, 1970). [1]

A variety of methods are being used in both the assessment of mental health and illness and the measurement of psychosocial variables. They include, *inter alia*, structured, non-structured, and guided interviews by psychiatrists and other mental health workers; psychological tests and projective techniques; questionnaires and rating scales; symptom check lists; and standardized reports and measurements of social adjustment and psychological impairment.

WHO has also embarked on a long-term programme for standardizing instruments and procedures for the assessment of mental disorders in different cultures (Lin, 1969; Sartorius et al., 1970).

It becomes apparent that satisfactory mechanisms are not yet available for the systematic collection of data on the incidence and prevalence of mental disorders: but this is true also of many physical disorders. Such mechanisms are, however, being developed and much effort is now being concentrated on establishing criteria for the classification and assessment of mental disorders and for the methodology of epidemiological studies.

REFERENCES

Amer. J. Psychiat., 1972, **128**, May Supplement, pp. 3-45

American Public Health Association (1962) *Mental disorders: a guide to control methods*, New York

Astrup, C. & Ødegaard, O. (1970) *Acta psychiat. scand.*, **46**, 180

Bagley, C. (1968) *Soc. Sci. Med.*, **2**, 1

Bovet, L. (1951) *Psychiatric aspects of juvenile delinquency*, Geneva, World Health Organization (*Monograph Series*, No. 1)

Brooke, E. M. (1960) *Eugen. Rev.*, **51**, 209

Brooke, E. M. (1963) *A cohort study of patients first admitted to mental hospitals in 1954 and 1955*, London, HM Stationary Office

Brooke, E. M. (in press) *Psychiatric morbidity statistics and their place in mental health information systems*, Geneva, World Health Organization (to be published in *Wld Hlth Stat. Rep.*)

---

[1] See also *Amer. J. Psychiat.*, 1972.

Czechoslovakia, Institute for Health Statistics (1968) [*Suicide* 1967], Prague (*Zdravotnická statistika ČSSR*, Vol. 11)

Densen, P. M., Balamuth, E. & Deardorff, N. R. (1960) *Milbank mem. Fd Quart.*, **38**, 48

Faris, R. E. L. & Dunham, H. W. (1939) *Mental disorders in urban areas: an ecological study of schizophrenia and other psychoses*, Chicago, University of Chicago Press

Gruenberg, E. M. (1964) *Epidemiology of mental retardation.* In: Stevens, H. A. & Heber, R., eds, *Mental retardation: a review of research*, Chicago, University of Chicago Press

Hare, H. E. & Wing, J. K., eds (1970) *Psychiatric epidemiology: Proceedings of the International Symposium, Aberdeen, 1969*, London, Oxford University Press

Hollingshead, A. B. & Redlich, F. C. (1958) *Social class and mental illness: a community study*, New York, Wiley

Jellinek, E. M. (1960) *The disease concept of alcoholism*, New Haven, Hillhouse Press

Kanno, C. K. (1971) *Eleven indices: an aid in reviewing state and local mental health and hospital programs*, Washington, D.C., Joint Information Service of the American Psychiatric Association and the National Association for Mental Health

Kessel, N. (1966) *J. psychosom. Res.*, **10**, 29

Kramer, M. (1969) *Applications of mental health statistics*, Geneva, World Health Organization

Leighton, A. M. et al. (1963) *Psychiatric disorder among the Yoruba*, New York, Cornell University Press

Leighton, D. C. et al. (1963) *The character of danger. The Stirling County study of psychiatric disorder and sociocultural environment*, New York & London, Basic Books

Lin, T. (1953) *Psychiatry*, **16**, 313

Lin, T. (1967) *Some epidemiological findings of suicides in youth.* In: Caplan, A. & Lebovici, S., eds, *Adolescents in a period of change*, New York, Basic Books

Lin, T. (1969) *Soc. Psychiat.*, **47**, 47

Lin, T. & Standley, C. C. (1962) *The scope of epidemiology in psychiatry*, Geneva, World Health Organization (*Publ. Hlth Pap.*, No. 16)

Lint, J. de & Schmidt, W. (1971) *Brit. J. Addict.*, **66**, 97

Mischler, E. G. & Scotch, N. A. (1963) *Psychiatry*, **26**, 315

Plunkett, R. & Gordon, J. (1960) *Epidemiology and mental illness*, New York, Basic Books

Primrose, E. J. R. (1962) *Psychological illness: a community study*, London, Tavistock

Reid, D. D. (1960) *Epidemiological methods in the study of mental disorder*, Geneva, World Health Organization (*Publ. Hlth Pap.*, No. 2)

Rennie, T. A. C. et al. (1957) *Amer. J. Psychiat.*, **133**, 831

Rutter, M. et al. (1969) *J. Child Psychol. Psychiat.*, **10**, 41

Sainsbury, P. (1955) *Suicide in London: an ecological study*, London, Chapman & Hall

Sainbury, P. (1968) *Suicide and depression.* In: Coppen, A. & Walk, A., eds, *Recent developments in affective disorders*, Ashford, Royal Medico-Psychological Association (*Brit. J. Psychiat. Special Publication*, No. 2), pp. 1-13

Sartorius, N., Brooke, E. & Lin, T. (1970) *Reliability of psychiatric assessment in international research.* In: Hare, E. & Wing, J., eds, *Psychiatric epidemiology*, London, Oxford University Press

Sells, S. B., ed. (1968) *The definition and measurement of mental health: a symposium sponsored by the National Center for Health Statistics*, Washington, D. C., US Government Printing Office (US Public Health Service Publication No. 1873)

Shepherd, M., Brooke, E.. M., Cooper, J. E. & Lin, T. (1968) *Acta psychiat. scand.*, Suppl. 201

Srole, L. et al. (1962) *Mental health in the metropolis: the Midtown Manhattan study*, New York, McGraw-Hill, Blakiston Division

Taylor, S. J. C. & Chave, S. (1964) *Mental health and environment*, London, Longmans

US Department of Health, Education and Welfare (1963) *Provisional patient movement and administrative data. Public mental hospitals. United States, 1961 and 1962*, Bethesda (Mental health statistics, current reports, Series MHB-H-7)

WHO Expert Committee on Mental Health (1968) *Fifteenth report. Organization of services for the mentally retarded*, Geneva (*Wld Hlth Org. techn. Rep. Ser.*, No. 392)

WHO Regional Office for Europe (1971a) *Trends in psychiatric care: day hospitals and units in general hospitals. Report on a symposium, Salzburg, 7-11 June 1971*, Copenhagen

WHO Regional Office for Europe (1971b) *Comprehensive psychiatric services and the community. Report on a working group, Opatija, 17-21 May 1971*, Copenhagen

WHO Regional Office for Europe (1971c) *Classification and evaluation of mental health service activities. Second interim report of a working group, Düsseldorf, 2-4 November 1970*, Copenhagen

Wing, L., Bramley, C., Haily, A. & Wing, J. K. (1968) *Soc. Psychiat.* 3, 16

World Health Organization (1968) *Prevention of suicide*, Geneva (*Publ. Hlth Pap.*, No. 35)

CHAPTER 28

OCCUPATIONAL GROUPS

Working populations provide excellent groups for epidemiological investigations aimed at uncovering effects of environmental factors on health. They constitute 25–60 % of the total population, depending on the country. Considerable numbers are concentrated in organized agricultural plantations and in mining and industrial enterprises that are reached by comprehensive occupational health programmes. These groups reflect the health and illness pattern of the total adult population of an area, and in addition they exhibit evidence of the effects of their employment. Also, occupational groups represent both sexes and different age groups and social standards. Workers in the developing countries, particularly in small enterprises, often live with their families in their workplaces, so that there may be no line of demarcation between the community and work environments.

Research in the area of occupational health has succeeded in developing sensitive criteria permitting the early detection of impaired health in certain instances. These include biological and clinical indices by which different stages of deviation from baseline "states of health" can generally be evaluated, and in many cases quantitatively measured. Examples are changes in the organic and inorganic sulfate ratio in the urine—an early indicator of absorption of benzene; enzymatic changes in blood serum resulting from exposure to different toxic substances (e.g., transaminase in the case of liver damage); changes in pulmonary expansion and forced expiratory volume following exposure to certain dusts; and early changes in higher nervous functions that can be sensitive indicators of stress situations. Some indices used in occupational medical practice can also be of value in estimates of health promotion; these include the evaluation of human efficiency and productivity at work, the calculation of sickness absenteeism, and various measurements of physical fitness.

Occupational health monitoring and standards contribute to the establishment of environmental quality standards in general, although there will obviously be differences between environmental standards used within the work environment (see Chapters 7 and 32) and those applicable to the community at large.

CHAPTER 29

DOMESTIC AND WILD ANIMALS

It is of interest to glance briefly at the potential advantages of the surveillance and monitoring of domestic and wild animals as a means of obtaining early warning of possible adverse environmental effects on man.

Farm animals can be used in this way. For example, when poison gas drifted dangerously on the wind in Utah, warning was given by mortality in sheep (Boffey, 1968). When an accident resulted in radioactive fallout in the United Kingdom in 1957, the analysis of cow's milk for radioactive iodine provided a useful measure of the contamination of the environment (United Kingdom, Atomic Energy Office, 1957).

Pet animals can also be used for this purpose. A classic example is the use in earlier days of canaries in mines and sewers as indicators of dangerous atmospheric conditions, and a more recent example is the examination of pet dogs as indicators of harmful air pollutants leading to chronic respiratory disease and cancer (Reif & Cohen, 1970, 1971).

Birds of prey have been seriously affected by DDE, a breakdown product of DDT that is even more stable than the parent compound. Their reproductive rate has fallen drastically because the shells of their eggs have become too fragile to allow them to hatch (Hickey & Anderson, 1968). When the sea becomes infested with the poisonous dinoflagellate that gives rise to the phenomenon called the "red tide", this is taken up by shellfish, which thereby become poisonous for man (McFarren et al., 1960). The shellfish also become poisonous for birds, mortality among which may give warning in time for man to avoid this hazard.

Epidemiological surveillance of domestic and wild animals can be useful in detecting carcinogens, teratogens and mutagens in the environment. Animals are of advantage for these studies in several ways. Mammals mostly live their whole life in a restricted area, and so are better indicators of localized hazards than man, who moves about and is exposed to various environments. Another advantage of animals is that, with their shorter life span, they respond to pollutants and other chemicals more quickly than man (Nielsen, 1971).

It has long been known, for example, that cattle develop bladder cancer in certain parts of the world. The cause has been found to be a carcinogen present in bracken (Pamukcu et al., 1967). The incidence of stomach cancer in man is high in some areas of the United Kingdom, and the possibility that this is due to the carcinogen that affects cattle is now being investigated.

Aflatoxin was brought into prominence by a disease in turkeys that appeared in the United Kingdom some years ago (Blount, 1961). This was traced to a particular batch of peanut meal in the feed.

During the last decade, animals have been much used in testing drugs for teratogenicity, but comparative studies of spontaneously occurring malformations have only recently been undertaken (Selby et al., 1970).

In some respects, knowledge of spontaneous birth defects is greater for animals than for man. It is not uncommon for epidemics of congenital malformations to occur in domestic animals. It is then often a straightforward matter to track down the cause to infection, intoxication, deficiency, or genetic or environmental factors.

Quite a number of viruses are known in animals that may affect the fetus without killing it. In sheep, natural infection with bluetongue virus in pregnant ewes, or vaccination with an attenuated strain, may result in congenital encephalopathy and other defects in 20 % of the lambs (Richards et al., 1971); in cats, certain parvoviruses produce cerebellar hypoplasia. Several viruses affect the fetus of pigs, cows and sheep, sometimes causing abortion or resorption of the fetus and sometimes various types of congenital abnormality, especially of the nervous system (Done, 1968; Barlow et al., 1970; Kahrs et al., 1970).

Outbreaks of congenital abnormalities sometimes occur in farm animals due to the ingestion of teratogens. Ewes grazing on pasture containing the plant *Veratrum californicum* may give birth to lambs of which as many as 15 % have brain and head deformities (Binns et al., 1963). Lupins fed to pregnant cows can produce cleft palate, arthrogryposis and other abnormalities in the fetus (Shupe et al., 1967).

Fluorosis resulting from toxic quantities of fluorides in drinking water, usually from deep wells, is often detected in animals before its effects in man are noticed. Selenium poisoning, indicative of seleniferous rocks and vegetation (locoweeds), is also noticed first in animals.

The presence of rabies in an area may be heralded by its appearance in wild-life (foxes, jackals), which, in turn, reflects ecological changes in the fauna of the district concerned.

The examples show the great potential value of studies of spontaneously occurring disease in animals as pointers to possible environmental effects on human health.

REFERENCES

Barlow, R. M., Gardiner, A. C., Storey, I. J. & Slater, J. S. (1970) *J. comp. Path.*, **80,** 635-643

Binns, W., James, L. F., Shupe, J. L. & Everett, G. (1963) *Amer. J. vet. Res.*, **24**, 1164-1175

Blount, W. P. (1961) *Turkeys*, **9**, 52

Boffey, P. M. (1968) *Science*, **162**, 1460-1464

Done, J. T. (1968) *Lab. Anim.*, **2**, 207-217

Hickey, J. J. & Anderson, D. W. (1968) *Science*, **162**, 271-273

Kahrs, R. F., Scott, F. W. & de Lahunta, A. (1970) *Teratology*, **3**, 181-184

McFarren, E. F., Schafer, M. L., Campbell, J. E., Lewis, K. H., Jensen, E. T. & Schantz, E. J. (1960) *Advanc. Food Res.*, **10**, 135-179

Nielsen, S. W. (1971) *J. Amer. vet. med. Ass.*, **159**, 1103-1107

Pamukcu, A. M., Göksoy, S. K. & Price, J. M. (1967) *Cancer Res.*, **27**, 917-924

Reif, J. S. & Cohen, D. (1970) *Arch. environm. Hlth*, **20**, 684-689

Reif, J. S. & Cohen, D. (1971) *Arch. environm. Hlth*, **22**, 136-140

Richards, W. P. C., Crenshaw, G. L. & Bushnell, R. B. (1971) *Cornell Vet.*, **61**, 336-348

Selby, L. A., Marienfeld, C. J., Heidlage, W., Wright, H. T. & Young, V. E. (1971) *Cornell Vet.*, **61**, 203-213

Shupe, J. L., Binns, W., James, L. F. & Keeler, R. F. (1967) *J. Amer. vet. med. Ass.*, **151**, 198-203

United Kingdom, Atomic Energy Office (1957) *Accident at Windscale No. 1 pile on 10th October, 1957*, London, HM Stationery Office

CHAPTER 30

DATA HANDLING AND ASSESSMENT

Introduction

Public health departments from their earliest beginnings have needed to develop systems for collecting and recording what were considered to be essential public health data. Initially, such systems were organized so as to facilitate the early identification and control of communicable diseases, but were soon enlarged to provide more extensive information on the populations they served so as to make possible a better understanding of the factors influencing the general state of health of the region. More recently, the attention paid to collecting and assessing data on sanitary and environmental conditions has increased considerably, and a number of national and international institutions and organizations are now gathering information on the human environment (Citron, 1970; Smithsonian Institution, 1970).

The data relevant to the environmental sciences currently being collected are more diverse than those for most other scientific disciplines, and their quality varies widely. The users of environmental information are correspondingly more diverse than those using information in other fields.

Furthermore, despite the many national and international efforts, current studies of the environment are being conducted in a fragmentary and piecemeal fashion. Taken together, these considerations have prompted demands for the immediate development of broad-based, long-term, multidisciplinary research, monitoring, and surveillance programmes (Citron, 1970; World Health Organization, 1971; Battelle Memorial Institute, 1970; US Department of Health, Education, and Welfare, 1970; Oak Ridge National Laboratory, 1970; International Council of Scientific Unions, 1970; Fawcett, 1970).

Because responsibilities have been fragmented, information centres or monitoring programmes have been specialized and data banks isolated, so that techniques for integrating environmental information have not yet been developed. Correspondingly, the methodology for assessing the health problems of the human environment is inadequately developed, particularly with respect to the global aspects and to the general problems of an integrated approach to the health effects of the environment. The development of this methodology can be furthered by the ideas and techniques of computer and systems sciences together with a modern computer facility.

The purpose of this and the succeeding chapter is to discuss: (i) the most important methods that have been, or could be, used; and (ii) the problems and difficulties with respect to research and planning needs in applying a systems approach to the assessment and control of environmental hazards. We shall be concerned mainly with the information flow from the system under control (the left-hand side of the figure on p. 335) and the processing of data in the control components of the system.

Since, in principle, every major human or economic activity contributes to some extent to pollution problems, the need to acquire sufficient relevant data poses a serious problem because the acquisition of such data is costly. Data are needed to provide the basis for decisions calling for control actions, and the types of data collected must be selected with this specific aim in mind. For the purposes of decision-making and control, the existing steady (or normal or initial) state of the system (base-lines) must first be determined. The relations between the control parameters and the states of the system must then be analysed and computed so that both short- and long-term hazards may be detected, and the effects of control actions predicted.

We shall deal here only with theoretical and technical methods and possibilities, and deliberately omit the discussion of economic, cultural, political, and social factors.

Acquisition, Integration, and Management of Data

Categories of data

It is necessary to categorize data by means of several different criteria, relevant both to the limitations of particular data-processing systems and to the operational needs of the users.

Since the number and volume of environmental health problems that can be identified will clearly always be greater than the funds available to find solutions to them, a rank-ordering of these problems and consequently of the types of data to be collected will be necessary (Battelle Memorial Institute, 1970).

A related type of data categorization is based on the partitioning of the human ecosystem into sub-systems, as indicated in the next chapter.

The system adopted for categorizing data will have an important influence on the efficiency and reliability of any complex information network. This is of vital importance to the problems of data collection and processing that arise out of the needs of a programme for assessing environmental hazards. Accordingly, studies on principles of categorization are needed, as are agreements on a preliminary categorization system on a world-wide basis. Success in meeting these requirements will depend very much on the extent to which the ecosystem to be controlled can be reasonably divided into sub-systems.

Standardization, classification, and cataloguing

If it is remembered that the same data will be needed by different groups of users and that one user may need data collected by several different agencies, it will be seen that adequate standardization, classification, and cataloguing of data is a question of major importance.

There are no general rules for standardization and there can be no comprehensive and inviolable classification and cataloguing schemes for all data in the field of environmental health. It would be wasteful to try to create such schemes, because the money and manpower employed might well have as its end-product a major impediment to the improvement or development of new methods for assessing the health problems of the environment. Standardization and classification, despite the fact that they are indispensable for any operating control programme, must be handled with great care. In particular, they must be carried out in such a way that changes, improvements, and extensions can easily be made in the future. This will call for the initiation of specific interdisciplinary research programmes, since there are as yet only a few special-purpose standardization and classification schemes in existence, and the problem of the intersystem compatibility of these schemes has rarely been tackled.

As regards the standardization of *numerical data*, an adequate system of rules for standardization and classification can be developed in the near future that will ensure that data measured in different regions or by different agencies are comparable, and that will permit the exchange of data between different groups of users for automatic processing and searching by computers. A considerable amount of work has already been done and a number of projects are being planned by WMO (World Meteorological Organization, 1969, 1970) and WHO (World Health Organization, 1968, 1970).

The problem is more or less the same for *qualitative data* as for numerical data, but it seems to be much harder to find a satisfactory solution. In certain restricted areas, universally accepted nomenclatures already exist, such as the International Classification of Diseases, the list of key words of the MEDLARS (National Library of Medicine, 1972), or the Standardized Nomenclature of Veterinary Diseases and Operations (SNVDO) (Epizootiology Section, National Cancer Institute, 1966), but the number of such nomenclatures is small. Standardized nomenclatures and synonym lists for many special fields of interest are required in order to achieve compatibility and to integrate special-purpose nomenclatures so as to cover the whole area of environmental health.   A closely related issue is the need to establish agreements on the indices of environmental change to be reported (Citron, 1970; Smithsonian Institution, 1970, World Health Organization, 1971; Battelle Memorial Institute, 1970; US Department of Health, Education, and Welfare, 1970; Oak Ridge National Laboratory, 1970; International Council of Scientific Unions, 1970; Fawcett, 1970).

All higher level categories of standardization depend heavily on the establishment of such nomenclatures and classifications, and on agreements on the list of health indices to be reported.   At the present time, only a few very specific standard reporting forms and procedures are available (e.g., the WHO forms for the surveillance of selected communicable diseases, and the reporting form for the WHO drug monitoring system; see Chapter 25).   It is obvious that there can be no universally applicable reporting form and procedure, but it is desirable that all special-purpose forms should be drawn up in accordance with the general principle of consistency with the classification scheme.   This will facilitate automatic comparison or combination of reports.   The importance of inter-specific report compatibility is exemplified in the surveillance of communicable diseases, in which the epidemiologist requires not only microbiological information, but also information on histopathology and biochemistry, and ecological knowledge of the vector-borne diseases.

International comparability of socio-cultural variables related to urbanization, migration, occupation, educational background and ethnic factors is difficult to achieve, and it will be necessary to face up to the possibility that standardization may never be achieved in some of these fields.   In air pollution control, for example, standard questionnaires may have limited applicability in international comparisons because of cultural differences and problems of translation (World Health Organization, 1970).

Acquisition, transmission, and dissemination

Despite the fact that "the problem in environmental data handling is not a technological one, but an institutional one where the legal, organizational and co-ordination problems between all the parties involved are the most important barriers" (Quelette et al., 1971), there are a number of purely technological problems, as well as others that are partly technological and partly institutional.

A great variety of automatic electromechanical and, in particular, automatic electronic data collection devices exist.   They vary from small electronic sensors to satellites for remote sensing by means of radar, aerial photography, and infrared multi-spectral sensors.   Very specialized monitors, e.g., automatic monitors for measuring the concentration of sulfur dioxides, nitrogen oxides, and ozone in the air, can be installed to gather much of the relevant environmental data.   Even the automatic general bacteriological monitoring of rivers and streams may be possible by adapting techniques used in breweries and the pharmaceutical industry. This is clearly an important aspect of data collection, but the highly technical and specialized character of sensing devices is beyond the scope of this publication and will not be discussed here in greater detail.

Some remarks on data collection techniques in general are nevertheless appropriate. A major distinction exists between automatic monitoring, i.e., the collection of data automatically and *a fortiori* regularly (continuously or at intervals), and non-automatic spot check or sampling monitoring, i.e., the collection of data at random points on the time scale and/or at random localities. As already mentioned, automatic monitoring appears to be technically possible for almost all physical and chemical environmental indices, and for some bacteriological data as well. The choice of the specific monitoring technique—continuous, short-period, or long-period—is made partly on technical grounds (availability of equipment, etc.), partly on the basis of cost-effect calculations, and partly on theoretical considerations (availability of analytical methods and their specificity and sensitivity, i.e., their ability to yield useful results from the measurements). Spot check monitoring is used mainly in biological systems (e.g., medical examinations in schools and undertakings, and tests in medical laboratories), but may also be appropriate to the measurement of environmental indices, since it is often impossible, useless, or too expensive to collect certain data regularly; in addition, methods are available for drawing valuable conclusions from the spot check monitoring of a parameter (Alt & Rubinoff, 1970; Katz, 1968; World Health Organization, 1968).

Integration of data

An important part of the activity of a monitoring and surveillance system will be to combine and integrate data of different types and from different sources, and even from sources outside the system under consideration. For example, a WHO monitoring and surveillance system for environmental health will need data from other organizations, such as WHO, FAO, UNESCO, and other agencies, and from existing national or regional systems (see Chapter 18). If standardization for each data group is adequate and the objectives of integration are well defined, the preparation of computer programmes for integration poses no great problems and it can be effected automatically by the use of computers. In this respect, the most important currently available technique for the integration of data is the so-called computerized data bank (Thomas, 1971). Data banks are conceived of as providing common meeting grounds for different users, each of whom makes his own data available to other interested users while himself benefiting from the data supplied by others.

At the base of all data bank activities lies the need to understand the interdependence between, and the relationships that link together, objects and problems of different types and origins. Intensive and long-range planning is crucial to the determination of the structure and scope of the data banks used in a control system, and the types of data and of users to be dealt with. Without such planning, data banks would grow indefinitely; large amounts of data in the bank would never be used, since they would be obsolete, and nobody would know that they were there or for what reason they were originally stored. The problems connected with the building and use of large data banks have been intensively studied (Thomas, 1971; CODASYL Data Base Task Group, 1971), but many difficulties remain and the solutions found so far are less than adequate. Most of the work in this field has been done for business and public administration purposes. However, experiments are in progress on constructing medical information banks (e.g., at the Hebrew University, Jerusalem, Israel) and environmental data banks (e.g., the national aerometric data bank of the Air Pollution Control Office of the USA).

One non-technical but important problem of large data banks is that of privacy (Niblett, 1971), which has to be considered in planning environmental monitoring systems, and for which solutions have to be developed on technical, political, and educational grounds. The problems of data confidentiality and privacy concern not only individuals but also, to a large extent, government and industry, since information on, for example, waste disposal, air pollution, or water contamination in a specific region where, for example, a chemical firm is located, may well reveal the trade secrets of this firm. It is necessary, therefore, in order to protect the confidentiality of the original source in a given region or country, to integrate the data from any such region with data from other regions before publication, and to restrict access to the original data.

REFERENCES

Alt, F. L. & Rubinoff, M. (1970) *Advances in computers*, Vol. 10, New York, Academic Press

Battelle Memorial Institute (1970) *Technical intelligence and project information system for the EHS*, Columbia, Ohio

Citron, R. (1970) *The establishment of an international environmental monitoring program*, Washington, D.C., Smithsonian Institution

CODASYL Data Base Task Group (1971) *Report*, New York, Association for Computing Machinery

Epizootiology Section, National Cancer Institute (1966) *Standard nomenclature of veterinary diseases and operations*, 1st ed. revised, Bethesda, Md

Fawcett, J. E. S. (1970) *Report to Anglo-American Conference on Environmental Control, 13-16 November 1970*, Ditchley Park, Enstone, Oxon., England, The Ditchley Foundation (*Ditchley Paper* No. 33)

International Council of Scientific Unions (1970) *Report of the Ad Hoc Committee of the ICSU on Problems of the Human Environment*, Paris

Katz, M., (1969) *Measurement of air pollutants: Guide to the selection of methods*, Geneva, World Health Organization

Klerer, M. & Korn, G. A. (1967) *Digital computer user's handbook*, McGraw-Hill, New York

National Library of Medicine (1972) *MEDLARS System used at National Laboratory of Medicine*, Bethesda, Md, National Institutes of Health

Niblett, G. B. F. (1971) *Digital information and the privacy problem*, Paris, Organisation for Economic Co-operation and Development (*OECD Informatics Studies* No. 2)

Oak Ridge National Laboratory (1970) *Proposal to National Science Foundation: The environment and technology assessment*, Oak Ridge, Tenn.

Quelette, R. B., Rosenbaum, D. M. & Greeley, R. F. (1971) *Datamation*, 15 April, pp. 30-33

Smithsonian Institution (1970) *National and international environmental monitoring activities*, Washington, D.C.

Thomas, U. (1971) *Computerized data banks in public administration*, Paris, Organisation for Economic Co-operation and Development (*OECD Informatics Studies* No. 1)

US Department of Health, Education, and Welfare (1970) *Man's health and the environment*, Washington, D.C.

World Health Organization (1968) *Research into environmental pollution. Report of five WHO Scientific Groups*, Geneva (*Wld Hlth Org. techn. Rep. Ser.*, No. 406)

World Health Organization (1970) *Air quality criteria and guides*, Geneva (unpublished document EP/71.3)

World Health Organization (1971) *Problems of the human environment*, Geneva (unpublished document A24/A/3)

World Meteorological Organization (1969) *Collection, storage and retrieval of meteorological data*, Geneva (*World Weather Watch Planning Report* No. 28)

World Meteorological Organization (1970) *Further planning of the storage and retrieval service*, Geneva (*World Weather Watch Planning Report* No. 32)

CHAPTER 31

SYSTEMS ANALYSIS AND CONTROL

The interactions (interdependencies) between human health and the environment will be considered here in the light of modern systems and control theory. An attempt will be made to present the principal ideas, main results, and major problems of a systematic approach to the problems of environmental health. It should be stressed that in this chapter we have adopted an operational standpoint and have used the term "control" with the meaning "to cause the magnitude of a variable to remain within defined limits". Thus, to control pulmonary tuberculosis would mean to restrict the frequency of its occurrence to the currently practicable minimum level.

There is no need to stress the complexity of the human ecosystem and the fragmentary character of our current knowledge concerning the nature and intensity of the interactions that govern it. It cannot be analysed at the present time; in consequence, the extent to which changes can be regulated is partial at best. Furthermore, attempts to control environmental change may very well have unpredictable consequences. The development of insect resistance to a particular insecticide is a consequence of this kind.

In such circumstances, it is customary to proceed to a synthesis of the control mechanisms of the given complex system by isolating the more restricted sub-systems for which available physical and physiological knowledge is sufficient to suggest that control is possible.

Thus sufficient information is available with respect to the spread of water-borne infection to enable the public health specialist to consider the problems of drinking-water supply within a separable sub-system, and to ascertain the strength of the interactions between this sub-system and others. For example, the water-supply sub-system is very strongly influenced by the waste-disposal sub-system.

One may then proceed to describe as exactly as possible the operation and behaviour of each sub-system, taking into account possible inputs from and outputs to other sub-systems, select the variables to be controlled (according to the desired aim), and then devise the observation and control mechanism. Finally, one can devise an integrated model or quantitative description of all the control sub-systems and of their interactions. This model can then be studied to see how changes in various control parameters or alternative methods of regulation might affect the performance of the several parts of the overall system so as to maximize the likelihood that the desired outcome will be achieved.

A preliminary methodological discussion is presented here whose purpose is to identify the basic principles to be used in describing a relatively autonomous *health sub-system* of the *total human ecosystem*. Some insight into the complexity of the task of separating out one sub-system from another can be gained by considering the interaction between health and nutrition. Any adequate description of the health sub-system must include detailed information on the state of nutrition of the population, and the control measures must make specific reference to the quality of food available. Nevertheless, the control of food production, the kinds of food produced, the modes of production, and even the quality fall within the agriculture, animal husbandry, and fisheries sub-systems. There are clear practical and theoretical reasons for considering each of these sub-systems separately, but careful subsequent description of the interactions and points of contact between sub-systems is essential.

From the operational point of view an initial distinction should be made between the structural aspects and the control variables of the system under scrutiny.

The *structure* of the health system exists and develops in large measure independently of the observations and control measures that might be taken within the system. Thus, every community, region, or country has an existing organizational structure for the delivery of health care. There are existing methods of supplying water, existing sewerage systems and sewage disposal plants, and existing railways and other transport networks. The cities and towns are already there, as are the factories and farms. The controls within the health system must take them into account in their present state. Changes in the structural components are in most instances made slowly and gradually.

The *control variables*, whether or not they are already being regulated or are liable to be brought into play in future health planning and possible control mechanisms, are the tools with which the authorities responsible for the health system can strive to achieve the desired outcome within the given structure.

In this way one may, in logical order and without prejudice to their relative importance, determine or define the laws of behaviour of the system, determine its status, follow its development, and direct the development towards the desired goal. It must be emphasized that *the choice of final aims*, whether in terms of their nature or their order of priority, is external to the system; only the set of all possible goals to which the system may be directed is determined by the system itself.

For example, and in outline, the water-control sub-system in a given geographical area or region depends on:

(1) the structure of the water supply; the patterns of consumption, purification, treatment, and discharge of sewage; and the interaction of quantitative and qualitative variables with public health;

(2) the observation and control mechanisms through which the performance of the system can be optimized, as judged by acceptable social and medical criteria. This includes the monitoring of outfalls, bacterial counts in the water supply, and legislative regulations. The criteria for optimization can be regarded as external constraints on the system, i.e., as variables in an economic or social sub-system.

It is important to realize that the distinction between the structural part of a sub-system and the control variables and mechanisms is a conceptual one. For example, outflow patterns are usually regarded as structural, but it is technologically possible to regulate the flow in disposal lines so that the outflow pattern becomes a control variable. Normally, when plans are being made to institute specific controls within a given locality according to some pre-established standards, norms, and objectives, a clear distinction between structural component and variable ceases to exist after some time, because the goals have changed or because it has been discovered that other factors need to be taken into account and that other structural relationships within the systems have become relevant.

The General Scheme

Two complementary modes of action need to be pursued in order to ameliorate the effects of the environment on man (or, conversely, the effects of man on the environment). The first is local, and is aimed at the protection of a given individual, family, or well-defined and geographically restricted community of individuals. It is characterized by the use of measures specific to each potential health problem: this is the approach of occupational health and environmental health, narrowly defined, and includes waste disposal, the supply of potable water, and many sanitation measures (see Part I). These actions may be regarded as part of a primary or direct control system. In such a primary control system, the response of the regulatory agent (whether an agency of the health authorities, or an automatic device) is rapid, and carefully defined or prescribed by the system planners. The second mode of action is global, and is aimed at applying to the environment preventive or corrective measures that are indirect and somewhat removed from the day-to-day activities of the primary control component. We shall refer to this mode of action as functioning within the *secondary* control system. The secondary control system will be guided by a set of general principles rather than by exact rules. The principal function of the secondary control component is to monitor the behaviour of the primary control system and adapt the performance of the latter to secular, long-term changes in the health sub-system. It must, in addition, evaluate the efficiency of the primary control system's performance and alter the direct control mechanisms in accordance with the overall objectives of the control of the human ecosystem.   Activities such as the development of campaigns of public education in good health practice or the evaluation of the relevance and validity of proposed criteria and guides are typical functions within the secondary control component.

An analysis of the current state of affairs in environmental health would largely be concerned with the methods of primary control, but since the secondary control system has not yet been developed to any great extent, we shall concentrate here on the latter.   The objective will be to stimulate and guide the implementation of overall programmes for the control and management of the interrelationships between the environment and human health.   We shall consider the human ecosystem primarily in terms of the potentialities for detection, analysis, warning, and control, as they apply to the field of public health.

A CONTROL SYSTEM : GENERAL SCHEME

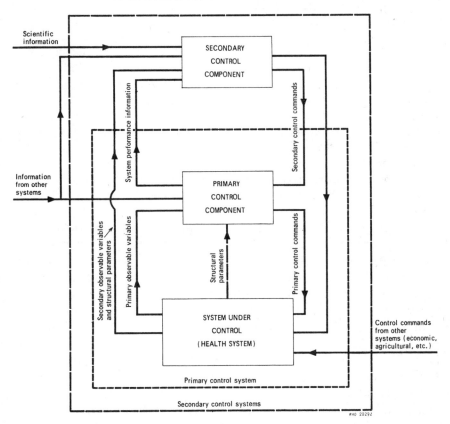

The general scheme discussed below is shown in the figure on p. 335 as comprising a set of information flows between the system to be controlled and two decision components, which are designated as the primary and secondary control components. The primary control component together with the system to be controlled and the flows between them, constitute the primary control system. The secondary control component together with the primary control system and their pattern of interconnections, constitute the secondary control system. It will be noted that the information arrows are of two kinds: information on the state of the system (on the left-hand side) and signals for action, technically known as "commands" (on the right-hand side).

For simple systems, and even for complex systems that are completely known, not only as regards their internal structure, but also as regards their possible behaviour (and consequently the set of all possible goals to which they may be directed), it is possible to synthesize a model for system optimization once and for all, with the assurance that the mathematical routine (algorithm) representing the dynamic behaviour of the model will guarantee optimum performance for any particular set of external goals and constraints. This will be true both for structurally deterministic systems and for systems subject to random variation as long as the underlying random process is thoroughly understood. The ecological systems under consideration here, however, cannot be characterized even as far as their deterministic components are concerned, and in many cases of existing or intended environmental control it is not known, or at least it is not certain, that the goal one would want the system to reach even lies within its range of behaviour. Furthermore, there are a number of attributes of ecological systems subject to major fluctuations whose statistical properties are poorly understood at best.

Under such circumstances it again appears to be important to distinguish between the primary and secondary control systems for the reasons considered below.

In order to direct the health system towards an externally chosen aim it is necessary to influence the state of the system by operating on the control variables by means of the established control mechanisms. This is accomplished almost exclusively within the primary control system. Because the workings of the health sub-system are so inadequately understood, the primary control component may be inadequate for this purpose. It may prove necessary, therefore, to operate on the system itself, e.g., to alter the distinction between the structural and control parts of the system, to modify components of the existing structures, and the primary and perhaps even the secondary control methods and mechanisms. It is the task of the secondary control component both to plan and to execute changes in the organization and operating procedures of both control components.

Even though the interactions of the many components of the health system are poorly understood, sufficient information is available to justify attempts to establish mathematical models whose behaviour can be studied and compared with the known facts—current and historical—concerning human health and the effects of environmental factors. First attempts at model making will almost certainly be simplistic. Formulation of plausible and useful models can be effected only by a series of successive approximations to the real world situation. The first attempt at describing a complicated system can be little more than a rudimentary outline, which will be improved over the course of years as additional knowledge about the real world is obtained. Thus, the strategy of improvement is best included within the model itself; a component of the complete control system should be specifically designed to make adjustments and to prescribe appropriate alterations in the control components on the basis of measurements of the performance of the overall system. This function is performed within the secondary control system. Although the strategy of adaptive control is widely used in certain industrial activities, notably in communications, it does not appear to be employed in public health practice.

It should be remembered that the criteria for deciding when and how to alter the primary controls are themselves subject to variation, as a result of changes in the priorities assigned to the final aims, changes in the structure or the structural parameters of the system under control, improvements in the technological tools for preventive and corrective intervention, and new advances in therapeutic medicine.

The information symbolized by the arrows on the right-hand side of the figure consists of commands or signals whose nature depends on the specific mechanisms by which control is mediated, e.g., whether a control command acts automatically on the system, as in the regulation of the flows of high sulfur and low sulfur fuels in a combustion process, or whether a verbal instruction is given, a notification sent by post, etc. A general methodological discussion is unjustified, since these command instructions are governed by the specific constraints or technology and institutional forms peculiar to the system under control.

The signals represented by the arrows on the left-hand side of the figure consist almost exclusively of information in the usual sense of the word. [1] It is this information flow that calls for the provision of special techniques for collection, sifting, and correlation.

Observable Variables

It is clear that in most systems the important phenomena that are the targets of optimization are not directly accessible; for example, the ameliora-

---

[1] Of course, these signals must also be transmitted and processed by specific technological devices, but problems as to choice of computer or whether transmission is best effected by cable or letter are not of concern to the present discussion.

tion of the health of all the individuals in a community cannot be observed or measured directly because of prohibitive costs and delays.   As a result, systems theory distinguishes a particular class of effectively observable variables from other variables.   *The observable variables* are the elements in the information flow by which the state of the system to be controlled is determined.   Most of the health or environmental indices discussed here are observable variables in the sense given above.   Indeed, a major and continuing task for health scientists is to find observable variables that represent adequately some underlying variable itself not directly observable (see Chapter 22).

The human ecosystem can undergo rapid changes that are unpredictable (at least with our present knowledge) as to time, place, and severity.   Floods, famines, and other catastrophes, the emergence of a virulent microbial or viral strain, large-scale population migrations, and urban growth are some of the changes that, on the basis of our current knowledge, can be expected to occur but cannot be anticipated with any degree of specificity until they are well advanced.   As a consequence, a set of observable variables is required to represent such events within the model, to predict their occurrence, and perhaps to prepare for action to be taken before the undesired events occur, with the aim of preventing or reducing their harmful consequences.

In the last analysis, the model must be seen for what it is, i.e., a model. The extent to which it is useful in dealing effectively and efficiently with environmental degradation will depend on the extent to which it reflects important elements and relationships in a world that exists independently of any particular descriptive formulation of it.   The fitness or correctness of any model, including this one, must be measured by its utility and fruitfulness in dealing with the problem at hand.

This same criterion holds true for the many possible applications of the model, whether the primary and secondary control systems describe national-international, state-federal, or the particular situation to be modelled, and upon the appropriateness of the formulation for that situation.   As presented, it is not meant to be restricted as far as the possible applications are concerned, but rather to serve as a conceptual framework within which monitoring and surveillance for environmental hazards could be carried out.

PART IV

PUBLIC HEALTH PRINCIPLES
AND PRACTICES OF INTERVENTION

CHAPTER 32

ENVIRONMENTAL HEALTH CRITERIA AND STANDARDS

The scientific criteria for establishing environmental health standards are the quantitative relationships between the intensity, frequency, and duration of exposure to various environmental influences, on the one hand, and the risk or magnitude of an undesirable effect on man or his environment, on the other hand. Such relationships are derived from toxicological, epidemiological, and environmental studies, and some of the problems encountered have been discussed in Chapters 11 and 20. In principle, the "dose-response" relationships can be established with fair precision if the exposure levels are high, as in certain occupational situations (see Chapter 7); with low-level, long-term exposure, however, the task becomes very complex, and such information is available only in a few cases. In the absence of precise information on the exposure-effect relationship, other criteria, based on experience or on intuitive guesses, have been and will continue to be used by public health administrators to set environmental health standards. The experience accumulated by using such standards will show whether or not the guesses were correct and how the standards should be modified. In many instances water, milk, and food were made safe for consumption by imposing standards of quality based on relatively general and vague rules.

Environmental health standards are "acceptable" or "permissible" limits of concentration (or of another index of the intensity of exposure) established to protect a defined population from the undesirable effects of a specified exposure to one or several environmental hazards, e.g., in the work environment (see Chapter 7). Such limits may be set for:

(1) *pollutants taken up by an organism or a population.* This is sometimes called a "primary protection standard" (Preparatory Committee for the United Nations Conference on the Human Environment, 1971). Examples are acceptable daily intakes (ADI) of toxic substances (Joint Meeting of the FAO Working Party of Experts on Pesticide Residues and the WHO Expert Group on Pesticide Residues, 1970) or the maximum permissible intakes (MPI) of radioactive substances. The maximum permissible dose for ionizing radiation (International Atomic Energy Agency, 1967) is a special case of a "primary protection standard" as it relates to the absorption of energy and not of a substance;

(2) *pollutants present in specified environmental media* (e.g., air, water) *or products* (e.g., food, consumer goods). Such limits are sometimes called "derived working levels" (Preparatory Committee for the United Nations Conference on the Human Environment, 1971) and include ambient air quality standards, water quality standards, maximum allowable concentrations for occupational exposure, and others. When applied to products such as food or chemical consumer goods (e.g., detergents), they are often called "product standards";

(3) *discharges or emissions from pollution sources* (e.g., effluent standards in water pollution control, emission standards in air pollution control) *or by a given design of product* (e.g., fumes from motor vehicles, noise from aircraft, or ionizing or non-ionizing radiation from an electronic device).

In order to meet emission or effluent standards, it may be necessary to establish various types of "technological standards" concerned with the performance and design of equipment in those technologies and operations leading to the release of pollutants.

These "limits" or "standards", if adopted by governments or other competent authorities, may have the force of law, but are otherwise used as guidelines to good practice in prevention and control programmes (WHO Expert Committee on the Planning, Organization, and Administration of National Environmental Health Programmes, 1970).

When "standards" are adopted, the technological feasibility and financial implications of their application must be taken into account. Thus, a calculated risk may be taken in drawing up some standards for environmental quality on the basis of cost/benefit analysis. The cost of applying standards, which is made up of the direct financial outlay, the higher prices of consumer goods due to the restrictions on industry, use of skilled manpower, etc., is balanced against the benefits obtained by applying them (reduction of morbidity, improvement in human health and the quality of the environment). A country therefore selects the standards it can best afford in the light of health, social, economic, and technological considerations (WHO Expert Committee on the Planning, Organization, and Administration of National Environmental Health Programmes, 1970; WHO Expert Committee on Air Quality Criteria and Guides, 1972).

In addition to basing "standards" on environmental quality criteria, such as exposure–effect relationships, several other approaches are possible. One is to take, for example, the quality of community air in some selected area as "standard". In this approach, the target to be achieved is the quality that already exists in the selected area. A second approach is to take existing levels of environmental quality as standard, and design the control programme in such a way that no deterioration of environmental quality will result from further economic development of the region in question.

A distinction is sometimes made between environmental quality standards and goals (Stern, 1968). "Goals" are the levels of pollutants or of other factors that it is ultimately intended to achieve, whereas "standards" are the levels that it is intended to achieve in the immediate future; they may fall short of goals, because consideration must be given to the feasibility of achieving them within the immediately foreseeable future. A similar distinction exists in some countries between "hygienic standards", which represent the optimum conditions for which we must strive although we know that they are not always and everywhere obtainable, and "sanitary standards", which represent a compromise between science and practice, and are necessarily provisional. As the technology and economy of a country develop and national income increases, "sanitary standards" must be revised periodically and brought closer and closer to hygienic standards (Rjazanov, 1965).

Legislation

Many countries are now tending to consolidate their various items of legislation on pollution control and to introduce laws of wide scope that cover the environment as a whole. Recent laws of this type include the Environmental Protection Law of 1969 of Sweden (*Int. Dig. Hlth Leg.*, 1970a), the Basic Law for Environmental Pollution Control of Japan (*Int. Dig. Hlth Leg.*, 1971) (enacted in 1967 and amended in 1970), and the Singapore Environmental Public Health Act, 1968 (*Int. Dig. Hlth Leg.*, 1970b). At the same time, a trend can be noted towards the establishment of central co-ordinating bodies or organizations, major authority being delegated in certain cases to the ministry responsible for public health, as in Jamaica, the Netherlands, and Austria. An Environmental Protection Agency and a Council on Environmental Quality have been established in the USA, and a Department of the Environment in the United Kingdom, while in France a minister has been given special responsibility for the protection of nature and the environment. An environmental agency has also been set up in Japan.

There can be no doubt that in certain cases the application of national legislation can produce spectacular effects at the local level, as was the case, for example, in the United Kingdom with the Clean Air Act of 1956 (*Int. Dig. Hlth Leg.*, 1958). Yet this Act had to be amended in 1968 in order to increase its effectiveness over the country as a whole (*Int. Dig. Hlth Leg.*, 1969). The need for legislation of general applicability is also evident in countries having a federal structure. Thus, to be really effective, such measures as making the use of low-sulfur fuel compulsory, or banning the use of soft coal, must cover the entire country.

As far as the control of environmental radioactivity is concerned, the responsibility for monitoring programmes is assigned to various national authorities—which, in certain cases, have organized collaborative pro-grammes based on international co-operation. In the USA, the monitoring of environmental radioactivity is undertaken mainly by the Environmental Protection Agency, through its Office of Radiation Programs. In Canada, this responsibility is assumed by the Radiation Protection Division of the Department of National Health and Welfare and, in Belgium, by the Ministry of Public Health and the Family. In the Netherlands, where various agencies have responsibilities in this field, a special commission has been established to ensure the necessary co-ordination. The policies adopt-ed by these different authorities, although varying from country to country, sometimes reflect the recommendations of the International Commission on Radiological Protection (1966).

Air Quality

There are at least two different approaches to air pollution control, namely "air quality management" and the "best practical means".

The *air quality management* approach relates control requirements to the desired air quality. Knowledge is therefore required not only of the desired air quality (expressed in terms of air quality standards) but also of the existing air quality and sources of pollution. A mathematical model can then be developed and used to forecast future air pollution levels resulting, for example, from increased urbanization, industrialization, and economic growth in general. The stringency of a control programme will depend on the difference between the existing or estimated future air quality and the desired air quality standards or goals. As soon as the necessary reduc-tions in emissions have been calculated, emission standards can be adopted. Effective use of the air quality approach requires adequate air monitoring networks and the services of specialist staff.

Air quality management is a logical approach. It encourages joint action by those concerned, e.g., with town planning, industrial development, and transport policies, in drawing up programmes designed to achieve or maintain the desired air quality. It has, however, a number of drawbacks. Our present knowledge of the effects of air pollution is incomplete, so that scientifically based air quality criteria and standards are difficult to formulate for many pollutants. There is also a certain lack of precision in the predic-tion of the air quality that can be achieved by control programmes, since a number of decisions have to be made on the basis of information that is necessarily incomplete and approximate, particularly as regards emission inventories and dispersion data. There is therefore a need for continuous reappraisal of the adequacy of the predictions made in the planning stages as additional information becomes available on the performance of control programmes.

Air quality standards are based on air quality criteria, where these are available (US Department of Health, Education, and Welfare, 1969).

In addition to the effects of air pollution, other considerations have to be taken into account in drawing up standards, such as the existing level of air pollution in a given region, the available technology, the costs of applying standards, and other specific local factors. It has also to be decided whether or not there should be one standard for an entire region or different standards for different areas within that region. Since the residential, commercial, and industrial zones of an urban area, for example, are all surrounded by the same air mass, different air quality standards would be difficult to administer (although in a number of countries different air quality standards have in fact been adopted for residential and industrial areas). Nevertheless, because of marked differences in land usage, each area or region of a given country may adopt its own air quality standards.

Emission standards are necessary for the control of pollution, irrespective of whether or not ambient air quality standards have been established. As the name implies, an *emission standard* is a limit placed on the amount or concentration of a pollutant emitted from a source (US Environmental Protection Agency, 1971a). The standard is most commonly expressed in terms of the concentration of a substance in a given volume of gaseous effluent (objective emission standards) or in terms of the opacity of a smoke plume (often assessed by subjective means). Some emission standards for five categories of stationary sources have recently been published in the USA (*Federal Register*, 1971b). Air quality criteria and standards may also be used in the setting of emission standards; the procedure is to calculate the concentration of a polluting substance in the effluent leaving a stack that—after dilution and dispersion—would be approximately equivalent to a desired level in the ambient air at ground level near the stack. Such a calculation must take into consideration the various relevant factors, such as stack height, topography, temperature and momentum of the gas plume, and local meteorological conditions.

Several countries have also adopted emission standards for moving sources, particularly motor vehicles. For example, in the USA a recent regulation (*Federal Register*, 1971a) has stipulated that by 1975-76 new automobiles produced will not be allowed to emit more than 3.4 g per mile of carbon monoxide, 0.41 g per mile of hydrocarbons and 0.4 g per mile of oxides of nitrogen. These are, in fact, "product or design standards" because, in addition to limits on emissions, they often also specify the kind of control devices that such moving sources should have.

The *best practical means* approach is based on the principle that pollution should be reduced to the greatest extent possible with the methods available in practice, but that the cost of doing so should not be unreasonable (*Int. Dig. Hlth Leg.*, 1963). Such an approach, however, presupposes the existence of an authority responsible for deciding, *in each case*, what constitutes the best practical means, and this in turn makes it necessary to investigate not only the methods used within a given industry but also those of other industries.   The decision as to what is or is not a reasonable cost will have to take into account the effects of air pollution on the environment and on human health, as well as the political climate and public opinion.   Indirectly, therefore, air quality is also considered to some extent in this approach. Because it is more expensive to instal gas-cleaning equipment in existing installations than in new plants, the adoption of the best practical means approach often leads in practice to the specification of different requirements for new and existing units.   Emission requirements or standards are often used to define the best practical means for single sources.

Alert levels are a special type of air quality standards.   When the ambient air concentrations of specific pollutants reach these levels, which can be related to various degrees of possible hazard to health (US Environmental Protection Agency, 1971b), the operation of certain industrial plants and of motor vehicles is restricted, or other procedures are set in motion.

Other standards have been developed in various countries, namely, *fuel standards* and *design standards* (the latter involve the establishment of sanitary or buffer zones around areas in which specific industries or trades are located).   Such standards are also related to the desired purity of the ambient air and may therefore be said to be related to air quality criteria, although the relationship is somewhat more tenuous (Berjušov & Perockaja, 1964; WHO Expert Committee on Environmental Health Aspects of Metropolitan Planning and Development, 1965).

Water Quality

Comparatively few studies on water quality criteria have been carried out (McKee & Wolf, 1963; Čerkinskij, 1967; US Department of the Interior, 1968); intensive research programmes are therefore in progress in several countries to provide the necessary information.   In the absence of such criteria, water quality standards have been based, e.g., on established practice, economic and technological feasibility, educated guesses, and mathematical models.

Various types of water quality standards exist, one of the most important being concerned with the quality of drinking-water.   Both national and international drinking-water standards have been drawn up (see Chapter 2) (World Health Organization, 1970, 1971).

Other standards refer to the quality of the water of rivers, lakes, and estuaries, and of coastal or sea water.   Such standards take into account the different uses for which the water is intended (e.g., for community water supply, fisheries, agriculture, industry, recreation).   It is impossible to draw up water quality standards that would cover all water uses and all types of water body.   In some countries, the legislation contains provisions governing the composition and characteristics of the water of streams and other water bodies, depending on the use for which it is intended.

Such legislation specifies the maximum permissible concentrations of a number of undesirable or harmful substances, and almost invariably includes some form of classification of rivers and other bodies of water.

The parameters used for the classification of streams, lakes, and other water bodies or for describing the water quality requirements vary widely in different countries. They may include temperature, pH-value, dissolved oxygen and coliform bacteria content, in addition to certain visual characteristics, as well as floating solids, oils and greases, phenols, taste and odour producing substances, potentially toxic substances, acids and alkalis, BOD_5 at 20°C, and many others (*Int. Dig. Hlth Leg.*, 1966). The use of water quality standards and effluent standards in water quality management is similar to the use of air quality standards.

Whether water quality standards and classifications exist or not, the control process invariably involves the setting up of *effluent standards*. Such standards depend on the number of pollution sources and on the capacity of a given water body to receive the wastes discharged. The setting up of standards for the discharge of effluents must be approached carefully, since it is difficult to ensure that the different discharges are allotted a fair share of the available self-purification capacity of the river or lake. Except in the simpler situations, it is impossible to set effluent standards that will be effective other than for a given river basin or other defined water body. The best practicable means approach, described earlier (see pp. 345-346), is also applicable to water pollution control.

Occupational Exposure

A basic principle of occupational health is that, despite the potential health hazards inevitably associated with toxic substances, there exists for each a definable and measurable level of human exposure at some point above zero, below which there is no significant threat to human health. [1] Such an acceptable level of exposure, expressed in appropriate terms of magnitude and duration, is variously called the "threshold limit value" (TLV), the "maximum allowable concentration" (MAC), the "permissible dose", etc. (see Chapter 7).

Initially, acceptable levels of exposure were designed to achieve limited health objectives and were based on rudimentary criteria for distinguishing between health and ill-health. The problem of developing more stringent criteria on which to base permissible levels has since been approached from two different directions (Hatch, 1970). The first starts from the high levels at which demonstrable ill-effects occur, and works downwards, using increasingly sensitive measures of pre-clinical, physiological, biological, and

---

[1] This may not be applicable to substances that are considered to be potential carcinogens or mutagens.

chemical disturbances (Stokinger, 1969).   The second starts from the opposite end, and works upwards from the assumed "normal values" for a healthy animal or man, using highly sensitive measures of behaviour or other forms of response.   The permissible limit established is just less than the lowest level of exposure needed to induce any statistically significant deviation from the normal state of the organism (Kurljandskaja & Sanockij, 1965).   Because of this major difference in approach, it is not at all surprising to find marked differences in the recommended permissible levels, which may differ by a factor of ten and even more.   Out of more than 400 substances for which permissible levels have been established, the Joint ILO/ WHO Committee on Occupational Health in its sixth report (1969) found only 24 on which agreement was close enough for them to be recommended for international use (see Chapter 7).

Permissible levels of exposure are used in two different ways in national occupational health programmes: (1) as legally binding standards for industrial codes that have to be met by the application of the necessary control measures; (2) as quantitative guide-lines in a technical assistance programme designed to help industries in their efforts to provide adequate health protection in all hazardous processes and occupations.   As legal standards they have two disadvantages: (1) they do not always make it possible to distinguish sharply between safe and unsafe working conditions; and (2) they are not suitable for practical use by factory inspectors, who are not specially trained in the manifold details of disease prevention.   Permissible levels of exposure can also be used to supplement specific design standards for control equipment.

REFERENCES

Berjušov, K. G. & Perockaja, A. S. (1964) *Basic principles of housing hygiene in the USSR.* In: *Housing programmes: the role of public health agencies*, Geneva, World Health Organization (*Publ. Hlth Pap.*, No. 25), pp. 47-52

Čerkinskij, S. N., ed. (1967) [*Industrial water pollution*], Moscow, Medicina

Federal Register, 1971a, **36**, 12 658

Federal Register, 1971b, **36**, 15 704

Hatch, F. T. (1970) *Prevention of occupational diseases through control of airborne toxic substances at the workplace, Part I, Establishment of permissible limits for human exposure to toxic agents*, Geneva, World Health Organization (unpublished document WHO/OH/70.3)

International Atomic Energy Agency (1967) *Basic safety standards for radiation protection*, Vienna (*Safety Series* No. 9)

International Commission on Radiological Protection (1966) *Principles of environmental monitoring relating to the handling of radioactive materials*, London, Pergamon Press (*ICRP Publication* 7)

Int. Dig. Hlth Leg., 1958, **9**, 181

Int. Dig. Hlth Leg., 1963, **14**, 187

Int. Dig. Hlth Leg., 1966, **17**, 643

Int. Dig. Hlth Leg., 1969, **20,** 499

Int. Dig. Hlth Leg., 1970a, **21,** 173

Int. Dig. Hlth Leg., 1970b, **21,** 838

Int. Dig. Hlth Leg., 1971, **22,** 480

Joint ILO/WHO Committee on Occupational Health (1969) *Sixth report. Permissible levels of occupational exposure to airborne toxic substances,* Geneva (*Wld Hlth Org. techn. Rep. Ser.*, No. 415)

Joint Meeting of the FAO Working Party of Experts on Pesticide Residues and the WHO Expert Group on Pesticide Residues (1970) *Report,* Geneva (*Wld Hlth Org. techn. Rep. Ser.*, No. 458)

Kurljandskaja, E. B. & Sanockij, I. V. (1965) *Gig. Tr. prof. Zabol.*, **9** (3), 3-9

McKee, J. E. & Wolf, H. W. (1963) *Water quality criteria,* 2nd ed., Sacramento, Calif., The Resources Agency of California, State Water Quality Control Board (Publication No. 3-A)

Preparatory Committee for the United Nations Conference on the Human Environment (1971) *Report of the Preparatory Committee on its third session,* New York, United Nations (unpublished document A/CONF.48/PC/13)

Rjazanov, V. A. (1965) *Bull. Wld Hlth Org.*, **32,** 389-398

Stern, A. C. (1968) *Air pollution,* Vol. III, 2nd ed., New York, Academic Press

Stokinger, H. E. (1969) *Introduction to threshold limit values,* Chicago, Ill., American Conference of Governmental Industrial Hygienists

US Department of Health, Education, and Welfare (1969) *Guidelines for the development of air quality standards and implementation plans,* Washington, D.C.

US Department of the Interior, Federal Water Pollution Control Administration (1968) *Report of the Committee on Water Quality Criteria,* Washington, D.C., US Government Printing Office.

US Environmental Protection Agency (1971a) *Background information—Proposed national emission standards for hazardous air pollutants: asbestos, beryllium, mercury,* Research Triangle Park, N.C.

US Environmental Protection Agency (1971b) *Guide for air pollution episode avoidance,* Research Triangle Park, N.C.

WHO Expert Committee on Air Quality Criteria and Guides (1972) *Report,* Geneva (*Wld Hlth Org. techn. Rep. Ser.*, No. 506)

WHO Expert Committee on Environmental Health Aspects of Metropolitan Planning and Development (1965) *Report,* Geneva (*Wld Hlth Org. techn. Rep. Ser.*, No. 297)

WHO Expert Committee on the Planning, Organization, and Administration of National Environmental Health Programmes (1970) *Report,* Geneva (*Wld Hlth Org. techn. Rep. Ser.*, No. 439)

World Health Organization (1970) *European standards for drinking-water,* 2nd ed., Geneva

World Health Organization (1971) *International standards for drinking-water,* 3rd ed., Geneva

CHAPTER 33

SANITATION TECHNOLOGY

Introduction

Fully a third of the world's population is infested by hookworm (CCTA/WHO African Conference on Ancylostomiasis, 1963) and possibly one out of four people are infected with *Ascaris lumbricoides* (roundworm) (WHO Expert Committee on the Control of Ascariasis, 1967). Enteritis, including diarrhoeas and dysenteries, is a major cause of morbidity and death in developing countries, especially among infants under one year and young children in the 1–4-year age group.

An estimated 250 million people are afflicted by filariasis (WHO Expert Committee on Filariasis (*Wuchereria* and *Brugia* Infections), 1967), while 180–200 million are infected with schistosomiasis (WHO Expert Committee on Bilharziasis,[1] 1965). Amoebic infection prevalence rates in a community are often inversely related to the level of sanitation (Hunter et al., 1960).

These diseases are all preventable, some more easily than others. The public health principle of intervention involves erecting barriers, at points of choice, in the cycle of transmission. For the group of diseases mentioned above, basic sanitation is the most economical, rational, and often the only method of prevention. No other single measure can make a comparable contribution to the improvement of health and standard of living (UNICEF-WHO Joint Committee on Health Policy, 1969). Many examples of the efficacy of basic sanitary measures can be cited in both the developed and developing countries.

In Japan in 1962, a survey of 30 rural areas showed that, after installation of safe water supplies, the number of cases of communicable intestinal diseases was reduced by 71.5 %, while the death rate for infants and young children fell by 51.7 % (Dieterich & Henderson, 1963).

A programme for the sanitary handling and disposal of excreta was carried out in Peru. Before the campaign, 99 % of the schoolchildren in the area were affected with internal parasites. Four years later, the percentage infected with hookworm had fallen to 58 % (Winslow, 1951).

---

[1] Following a recommendation of a WHO Expert Committee, the name "schistosomiasis" is now used in preference to "bilharziasis".

In 78 cities in the United States, the decline in the incidence of typhoid fever, due largely to the elimination of unsafe drinking water between the years 1910 and 1946, led to a reduction in the death rate per 100 000 population from 20.54 to 0.15 (American Water Works Association, 1950).

Sanitation is thus fundamental to individual and community health. The technology is well-established. It provides protection against disease transmitted by contaminated water or food, or by insect vectors.

REFERENCES

American Water Works Association (1950) *Water quality and treatment*, 2nd ed., New York

CCTA/WHO African Conference on Ancylostomiasis (1963) *Report*, Geneva (*Wld Hlth Org. techn. Rep. Ser.*, No. 255), p. 5

Dieterich, B. H. & Henderson, J. M. (1963) *Urban water supply conditions and needs in seventy-five developing countries*, Geneva, World Health Organization (*Publ. Hlth Pap.*, No. 23)

Hunter, G. W., Frye, W. W. & Swartzwelder, J. C. (1960) *A manual of tropical medicine*, 3rd ed., Philadelphia, Penn., Saunders

UNICEF-WHO Joint Committee on Health Policy (1969) *Assessment of environmental sanitation and rural water supply programmes assisted by the United Nations Children's Fund and the World Health Organization (1959-1968)*, Geneva (unpublished document JC16/UNICEF-WHO/69.2)

WHO Expert Committee on Bilharziasis (1965) *Third report*, Geneva (*Wld Hlth Org. techn. Rep. Ser.*, No. 299)

WHO Expert Committee on the Control of Ascariasis (1967) *Report*, Geneva (*Wld Hlth Org. techn. Rep. Ser.*, No. 379) p. 6

WHO Expert Committee on Filariasis (*Wuchereria* and *Brugia* Infections) (1967) *Second report*, Geneva (*Wld Hlth Org. techn. Rep. Ser.*, No. 359)

Winslow, C.-E. A. (1951) *The cost of sickness and the price of health*, Geneva, World Health Organization (*Monograph Series*, No. 7)

A. Community Water Supplies

Basic sanitation measures

A community water supply system must serve more than the bare minimum needs of safe water for drinking and culinary purposes. For health, comfort, and convenience, additional quantities for bathing, washing, and public cleansing are necessary. The ultimate goal is the provision of safe water of acceptable quality, and in adequate quantity, for home use and for public, industrial, and recreational uses. To attain this goal, attention must be paid to a number of activities.

Source selection and water-use allocation

Ever increasing demands on finite resources compel the re-use of treated waste waters in some places. Water of high quality should not be used where water of lower quality would suffice, unless the supply exceeds requirements (United Nations Economic and Social Council, 1958). The best quality water should be reserved for human consumption.

Treatment

Turbidity is generally removed by coagulation and flocculation and by settling suspended matter with the aid of aluminium sulfate (alum) or ferric chloride. Filtration through sand is an economical treatment process for the removal of residual turbidity and biological contaminants. Slow sand filtration and infiltration galleries are more suited to rural areas than rapid sand filtration. Slow sand filtration can reduce total bacterial counts by a factor of 1000–10 000 and *E. coli* counts by a factor of 100–1000. Water of drinking quality (with *E. coli* mostly absent in 100 ml) can be produced from sources that are not too highly contaminated. The general adoption of rapid sand filtration in industrialized countries has been due mainly to the resulting savings in labour, land, and initial cost.

Treatment with chemicals, other than simple chlorination, is not practicable in rural areas, especially in developing countries. Generally, groundwater is free of bacterial pollution while surface waters are subject to high bacterial contamination, but some groundwaters may have a high mineral content. Groundwater is generally sought in rural areas, since as a rule it does not need treatment.

Disinfection

Iodine, bromine, ozone, ultra-violet rays, and boiling have been used for disinfection. Chlorine, however, remains the most widely used disinfectant for community water supplies, by virtue of its germicidal properties and the comparatively low cost and ease of application. Relative germicidal efficiencies of different forms of chlorine and ozone are shown in the accompanying table. The technical problems connected with the chlorination of water supplies in rural areas have been receiving greater attention in recent years, and many methods such as the double pot, drip-feed, and mechanical proportioning devices are now either commercially available or can be fabricated (India, Central Public Health Engineering Research Institute, 1970). In an emergency, chlorination can give encouraging results even in a city raw water supply, as was found when it was applied in Calcutta for cholera control (Bhaskaran et al., 1965).

RELATIVE GERMICIDAL ACTIVITIES OF DISINFECTING MATERIALS *

Germicide	Concentration, in mg/litre, required to kill or inactivate 99 % of: [a]			
	Enteric bacteria	Amoebic cysts	Viruses	Bacterial spores
O_3	0.001	1.0	0.10	0.20
HOCl as Cl_2	0.02	10	0.40	10
OCl⁻as Cl_2	2	10^3	> 20	> 10^3
NH_2Cl as Cl_2	5	20	10^2	4×10^2
Free Cl, pH 7.5	0.04	20	0.8	20
Free Cl, pH 8	0.1	50	2	50

* After Morris (1970).

[a] Within 10 minutes at 5°C.   The figures are accurate to within a factor of 2-10, depending upon the specific micro-organism concerned.

Distribution

Conveyance of water under pressure by pipes is the most economical and safe method of transporting water from source or treatment plant to consumer.   The handling of water after treatment and disinfection poses a fresh threat of contamination.   It is for this reason that the supply of safe piped water to each house through house connexions is the ultimate public health objective.   However, the supply of safe water through public stand-posts or by sanitary wells has to be accepted as an interim measure for economic reasons.

Advanced technology

Technology has advanced to such an extent that there is virtually no source of water supply, ground or surface, even if brackish or heavily contaminated, that cannot be treated, at a price, in such a way as to make it safe for human consumption.

The multipurpose concept of water resource management is being increasingly adopted.   Reservoirs are therefore being constructed that will serve not only as sources of supply but also for flood regulation, to augment dry-weather flow, or as recreational facilities.   Mathematical models and computer techniques are being used to evaluate the resources of particular catchments, and the accuracy of rainfall predictions is being improved by the use of weather satellites and radar.

The efficiency of unit processes in water treatment is constantly being improved and automation is being increasingly adopted.   New aids to coagulation (such as polyelectrolytes) have been introduced.   Increasing use is being made of activated carbon for taste and odour removal, and of ion-exchange resins for the removal of trace impurities (Fair et al., 1966). Chlorine continues to be the most commonly used sterilizing agent, but ozone is being increasingly adopted and is more effective in the destruction of viruses.

The removal of excess salinity, fluorides, iron/manganese, etc., may call for softening, defluoridation, coke-aeration, and similar additional treatment. Multilayer filtration with anthracite permits higher filtration rates. In India, where no anthracite is available, certain grades of bituminous coals have been found suitable (India, Central Public Health Engineering Research Institute, 1971).

Desalination of brackish and salt waters is now practicable, but is still more costly than conventional treatment, so that its application has so far been limited to special situations where fresh water is not available, e.g., on small islands lacking adequate gathering grounds. Major efforts are being made to increase operating efficiencies and to reduce costs. As fresh-water sources become exhausted, the desalination of sea-water is likely to become more generally justifiable on economic grounds (Burley & Mawer, 1967).

REFERENCES

Bhaskaran, T. R. et al. (1965) In: *Proceedings of a Symposium on Problems in Water Treatment, 1964*, Nagpur, Central Public Health Engineering Research Institute

Burley, M. J. & Mawer, P. A. (1967) *Desalination as a supplement to conventional water supply*, vol. 2, Medmenham, Water Research Association (*Technical paper* TP 60), p. 149

Fair, G. M., Geyer, J. C. & Okun, D. A. (1966) *Water and wastewater engineering*, New York, Wiley

India, Central Public Health Engineering Research Institute (1970) *Disinfection of small water supplies*, Nagpur

India, Central Public Health Engineering Research Institute (1971) *Technical Digest No. 18*, Nagpur

Morris, J. C. (1970) In: *Proceedings of a Symposium on Water Treatment in the Seventies*, London, Society for Water Treatment and Examination

United Nations Economic and Social Council (1958) *Water for industrial use*, New York (Report B/3058 ST/ECA/50)

B.   Excreta and Waste-Water Disposal [1]

Basic sanitation measures

The prevention of infections of faecal origin is the most important objective. Human excreta and waste water should be disposed of in such a manner as to avoid direct or indirect contact with man. The following are essential requirements: (1) there should be no contamination of soil, of groundwater, or of surface water; (2) excreta should not be accessible to flies or animals; and (3) there should be no odours or unsightly conditions.

---

[1] Radioactive wastes are not dealt with here. See: International Atomic Energy Agency, 1967, 1968a, 1968b; International Atomic Energy Agency/World Health Organization, 1971.

When no water-borne system is available, the only satisfactory procedure is to dispose of human excreta in household or public installations under proper supervision. The sanitary pit privy, the aqua privy, and the water-seal latrine are three types of installation that, when properly designed and maintained, fulfil the essential sanitary requirements.

When a piped water supply is available, a water-borne system of excreta collection and disposal is the most satisfactory method of sanitation. A waste-water system comprises a network of facilities and services such as: (1) the household sanitary plumbing installation, including sanitary apparatus and a house-sewer connexion; (2) a network of laterals, main and trunk sewers for the collection and transportation of waste water; (3) treatment facilities for removing the waste matter transported by the water; and (4) outfall or disposal works for discharging the treated waste water into receiving bodies of water. The degree of purification required will depend upon the subsequent uses of the effluent and/or the receiving body of water (Wagner & Lanoix, 1958; WHO Scientific Group on the Treatment and Disposal of Wastes, 1967).

Advanced technology

Methods are available for the treatment of domestic sewage to high standards of purity, although the nature of sewage has changed due, for example, to the introduction of synthetic detergents. These reduced the efficiency of treatment plants, caused foaming problems, and contaminated drinking-water withdrawn from points downstream of sewage outfalls. Biodegradable detergents have now been introduced, and the magnitude of the problem has thereby been reduced—a good example of how product change can reduce water pollution.

Industrial wastes more commonly contain substances that are difficult or unduly costly to remove, and it has sometimes been necessary, as a result, to change industrial processes or to prevent or restrict their operation. The extent of waste-water discharges from industrial processes may be reduced by such techniques as recirculation of water or the use of counter-current washing procedures. Considerable advances are being made in the recovery of by-products. Even if such a process is not wholly economic, it may be less expensive than treating waste waters containing the material in question.

Waste waters may be treated and discharged to a stream or the effluent may be reclaimed for further use or used to recharge groundwater (Kneese & Bower, 1968). River basin authorities now commonly place constraints on the quantity and quality of effluents that may be discharged (US National Academy of Sciences, 1966). This is an incentive towards more effective water usage and the recovery of by-products.

The purity of receiving waters can be increased by augmenting their dry-weather flow or in some cases by direct re-aeration either by mechanical means or by the use of diffused air (Kneese & Bower, 1968).

There is a growing realization that an important consideration in the siting of new communities or industries is the problem of effluent disposal. In the case of the chemical industry, for example, this is increasingly restricting the areas in which development is acceptable.

Treatment of waste waters may merely involve the removal of settleable solids, or it may be more comprehensive. In the case of biologically degradable wastes, such as sewage, the second stage is normally aerobic treatment, either in trickling filters or by the activated sludge process. Waste stabilization ponds provide a useful method of waste-water treatment and disposal, particularly for communities where both funds and trained personnel are in short supply. They are most suitable where land is inexpensive and organic loadings fluctuate (Gloyna, 1971).

Tertiary treatment is being increasingly required, due either to the limited dilution provided by receiving waters or the need for intensive re-use. The water-treatment system used at any given site will depend on the nature of the wastes. Possible contaminants fall into four broad classes: (1) suspended solids; (2) dissolved organic componds; (3) dissolved inorganic compounds; and (4) the plant nutrients, nitrogen and phosphorus (American Chemical Society, 1969). The materials removed from the water must also be disposed of.

Suspended solids often account for a high proportion of the biochemical oxygen demand of an effluent. They may be substantially removed by filtration, microstraining or by chemical coagulation followed by filtration, often through sand. This latter process has the advantage that it removes a high proportion of the phosphates.

The small amounts of soluble refractory organic compounds that remain in secondary effluents after suspended solids removal can cause tastes and odours, and may be toxic to animal or plant life. Activated carbon is now being used to remove such impurities, in either a fixed or fluidized bed. Spent carbon is regenerated by heating it to about 930°C in an atmosphere of air and steam to burn off the adsorbed organic substances. Work is now in progress on the chemical oxidation of dissolved organic impurities, by the use of oxidizing agents such as ozone, hydrogen peroxide, chlorine, and potassium permanganate.

Demineralization of secondary effluents to remove dissolved inorganic materials is being achieved by means of ion exchange, reverse osmosis, and electrodialysis. The liquid wastes from these processes may be difficult to dispose of: solar evaporation ponds have been suggested in certain areas.

During the last few years, increasing emphasis has been placed on the need to control the discharge of nitrogen and phosphorus in view of their role as algal nutrients (Sawyer, 1968). A high proportion of phosphorus in sewage can be removed by precipitation with aluminium sulfate, lime, and other coagulants. A generously designed activated sludge plant will oxidize the nitrogen present in sewage. The effluent can then be treated with denitrifying bacteria, which at low levels of dissolved oxygen reduce nitrite and nitrate to gaseous nitrogen. A carbonaceous nutrient, such as methanol, is added to support the denitrifying bacteria. Ammoniacal nitrogen in a secondary effluent may be removed by air stripping at a pH of about 11.5: lime is added, and the water passed through a forced-draught counter-current air-stripping tower.

The commonest method of removing bacteria from reclaimed water is by chlorination. Viruses can be a serious problem in water re-use (Coin et al., 1965); the methods suggested for their removal include the use of ozone, adsorption, ion exchange, filtration and gamma irradiation.

A water reclamation plant with a capacity of 7.5 million gallons (28 000 m³) per day came into operation in 1965 at Lake Tahoe, California, USA (Slechton & Culp, 1967), comprising conventional primary and secondary treatment, flocculation and phosphate removal with lime, nitrogen removal by ammonia stripping, multimedia filtration, organic removal by adsorption on activated carbon, and chlorination.

Industrial waste waters are often less amenable to conventional treatment than domestic sewage, and may contain toxic or bioresistant components. Incineration is increasingly being applied to the more intractable wastes, and deep well injection is also being used (Amphlett, 1961).

REFERENCES

American Chemical Society (1969) *Cleaning our environment: the chemical basis for action*, Washington, D.C., p. 123

Amphlett, C. B. (1961) *Treatment and disposal of radioactive wastes*, Oxford, Pergamon, p. 209

Coin, L., Menetrier, M. L., Labonde, J. & Hannoun, M. C. (1965) *Modern microbiological and virological aspects of water pollution*. In: Jaag, O., ed., *Advances in water pollution research. Proceedings of the Second International Conference, Tokyo, August 1964*, vol. 1, Oxford, Pergamon, p. 1

Gloyna, E. F. (1971) *Waste stabilization ponds*, Geneva, World Health Organization (*Monograph Series*, No. 60)

International Atomic Energy Agency (1967) *Basic factors for the treatment and disposal of radioactive wastes*, Vienna (*Safety Series* No. 24)

International Atomic Energy Agency (1968a) *Treatment of airborne radioactive wastes*, Vienna (*Proceedings Series*)

International Atomic Energy Agency (1968b) *Treatment of low- and intermediate-level radioactive waste concentrates*, Vienna (*Technical Report Series* No. 82)

International Atomic Energy Agency/World Health Organization (1971) *Disposal of radioactive wastes into rivers, lakes and estuaries*, Vienna, IAEA (*Safety Series* No. 36)

Kneese, A. K. & Bower, B. T. (1968) *Managing water quality: economics, technology, institutions*, Baltimore, Md, Johns Hopkins

Sawyer, C. N. (1968) *J. Wat. Pollut. Control Fed.*, **40,** 363

Slechton, A. F. & Culp, G. L. (1967) *J. Wat. Pollut. Control Fed.*, **39,** 787

US National Academy of Sciences (1966) *Waste management and control. A report to the Federal Council for Science and Technology*, Washington, D.C. (US National Research Council Publication 1400), p. 205

Wagner, E. G. & Lanoix, J. N. (1958) *Excreta disposal for rural areas and small communities*, Geneva, World Health Organization (*Monograph Series*, No. 39)

WHO Scientific Group on the Treatment and Disposal of Wastes (1967) *Report*, Geneva (*Wld Hlth Org. techn. Rep. Ser.*, No. 367)

C. Disposal of Solid Wastes [1]

Introduction

Solid wastes include domestic refuse and other discarded solid materials, such as those from commercial, industrial, and agricultural operations; they contain increasing amounts of paper, cardboard, plastics, glass, and other packaging materials, but decreasing amounts of ash (WHO Scientific Group on the Treatment and Disposal of Wastes, 1967). The amounts produced are increasing throughout the world; urban wastes alone amount to about 600 kg *per capita* annually, and for industrialized countries probably at least 700 kg *per capita*, with an annual increase of 1–2 % (WHO Scientific Group on the Treatment and Disposal of Wastes, 1967). As the density of domestic waste is decreasing, annual *per capita* volumes of up to 5 cubic metres are common. These figures do not include the additional solid wastes produced by agricultural and industrial operations, and as a by-product of sewage treatment.

The insanitary collection and disposal of solid wastes creates serious health hazards, e.g., by encouraging the breeding of flies, mosquitos, rodents, and other vectors of disease. It may also contribute to water pollution, air pollution, and soil pollution. It has adverse effects on land values, constitutes a public nuisance, and thus contributes to the deterioration of the environment.

The appropriate intervention and control measures are the rapid removal of refuse from premises by an efficient collection system and the proper processing of refuse before final disposal or re-use.

A refuse disposal system includes essentially: (1) the transportation system, using automotive vehicles, railway transport, pneumatic transport in pipelines under vacuum, and liquid transport in trunk sewers. Transfer stations for changing from one method of transport to another (e.g., truck hauling to railway hauling) are also necessary; (2) facilities for the processing of solid wastes, possibly using one or more of the following techniques: segregation of refuse components, incineration, composting, pul-

---

[1] Radioactive wastes are not dealt with here. See: International Atomic Energy Agency, 1967, 1968a, 1968b; International Atomic Energy Agency/World Health Organization, 1971.

verization, compaction, and grinding; and (3) facilities for the sanitary discharge of residues into the environment, e.g., sanitary landfill, controlled discharge into bodies of water, and discharge into the air of combustion gases and particulate matter.

There are numerous alternatives for the handling and disposal of solid wastes. In selecting the best, consideration must first be given to the protection of the health of the community and the prevention of public nuisances. The salvaging of constituents of refuse, such as paper, glass, steel, etc., for re-use by industry must also be considered (WHO Expert Committee on Solid Wastes Disposal and Control, 1971).

Methods of collection and disposal

The rapid increase in the production of wastes is causing storage, collection, and transportation difficulties, as well as problems of treatment and final disposal.

Storage is largely a local problem; it becomes acute in housing developments and apartment blocks where adequate provision for storage has not been made. Home incinerators and garbage grinders help to reduce volume, but are not widely used.

The collection and disposal of solid wastes was discussed recently by the WHO Expert Committee on Solid Wastes Disposal and Control (1971). In its report, the Committee reviews existing knowledge of the health and socio-economic aspects of incorrect handling of solid wastes and assesses present knowledge and technology concerning the collection, treatment, and disposal of such wastes, including the planning and operational aspects. Collection and transportation have recently been intensively studied in various parts of the world, using operations research techniques, with a view to improving efficiency and lowering costs. Unconventional systems, such as hydraulic or pneumatic transport in pipes, are being developed, especially for new towns and residential areas. These developments, which are very promising, will eventually reduce collection costs and minimize human contact with solid wastes.

Collection and transportation costs vary widely, depending on population density, route planning, the location of disposal sites, labour costs, etc.; representative figures varied from $7.50 to $30.00 a ton in the USA in 1965, but have increased substantially since that time (American Public Works Association, Committee on Solid Wastes, 1966). Careful planning of routes and of pick-up procedures should make significant savings possible.

Farm wastes pose a special problem that was not recognized until recently; it has been seriously exacerbated in recent years because of the high concentration of farm animals in small spaces resulting from the use of feed lots for cattle, new designs of pig-rearing facilities, chicken pens, etc.

Substantial savings in handling costs can be achieved by conservation (reducing the volume of waste), land disposal and on-site treatment, both anaerobically or through the use of oxidation ponds or aeration ditches (Institute of Water Pollution Control/University of Newcastle upon Tyne, 1970).

The most difficult problem, however, remains that of disposal. Because of the potential nuisance involved, the choice of disposal sites is often a source of serious controversy. Ideally, the site should be selected on the basis of regional studies. The disposal methods of choice are incineration, sanitary landfill, and composting. Unfortunately, indiscriminate dumping is still practised, both on land and on sea. Incinerator design is improving as combustion efficiency improves and greater control is obtained over gaseous emissions; even after incineration, however, a sizeable volume of ash remains.

Composting, although it has widespread popular appeal, has become increasingly uneconomical as a means of disposal, both because of the changing nature of refuse and the difficulty in disposing of the compost itself (Gotaas, 1956).

Sanitary landfill is everywhere the most popular method of disposal. While it requires the use of relatively large areas, it can be used effectively for land reclamation purposes; when properly managed it can be inoffensive, and avoid both air pollution and, to a large extent, leaching and resulting water pollution. A modification of the process is being developed in certain areas; refuse is hauled relatively long distances by rail, and disposal is combined with strip-mining operations.

Other processes, still at the experimental stage, include pulverization into a dense, homogeneous, and relatively inoffensive material. This process reduces transport costs and land area requirements for sanitary landfill. Investigations are also being carried out on the high-pressure compaction of refuse into blocks of high density. These blocks could be used as a filling material and for the reclamation of derelict land.

The importance of recycling in refuse disposal has been emphasized by the conservation-minded. It is almost always a marginal operation from an economic point of view, although aluminium, glass, iron, paper, and other materials can be reclaimed.

As far as disease transmission is concerned, garbage and refuse are relatively unimportant, but they contribute as much as any other factor to the unaesthetic and degrading environment in slum areas. The control of these wastes is therefore relevant to community health.

REFERENCES

American Public Works Association, Committee on Solid Wastes (1966) *Refuse collection practice*, 3rd ed., Chicago, Ill., Public Administration Service

Gotaas, H. B. (1956) *Composting: sanitary disposal and reclamation of organic wastes,* Geneva, World Health Organization (*Monograph series,* No. 31)

Institute of Water Pollution Control/University of Newcastle upon Tyne (1970) *Farm wastes. Proceedings of a Symposium*

International Atomic Energy Agency (1967) *Basic factors for the treatment and disposal of radioactive wastes,* Vienna (*Safety Series* No. 24)

International Atomic Energy Agency (1968a) *Treatment of airborne radioactive wastes,* Vienna (*Proceedings Series*)

International Atomic Energy Agency (1968b) *Treatment of low- and intermediate-level radioactive waste concentrates,* Vienna (*Technical Report Series* No. 82)

International Atomic Energy Agency/World Health Organization (1971) *Disposal of radioactive wastes into rivers, lakes and estuaries,* Vienna, IAEA (*Safety Series* No. 36)

WHO Expert Committee on Solid Wastes Disposal and Control (1971) *Report,* Geneva (*Wld Hlth Org. techn. Rep. Ser.,* No. 484)

WHO Scientific Group on the Treatment and Disposal of Wastes (1967) *Report,* Geneva (*Wld Hlth Org. techn. Rep. Ser.,* No. 367)

D. Vector Control

In current public health practice, vector control is chiefly concerned with insects and rodents. The technical procedures and problems have recently been reviewed (WHO Expert Committee on Insecticides, 1970; World Health Organization, 1972). Conventional methods of control include environmental control, which implies modification of the environment to a point where it is no longer suitable for the breeding or development of insect vectors or of rodent reservoirs of disease, e.g., improved drainage for the control of mosquitos, and proper refuse disposal to prevent the breeding of flies and rodents.

Chemical control is used where environmental control is not feasible or where rapid reductions in the vector populations are desired. Chemical control may be directed either against the larvae of insects (larvicides) or against the adult stages (adulticides). Adulticides can be applied either as long-acting residual sprays to the interior of buildings where the target insect is likely to come into contact with them, or as space sprays with the purpose of achieving immediate knock-down of those insects with which the droplets come into contact. Insecticidal dusts are used for the control of certain vectors, e.g., body lice, when the insecticide is mixed with talc, or fleas in rodent burrows, when the dust is applied directly to the burrows.

In addition to studies aimed at improving present methods of insect vector control, a number of methods that would reduce dependence on insecticides, such as genetic and biological control, are being investigated.

Genetic control of insects of agricultural importance has so far been effected by the release of insects sterilized by ionizing radiation or with chemosterilants (LaChance et al., 1967). In 1966, *Culex pipiens fatigans,* an important vector of filariasis, was eliminated from an isolated village in Burma by the release of a genetically incompatible strain of this species. Since then, a number of other genetic factors, such as translocations, sex distorting factors and hybrid sterility, have been discovered that can be introduced to control or eliminate natural populations, and these have the additional advantage of being more or less self-propagating (Knipling et al., 1968).

The feasibility of the genetic control of *C. p. fatigans, Aedes aegypti* and *Anopheles stephensi* on an operational scale is at present under investigation in a WHO field research unit. Other insects of public health importance under study are houseflies and tsetse-flies, *Anopheles gambiae, Anopheles albimanus,* and ticks.

These new methods are selective in their control of a species and are not a hazard to any other living creature in the area. A number of factors remain to be studied before any of them can be used on an extended scale, but the results of preliminary experiments have been encouraging.

As biological control agents for mosquitos, the use of small fish that prey on the larvae has been revived (Bay, 1967). Some success has been obtained against anopheline mosquitos in Iran and Greece, and against culicine mosquitos in Hawaii and California. The extent of control is not as complete as with insecticides, but increasing insecticide resistance demands that larvivorous fish be used, at least as an alternative. Research in the field is proceeding, much of it under WHO auspices, on the use of the following biological control agents: predacious *Toxorhynchites* mosquitos for mosquito control; parasitic *Reesimermis* nematodes for mosquito and blackfly control; *Nosema* protozoa and *Coelomomyces* fungi for mosquito control; and parasitic *Gryon* wasps for *Triatoma* control. The possible use of bacteria and entomo-viruses for the control of mosquito larvae is under review (*WHO Chronicle*, 1971).

In the control of rodents of public health importance, consideration has been given to the possible use of chemosterilants (Marsh & Howard, 1970); their use seems unlikely to develop further in the immediate future, and in urban situations the most fundamental approach remains the denying of food and harbourage to rats through improvement of the environment, followed by the judicious use of rodenticides to control residual rodent populations. Unfortunately, the development of resistance to anti-coagulant rodenticides (Greaves, 1971) represents a growing impediment to the safe and effective use of these agents, and WHO is encouraging the development of new groups of rodenticides, particularly those whose action is specific to rodents, and is arranging field trials for the most promising agents.

REFERENCES

Bay, E. C. (1967) *WHO Chronicle*, **21**, 415-423

Greaves, J. H. (1971) *Pestic. Sci.*, **2**, 276-279

Knipling, E. F., Laven, H., Craig, G. B., Pal, R., Kitzmiller, J. B., Smith, C. N. & Brown A. W. A. (1968) *Bull. Wld Hlth Org.*, **38**, 421-438

LaChance, L. E., Schmidt, C. H., Bushland, R. C. & Kilgore, W. W. (1967) In: Kilgore, W. W. & Doutt, R. L., eds, *Pest control: biological, physical and selected chemical methods*, New York and London, Academic Press, pp. 147-239

Marsh, R. E. & Howard, W. E. (1970) *Proceedings of the 4th Conference on Vertebrate Pests*, pp. 55-63

WHO Chronicle, 1971, **25**, 230-235

WHO Expert Committee on Insecticides (1970) *Insecticide resistance and vector control*, Geneva (*Wld Hlth Org. techn. Rep. Ser.*, No. 443)

World Health Organization (1972) *Vector control in international health*, Geneva

E. Food Sanitation

Sanitation measures for preventing food infection and poisoning include: (1) protection of food at all times from insects and vermin; (2) employment of food handlers who are free from infection and clean in their habits; (3) storage of food subject to infection at temperatures of 7°C or below, or 60°C or above, the latter applying to foods kept on steam tables during serving; (4) cleansing and bactericidal treatment of utensils and equipment used in the preparation and serving of food; (5) proper sanitary facilities and controls, such as the supply of safe hot and cold water and the provision of proper waste-water and garbage disposal facilities; and (6) continuous inspection and enforcement of codes and regulations pertaining to food sanitation (WHO Expert Committee on the Microbiological Aspects of Food Hygiene, 1968; Joint FAO/WHO Codex Alimentarius Commission, 1969).

The advanced technology of food sanitation presents certain problems that are discussed briefly below.

Irradiation

Ionizing radiation in food processing has been under study for over 20 years, and there is increasing evidence of its usefulness in the control of micro-organisms that give rise to food spoilage and constitute potential health hazards. The sources of radiation used at present are ^{60}Co, ^{137}Cs–accelerated electrons having energies up to 10 million electron volts (MeV), and X-rays from sources of energy up to 5 million volts. It has been shown that when the energy level is 10 MeV, none of the major elements present in foods consumed by man or in animal feeding-stuffs become radioactive (Joint FAO/IAEA/WHO Expert Committee on the Technical Basis for Legislation on Irradiated Food, 1965; WHO Expert Committee on the Microbiological Aspects of Food Hygiene, 1968). Higher levels may be associated with the hazards discussed in Chapter 14.

Radiation processing is advantageous for several reasons.   For example, it will kill micro-organisms in foods that are in hermetically sealed packages or in the frozen state.   Moreover, the treatment can be carried out at room temperature without substantially raising the temperature of the product. However, there are certain disadvantages: viruses and enzymes are highly resistant to radiation and the normal dosage used to control micro-organisms does not inactivate them.   If the radiation dose is increased so as to inactivate viruses and enzymes, the product may undergo changes in flavour, colour, and texture.

Milk treatment

The theoretical basis of milk sterilization outlined some years ago (Burton et al., 1965; Abdussalam et al., 1962) has remained essentially unchanged.   However, wider use is now made of modern heat treatment processes, particularly ultra-high-temperature (UHT) treatments.

UHT processes may be of the direct heating type, in which steam is injected into milk or milk into steam, or of the indirect heating type, in which the milk is heated by means of tubular or plate-type heaters that are basically similar to those used in pasteurization, but heated by steam instead of hot water.   In direct methods a temperature of 140–145°C, which is attained almost instantaneously, is applied for 1–4 seconds.   Existing types of indirect heater employ slightly lower temperatures for slightly longer times.   However, the UHT process can be applied only to bulk milk in continuous flow, and the sterile product must be protected from recontamination during packaging operations.   The process is of limited value unless it is combined with aseptic packaging, either on the spot or in another plant to which the milk is transported in bulk in sterile containers.

Aseptic filling of milk into sterile cartons on a large scale has been developed commercially.   New types of container made of plastics are becoming available, including rigid cartons formed at the dairy from precut blanks and sachets made from sheet film that can be sterilized.   There will undoubtedly be considerable development of alternative packages during the next few years.

All cartons and sachets are single-service containers having the advantages of light weight and ease of disposal, but they may create problems of environmental pollution if they are not biologically degradable.

Packaging

The introduction of new packaging materials into the food processing industry has created new areas of public health concern.   Packaging materials can be a possible source of contamination of foods with micro-organisms, but ordinarily they harbour only small numbers of innocuous micro-organisms or no organisms. Wrappers may be treated or impregnated with bacteriostatic or fungistatic compounds to make them safer, e.g., sorbic or caprylic acid. Paper products used for milk cartons contain mostly bacilli and micrococci, and occasionally other rod-shaped micro-organisms, actinomycetes, and mould spores, but no organisms ordinarily considered to be of public health significance. Treatment with hot paraffin kills most of the organisms present, provides an almost sterile surface, and prevents bacteria within the cardboard from reaching the food. Wax paper is practically sterile as produced, as indeed are most packaging materials (Frazier, 1967).

Unless the food is sterile in the sealed package it will eventually spoil, and the plastic anaerobic packaging of non-sterilized and inadequately heat-treated products may produce unique problems of special risk, e.g., smoked fish sealed in plastic bags and held at a certain temperature before consumption may be the cause of outbreaks of botulism (*Morbidity and Mortality*, 1963).

A major problem with the use of plastic films for packaging purposes arises from the lack of information about the migration of their components into the food, and from the lack of toxicological data on these substances. Plastic films contain small amounts of monomers, catalysts, stabilizers, plasticizers, anti-oxidants, siccatives, slimicides, adhesives, antistatic agents, and other compounds. It is practically impossible to find a plastic material that is completely resistant to slow chemical or physical attack by foodstuffs; consequently, the contamination of food by traces of a wide variety of complex chemical compounds is inevitable. This problem is not restricted to plastic packaging materials, but applies to all substances coming into contact with food, such as paper and paperboard, tin-plated cans, glass, wood, textiles, nylon, resins, and cellophane. Although these materials are not manufactured by polymerization processes and are not as complex in composition as plastics, they are nevertheless composed of substances that migrate into foodstuffs, and most of these substances have not been toxicologically evaluated (Aldershoff, 1971).

REFERENCES

Abdussalam, M. et al. (1962) *Milk hygiene*, Geneva, World Health Organization (*Monograph Series*, No. 48)

Aldershoff, W. G. (1971) *Report on the fact-finding symposium concerning packaging materials for foodstuffs, Noordwijk-aan-Zee, 1971*, Leidschendam, Ministry of Social Affairs and Public Health

Burton, H. et al. (1965) *Milk sterilization*, Rome (*Food and Agriculture Organization: Agricultural Studies*, No. 65)

Frazier, W. C. (1967) *Food microbiology*, 2nd ed., New York, McGraw-Hill

Joint FAO/IAEA/WHO Expert Committee on the Technical Basis for Legislation on Irradiated Food (1966) *Report*, Geneva (*Wld Hlth Org. techn. Rep. Ser.*, No. 316)

Joint FAO/WHO Codex Alimentarius Commission (1969) *Recommended international code of practice: general principles of food hygiene*, Rome, FAO

Morbidity and Mortality (1963), **12**, No. 40

WHO Expert Committee on the Microbiological Aspects of Food Hygiene (1968) *Report*, Geneva (*Wld Hlth Org. techn. Rep. Ser.*, No. 399)

F. Air Pollution

There are, broadly, four different methods for the control of atmospheric pollution; namely, containment, dispersion, replacement of technological processes by new ones that produce less air pollution, and appropriate siting of potential sources of pollution.

Containment

This is usually interpreted to mean the control of an individual source by the installation of a properly engineered gas-cleaning device.

Increasingly rigorous controls have been applied to emissions from industrial processes in recent years, and there have been corresponding developments in gas-cleaning equipment. The equipment available for collecting solid and liquid particles, for example, includes fabric filters, electrostatic precipitators, cyclones, other mechanical devices, and high- and low-energy wet scrubbers. The choice of the type of equipment to be installed depends on such variables as the nature and concentration of the pollutant, the effluent flow-rate and temperature, and the degree of cleaning required.

Although considerable progress has been made in the reduction of particulate emissions and smoke from the combustion of fossil fuels, both by the use of high-efficiency (over 98 %) collection devices, such as electrostatic precipitators, and by advances in combustion technology (Stern, 1968), a good deal remains to be done, particularly as regards the removal of sulfur dioxide and nitrogen oxides from stack gases.

Smokeless, i.e., low volatile, fuels have been used very effectively in some urban areas, e.g., in London, but in a number of developing countries, where the cheapest available fuel is used, pollution from domestic heating or cooking remains a problem.

The processes now being studied for the removal of sulfur dioxide from stack gases include dry absorption reactions with alkaline powders (limestone or dolomite), alkalized alumina or manganese oxides, adsorption on specially activated carbons, and catalytic oxidation using vanadium oxide. Unfortunately, these processes are still too costly to be generally applicable (Leithe, 1968).

Less work has been done on the abatement of discharges of nitrogen oxides from power plants and other large combustion sources; the development of methods for dealing economically with large volumes of exhaust gas containing a small proportion of nitrogen oxides, therefore, is still a task for the future. For higher concentrations and low flow-rates, two-stage catalytic reduction has been proposed (Teske, 1968).

A number of countries now have legislation imposing limits on at least some of the pollutants emitted by petrol-powered motor vehicles. The control techniques used include recycling of crankcase vent gases, much finer adjustment of ignition and carburation, insulation of petrol tanks, and provision for the collection and recovery of carburettor evaporative losses (WHO Expert Committee on Urban Air Pollution, 1969).

However, in order to be able to satisfy the stricter exhaust requirements that will be in force in countries such as the USA in the next decade (*Federal Register*, 1971), additional control measures will be necessary. These include the use of thermal or catalytic after-burners and by-pass converters for oxides of nitrogen (Stern, 1968). The amount of smoke emitted by diesel vehicles depends to a large extent on the mechanical condition of the engine and auxiliary equipment, together with the method of operation. Worn and incorrectly timed fuel pumps, faulty injectors, and an open setting of the maximum fuel stop are all important causes of smoke. Diesel vehicles, when properly maintained and operated, are capable of virtually smoke-free operation (Cleary, 1970).

In the longer term, it is likely that alternative types of vehicle will be developed. These may include more efficient electrically driven or petrol-electric hybrid vehicles, or vehicles driven by gas turbines or other power sources, e.g., fuel cells, engines using liquefied petroleum gas (LPG), or steam engines. It is also possible that the development of highly efficient urban transport systems may obviate the necessity for cars in inner city areas (Irens, 1966).

With regard to aircraft emissions, reductions in the amounts of aerosols, hydrocarbons, oxides of nitrogen, and carbon monoxide, together with a significant reduction in visible smoke, should result from the improvements in combustion design and combustion technology at present being under-taken (Cleary, 1970).

Dispersion

This procedure relies on atmospheric diffusion phenomena to dilute the contaminant to such an extent that ground-level concentrations are innocuous. It has been shown that, in the absence of appreciable momentum and temperature in a gas plume, the maximum ground-level concentration of a pollutant is directly proportional to the emission rate of the effluent gas, and inversely proportional to the wind velocity and the square of the effective stack height. A number of empirical formulae have been put forward on the basis of this generalized relationship (Strom, 1968). For large gas flows and high-temperature emissions (e.g., from large power plants), special corrections must be made for the buoyancy due to the momentum and temperature of the plume.

As a general rule, in the absence of atmospheric stability, the point of maximum ground-level concentration is located 5–20 stack heights from the chimney.

In fixing stack heights for industrial plants, allowance must be made for the occurrence of tall vertical eddies downwind of the stack; discharged gases tend to be drawn into these eddies, thereby reducing the effective stack height. To minimize the effects of this "downwash", the discharge velocity from chimneys serving large plants should, wherever possible, be about 16 m/sec at full load; even for small plants, the minimum velocity should be about 8 m/sec. Special correction factors should also be applied to allow for the effect of nearby buildings. Other factors that should be considered include the normal atmospheric conditions near the plant site (lapse rates, wind velocity and directional frequency), the nature of the surrounding terrain, and the presence of other sources of pollution in the vicinity (Pasquill & Smith, 1971).

Dispersion is generally used for control purposes on economic grounds, as in the case of the sulfur dioxide emissions from power stations.

Replacement

This comprises the replacement of a technological process that causes air pollution by a new one that does not, which is not always easy to achieve in practice. The new process has not only to be technologically equivalent to the old one in all essentials (such as the quality of the final product), but must also be equally satisfactory as regards the cost of production. These requirements are not always compatible.

Siting of potential pollution sources

In the past, this problem has received scant consideration in planning, either at regional or local government levels, in many parts of the world. Indiscriminate siting of dwellings and factories discharging pollutants has produced conditions under which people are exposed to air pollution that could have been avoided by intelligent planning. Much stricter control measures have to be employed under such conditions than would otherwise have been necessary. Many other factors must be taken into account in selecting a site, such as the availability of raw materials and other resources, fuels and power, labour supply, proximity to related industries and to markets, and transportation facilities. Restrictions on the location of industry must therefore be reasonable, otherwise many factories will be unable to operate, with consequent detriment to the economy.

From an air pollution viewpoint, site selection should take into consideration the nature of the air contaminants; the efficiency of available control devices; pertinent meteorological factors and the dispersive ability of the air at each possible site; the present quality of the environment at that site; and the potential effects on the surrounding areas.

It is now appreciated that good practice consists in physically separating people from polluting industries. This is usually accomplished by the provision of suitable buffer zones, consisting either of parklands or of areas in which light, non-polluting industries are located. The extent of the buffer zone depends on the type and magnitude of the industry concerned and its pollution potential.

REFERENCES

Cleary, G. J. (1970) *Preliminary assessment of air pollution in Singapore. WHO assignment report to the Government of Singapore*, Geneva, World Health Organization (unpublished document WPR/141/70)

Federal Register, 1971, **36**, 12 658

Irens, A. N. (1966) *Tomorrow's town transport—the advantage of electric traction.* In: *Proceedings of the International Clean Air Congress, London, 4-7 October 1966*, London, National Society for Clean Air (paper VI/4), pp. 168-171

Leithe, W. (1968) *Chem. Engr (Lond.)*, **46**, 262-263

Pasquill, F. & Smith, B. H. (1971) *The physical and meteorological basis for the estimation of the dispersion of windborne material.* In: *Proceedings of the Second International Clean Air Congress, Washington, D.C., December 6-11, 1970*, New York, Academic Press, pp. 1067-1072

Stern, A. C., ed. (1968) *Air pollution*, vol. III, 2nd ed., New York, Academic Press

Strom, G. H. (1968) *Atmospheric dispersion of stack effluents.* In: Stern, A. C., ed., *Air pollution*, vol. I, 2nd ed., New York, Academic Press, pp. 227-274

Teske, W. (1968) *Chem. Engr (Lond.)*, **46**, 263-266

WHO Expert Committee on Urban Air Pollution (1969) *Report*, Geneva (*Wld Hlth Org. techn. Rep. Ser.*, No. 410)

CONTRIBUTORS AND REVIEWERS

Grateful acknowledgement is made to the temporary advisers, consultants, and reviewers who assisted in the preparation of this publication. Since they represent a wide range of scientific viewpoints, their inclusion in this list does not necessarily imply their endorsement of all the opinions expressed. Primary responsibility for the content rests with the technical staff of WHO. Work on this publication was coordinated by the Organization's Office of Science and Technology.

Dr M. Abdussalam, Chief Veterinarian, Veterinary Public Health, WHO, Geneva, Switzerland

Dr C. Agthe, Senior Scientist, Unit of Chemical Carcinogenesis, International Agency for Research on Cancer, Lyon, France

Dr N. Ansari, Chief Medical Officer, Parasitic Diseases, WHO, Geneva, Switzerland

Mr J. de Araoz, Scientist, Development of Institutions and Services, WHO, Geneva, Switzerland

Dr I. Barrai, Chief Medical Officer, Human Genetics, WHO, Geneva, Switzerland

Dr V. Beneš, Chief, Department of Toxicology, Institute of Hygiene and Epidemiology, Prague, Czechoslovakia

Dr J. Bengoa, Chief Medical Officer, Nutrition, WHO, Geneva, Switzerland

Dr Viola W. Bernard, Director, Division of Community and Social Psychiatry, Columbia University, New York, USA

Dr P. E. Berteau, Scientist, Vector Biology and Control, WHO, Geneva, Switzerland

Professor W. I. B. Beveridge, Head, Department of Animal Pathology, School of Veterinary Medicine, University of Cambridge, England

Mr P. Bierstein, Chief Sanitary Engineer, Pre-Investment Planning, WHO, Geneva, Switzerland

Mr W. Binks, *formerly* Director, Radiological Protection Service, Department of Health and Medical Research Council, Sutton, Surrey, England

Professor N. P. Bočkov, Director, Institute of Medical Genetics, Moscow, USSR

Professor F. Bourlière, Professor of Physiology, Faculty of Medicine, Paris, France

Professor W. Brauer, Institute for Information and Computer Science, University of Hamburg, Federal Republic of Germany

Dr A. W. A. Brown, Scientist, Vector Biology and Control, WHO, Geneva, Switzerland

Professor K. A. Buštueva, Department of Community Hygiene, Central Institute for Advanced Medical Training, Moscow, USSR

Mr M. Carrera, Sanitary Engineer, Community Water Supply and Sanitation, WHO, Geneva, Switzerland

Dr G. Castellanos, Medical Officer, Mental Health, WHO, Geneva, Switzerland

Dr G. J. Cleary, Scientist, Environmental Pollution, WHO, Geneva, Switzerland

Dr J. F. Copplestone, Scientist, Vector Biology and Control, WHO, Geneva, Switzerland

Professor R. Cruickshank, Emeritus Professor of Microbiology, University of Edinburgh, Scotland

Dr J. L. Cutler, Medical Officer, Division of Strengthening of Health Services, WHO, Geneva, Switzerland

Mr J. M. Dave, Ministry of Health and Family Planning, New Delhi, India

Dr B. H. Dieterich, Director, Division of Environmental Health, WHO, Geneva, Switzerland

Professor B. Dinman, Director, Institute of Environmental and Industrial Health, University of Michigan, USA

Dr A. L. Downing, Director, Water Pollution Research Laboratory, Stevenage, Herts, England

Professor M. Eden, Research Laboratory for Electronics, Massachusetts Institute of Technology, Cambridge, Mass., USA

Dr M. A. M. El Batawi, Chief Medical Officer, Occupational Health, WHO, Geneva, Switzerland

Dr H. L. Falk, Associate Director for Program, National Institute of Environmental Health Sciences, US Public Health Service, Research Triangle Park, N.C., USA

Professor R. B. Fisher, Dean, University of Edinburgh Medical School, Edinburgh, Scotland

Professor S. Forssman, Scientific Adviser, Swedish Work Environment Fund, Stockholm, Sweden

Dr L. Friberg, Professor and Chairman, Department of Environmental Hygiene, Karolinska Institute, Stockholm, Sweden

Dr H. Friebel, Chief Medical Officer, Drug Efficacy and Safety, WHO, Geneva, Switzerland

Professor G. F. Gause, Director, Institute of New Antibiotics, Academy of Medical Sciences, Moscow, USSR

Dr J. R. Goldsmith, Head, Environmental Epidemiology Unit, Bureau of Occupational Health and Environmental Epidemiology, State Department of Public Health, Berkeley, Calif., USA

Dr N. G. Gratz, Scientist, Vector Biology and Control, WHO, Geneva, Switzerland

Dr M. Gross, Laboratory for Automation and Communications Science, University of Paris VIII, France

Professor E. M. Gruenberg, Director, Psychiatric Epidemiology Research Unit, Department of Psychiatry, Columbia University, New York ,USA

Dr F. W. J. van Haaren, Head, Laboratories of the Municipal Waterworks, Amsterdam, Netherlands

Dr L. D. Hamilton, Head, Division of Microbiology, Medical Research Center, Brookhaven National Laboratory, Upton, N.Y., USA

Professor T. F. Hatch, Professor Emeritus of Industrial Health Engineering, Graduate School of Public Health, University of Pittsburgh, Pa., USA

Dr A. Hollaender, Biology Division, Oak Ridge National Laboratory, Oak Ridge, Tenn., USA

Dr A. R. Kagan, Medical Officer, Division of Strengthening of Health Services, WHO, Geneva, Switzerland

Dr M. M. Kaplan, Director, Office of Science and Technology, WHO, Geneva, Switzerland

Dr E. I. Komarov, Medical Officer, Radiation Health, WHO, Geneva, Switzerland

Dr R. E. C. Kratel, Scientist, Occupational Health, WHO, Geneva, Switzerland

Professor A. R. M. Lafontaine, Director, Institute of Hygiene and Epidemiology, Ministry of Public Health and Family Affairs, Brussels, Belgium

Dr M. Laird, Professor and Head, Department of Biology, Memorial University of Newfoundland, St. John's, Newfoundland, Canada

Dr G. Lambert, Environmental Physiologist, Occupational Health, WHO, Geneva, Switzerland

Mr J. Lanoix, Chief Sanitary Engineer, Development of Institutions and Services, WHO, Geneva, Switzerland

Mr H. Le Bras, National Institute for Demographic Studies, Ministry of Labour, Employment, and Population, Paris, France

Dr L. Levi, Director, Laboratory for Clinical Stress Research, Karolinska Institute, Fack, Stockholm, Sweden

Dr J. Logan, President, Rose-Hulman Institute of Technology, Terre Haute, Ind., USA

Dr F. C. Lu, Chief, Food Additives, WHO, Geneva, Switzerland

Dr R. MacLennan, Epidemiologist, Unit of Epidemiology and Biostatistics, International Agency for Research on Cancer, Lyon, France

Dr P. Macúch, Medical Officer, Office of Science and Technology, WHO, Geneva, Switzerland

Dr E. L. Margetts, Medical Officer, Mental Health, WHO, Geneva, Switzerland

Dr A. E. Martin, Principal Medical Officer, Department of Health and Social Security, London, England

Professor Z. Matyáš, Department of Food Hygiene and Technology, School of Veterinary Medicine, Brno, Czechoslovakia

Professor M. Meselson, Biological Laboratories, Harvard University, Cambridge, Mass., USA

Dr J. de Moerloose, Chief, Health Legislation, WHO, Geneva, Switzerland

Dr R. H. Mole, Medical Research Council Radiobiology Unit, Harwell, England

Dr R. Montesano, Unit of Chemical Carcinogenesis, International Agency for Research on Cancer, Lyon, France

Dr B. Moore, Public Health Laboratory, Heavitree, Exeter, England

Mrs J. Moser, Scientist, Mental Health, WHO, Geneva, Switzerland

Dr N. Napalkov, Chief Medical Officer, Cancer, WHO, Geneva, Switzerland

Professor N. Nelson, Director, Institute of Environmental Medicine, New York University, New York, USA

Dr V. A. Newill, Office of Research and Monitoring, Environmental Protection Agency, Washington, D.C., USA

Mr L. Orihuela, Chief Sanitary Engineer, Community Water Supply and Sanitation, WHO, Geneva, Switzerland

Dr H. Oyanguren, *formerly* Director, Institute of Occupational Health and Air Pollution Research, Santiago, Chile

Dr D. Ozonoff, Research Laboratory of Electronics and Department of Nutrition and Food Science, Massachusetts Institute of Technology, Cambridge, Mass., USA

Mr R. Pavanello, Chief Sanitary Engineer, Environmental Pollution, WHO, Geneva, Switzerland

Dr L. Reinius, Food Hygienist, Veterinary Public Health, WHO, Geneva, Switzerland

Mr J. P. Robinson, Science Policy Research Unit, University of Sussex, Brighton, England

Dr E. Roelsgaard, Chief Medical Officer, Epidemiological Surveillance of Communicable Diseases, WHO, Geneva, Switzerland

Dr A. Rossi-Espagnet, Epidemiologist, Strengthening Health Services, WHO, Geneva, Switzerland

Professor J. Rotblat, Department of Physics, St Bartholemew's Hospital Medical College, London, England

Dr D. D. Rutstein, Ridley Watts Professor of Preventive Medicine, Harvard University School of Medicine, Boston, Mass., USA

Dr R. Rylander, Department of Environmental Hygiene, Karolinska Institute, Stockholm, Sweden

Dr N. Sartorius, Medical Officer, Mental Health, WHO, Geneva, Switzerland

Professor M. Schaefer, Department of Health Administration, University of North Carolina, USA

Dr A. Schoen, University of Berlin, Federal Republic of Germany

Professor M. P. Schutzenberger, Mathematics Teaching and Research Unit, University of Paris VII, France

Professor N. S. Scrimshaw, Head, Department of Nutrition and Food Science, Massachusetts Institute of Technology, Cambridge, Mass., USA

Dr W. H. P. Seelentag, Chief Medical Officer, Radiation Health, WHO, Geneva, Switzerland

Mr F. Sella, Secretary, United Nations Scientific Committee on the Effects of Atomic Radiation, United Nations, New York, USA

Dr E. Shalmon, Scientist, Environmental Pollution, WHO, Geneva, Switzerland

Professor P. Shubik, Eppley Institute, University of Nebraska, USA

Professor H. Shuval, Director, Environmental Health Laboratory, Department of Medical Ecology, Hebrew University—Hadassah Medical School, Jerusalem, Israel

Dr Katharine B. Sturgis, Wynnewood, Penn., USA

Mr D. V. Subrahmanyam, Sanitary Engineer, Community Water Supply and Sanitation, WHO, Geneva, Switzerland

Dr T. Suzuki, Chief, Department of Industrial Hygiene, Institute of Public Health, Tokyo, Japan

Dr L. Tomatis, Chief, Unit of Chemical Carcinogenesis, International Agency for Research on Cancer, Lyon, France

Professor R. Truhaut, Faculty of Pharmacy, University of Paris, France

Dr J. C. Villforth, Director, Bureau of Radiological Health, US Public Health Service, Washington, D.C., USA

Dr V. B. Vouk, Scientist, Environmental Pollution, WHO, Geneva, Switzerland

Dr Dora Wassermann, Department of Occupational Health, Hebrew University—Hadassah Medical School, Jerusalem, Israel

Professor M. Wassermann, Department of Occupational Health, Hebrew University—Hadassah Medical School, Jerusalem, Israel

Dr E. Windle-Taylor, Director of Water Examination, Metropolitan Water Board Laboratories, London, England

INDEX

INDEX